# Hearing Aids: Standards, Options, and Limitations

# Hearing Aids: Standards, Options, and Limitations

edited by

**Michael Valente, Ph.D.**

*Associate Professor*
*Director of Adult Audiology*
*Washington University School of Medicine*
*St. Louis, Missouri*

1996
**THIEME MEDICAL PUBLISHERS, INC.** New York
**GEORG THIEME VERLAG** Stuttgart · New York

Thieme Medical Publishers, Inc.
381 Park Avenue South
New York, New York 10016

HEARING AIDS:
STANDARDS, OPTIONS, AND LIMITATIONS
Michael Valente

**Library of Congress Cataloging-in-Publication Data**

Hearing aids: Standards, Options, and Limitations / [edited by]
   Michael Valente.
       p.   cm.
     Includes bibliographical references and index.
     ISBN 0-86577-576-1 (TMP : New York).— ISBN 3-13-102731-2 (GTV :
Stuttgart)
     1. Hearing aids.   I. Valente, Michael.
     [DNLM:   1. Hearing Aids.   WV 274 H4352 1995]
RF300.H43   1995
617.8′9—dc20
DNLM/DLC
for Library of Congress                                   95-32782
                                                             CIP

*Important note:* Medicine is an ever-changing science. Research and clinical experience are continually
broadening our knowledge, in particular our knowledge of proper treatment and drug therapy.
Insofar as this book mentions any dosage or applications, readers may rest assured that the authors,
editors, and publishers have made every effort to ensure that such references are strictly in accordance
with the state of knowledge at the time of production of the book. Nevertheless, every user is requested
to carefully examine the manufacturers' leaflets accompanying each drug to check on his own
responsibility whether the dosage schedules recommended therein or the contraindications stated by
the manufacturers differ from the statements made in the present book. Such examination is particularly
important with drugs that are either rarely used or have been newly released on the market.

Some of the product names, patents, and registered designs referred to in this book are in fact registered
trademarks or proprietary names even though specific reference to this fact is not always made in the
text. Therefore, the appearance of a name without designation as proprietary is not to be construed as
a representation by the publisher that it is in the public domain.

Printed in the United States of America.

5 4 3 2 1

TMP ISBN 0-86577-576-1
GTV ISBN 3-13-102731-2

# Contents

# *Preface*

Upon completing *Strategies for Selecting and Verifying Hearing Aid Fittings* (Thieme Medical Publishers, 1994), I realized it might be beneficial to edit a second text that addressed the issues to consider when ordering hearing aids. That is, *Strategies for Selecting and Verifying Hearing Aid Fittings,* addressed the issues related to "what to do with hearing aids after they have been received," but it did not consider the numerous issues involved in ordering hearing aids. This text was completed because I felt it was important for dispensing audiologists to spend as much time in considering the many issues involved when ordering hearing aids as they do when selecting and verifying the performance of hearing aids.

This textbook is divided into three sections and is intended for audiology graduate students as well as the practicing dispensing audiologist.

The first section examines the issues involved in measuring the performance of hearing aids. It is important for the dispensing audiologist to have a strong knowledge of the performance of hearing aids using standardized methods as well as how the performance of the hearing aids may change when they are placed in the ear canal and on the head.

The second section highlights the numerous options that are available to the dispensing audiologist when they are in the process of ordering hearing aids. This section is intended to help the dispensing audiologist have a clearer understanding of the advantages and disadvantages of the numerous microphones, receivers, telecoils, amplifiers, potentiometers, switches, and transmission line modifications that are available when ordering earmolds and hearing aids. Hopefully, the information contained within this section may provide guidelines to help the audiologist make better choices of these options for their patients.

The final section deals with the problems of distortion, noise, and the central nervous system and how these problems continue to interface with the goal of providing optimum benefit with amplification.

No project of this magnitude can be completed without the help of many friends. First, I would like to express my deepest gratitude to all the authors for the time and energy they placed into each chapter. Their skills and knowledge are the basis of the success of this text. Second, each chapter was reviewed by two external reviewers. I would like to thank Jerry Agnew, James Kates, Robert Keith, Francis Kuk, Edward Lybarger, Samuel Lybarger, Bowen Marshall, Eugene McHugh, David Preves, Wayne Olsen, Carol Sammeth, Brad Stach, Paul Stypulkowski, and Robert Sweetow for expending considerable time and effort in reviewing the chapters and providing numerous helpful suggestions to each author. Their efforts resulted in chapters that were expanded and made clearer. Third, I would like to thank Philip van Tongeren, Vice President and Publisher, and Tina Galka at Thieme Medical Publishers for their assistance from our initial contact to the completion of this text. Fourth, I would like to thank Margaret Juelich, Judy Peterein, Belinda Sinks, Diane Duddy, Tracy Wilson-Holden, Robert Loomis, Kathy Vander Werff, and Lisa Potts. These kind and very talented audiologists allowed me the time and freedom that was necessary to complete this project. Fifth, I would like to thank Kathy Swan, our secretary, who graciously arranged my schedule so that I could have the necessary time to complete this book.

Finally, and most importantly, I would once again like to thank my wife Maureen and our daughters Michelle and Anne. Their love, understanding, and support was once again essential for the successful completion of this project. I know they are as proud of me as I am of them.

*Michael Valente, Ph.D.*

# Contributors

**Jeremy Agnew, Ph.D.**
Director of Product Development
Starkey Laboratories, Inc.
Eden Prairie, MN

**Jane Baran, Ph.D.**
Associate Professor
Department of Communication
  Disorders
University of Massachusetts
Amherst, MA

**Robert de Jonge, Ph.D.**
Professor of Audiology
Department of Speech Pathology and
  Audiology
Central Missouri State University
Warrensburg, MO

**Todd Fortune, Ph.D.**
Research Audiologist
Argosy Electronics
Eden Prairie, MN

**Francis K. Kuk, Ph.D.**
Division of Audiology
Department of Otolaryngology
University of Illinois at Chicago
Chicago, IL

**Edward H. Lybarger, B.A.**
President
Allegheny Hearing Association, Inc.
Pittsburgh, PA

**Peter L. Madaffari, B.S., M.S.**
Vice President, Transducer Development
Tibbetts Industries, Inc.
Camden, ME

**Frank E. Musiek, Ph.D.**
Professor
Departments of Otolaryngology and
  Neurology
Dartmouth-Hitchcock Medical
  Center
Lebanon, NH

**Lisa G. Potts, M.S.**
Research Audiologist
Washington University School of
  Medicine
St. Louis, MO

**David A. Preves, Ph.D.**
Vice President, Research and
  Development
Argosy Electronics
Eden Prairie, MN

**Donald J. Schum, Ph.D.**
University of Iowa
Hospitals and Clinics
Iowa City, IA

Oticon A/S
58, Strandvejen
DK-2900
Hellerup, Denmark


**W. Kent Stanley, B.S.**
Senior Vice President and Senior
 Design Engineer
Tibbetts Industries, Inc.
Camden, ME

**Maureen Valente, M.A.**
Department of Communication
 Disorders
St. Louis University
St. Louis, MO


**Michael Valente, Ph.D.**
Associate Professor
Director of Adult Audiology
Washington University School of
 Medicine
St. Louis, MO

# Standardizing Hearing Aid Measurement Parameters and Electroacoustic Performance Tests

## David A. Preves

## Introduction

Fine contributions to the literature on the standardization of electroacoustical performance measurements for hearing aids can already be found in other audiological texts (e.g., Lybarger, 1985; Kasten and Franks, 1986). This chapter, however, has a somewhat different purpose: besides presenting details of several hearing aid-related standards, this chapter is written to provide the interested reader a closer look at the inner workings of standards committees as they formulate and draft standards. Procedural steps required to develop and obtain approval of new and revised standards are discussed. Several American National Standards Institute (ANSI) hearing aid-related standards are reviewed in light of how they differ from comparable international standards on hearing aids. First, a brief overview is presented regarding some general aspects of standardization activities.

## Organization of Standards Committees

The *Acoustical Society of America* (ASA) is the Standards Secretariat for the following accredited *American National Standards Institute (ANSI)* Committees: *S1—Acoustics; S2—Mechanical Shock and Vibration; S3—Bioacoustics;* and *S12—Noise.* These four committees operate as specified by the ANSI Procedures for Accredited Standards Committees (ANSI, 1993). Each committee has a formal title and a definition of scope. Within each of these committees are many working groups that have their own titles and scopes. The committee Chairs appoint working group Chairs and, in turn, the working group Chairs appoint working group members. Working groups may also have corresponding members. Interested observers that might be directly or materially affected by the standards being developed are welcome to attend full committee meetings and working group meetings.

Hearing aid standards come under the aegis of the S3 Bioacoustics committee. The rather formidable scope of the S3 committee is: Standards, specifications, methods of measurement and test, and *terminology* in the fields of mechanical shock and physiological acoustics, including aspects of general acoustics, shock, and vibration that pertain to biological safety, tolerance, and comfort (ASA, 1994). Among the working groups within the S3 committee, there are a number whose scopes are related to hearing aids. They are *S3-48, Hearing Aids; S3-80, Probe Tube Measurements of Hearing Aid Performance; S3-37, Coupler Calibration of Earphones;* and *S3-81, Assistive Listening Devices.* Most of this chapter will focus on standards developed by the S3-48 working group.

## Working Group S3-48, Standardization of Hearing Aid Measurements

Formal standards activity undertaken by writing groups of the Acoustical Society of America in the United States for hearing aid measurement date back to the 1950s (Lybarger, 1994). An excellent historical summary can be found in Skafte (1994). For many years, the scope for the S3-48 working group on hearing aids standards has been "(a) all aspects of hearing aid measurement except couplers; and (b) review of related international documents" (ASA, 1994). In recent years, this working group developed the S3.22 standard on specifying toleranced hearing aid characteristics with pure tone signals; the S3.35 standard for measuring the performance characteristics of hearing aids on a manikin; and the S3.42 standard on measuring the performance of hearing aids with a broad-band noise signal.

The Chair of the S3-48, working for many years, was Sam Lybarger. The roots of this working group grew from his early participation as Chairman in the 1950s and 1960s of such standards committees as the ASA Z24-W-10 and S3-W-34 writing groups (Lybarger, 1994). In his long-running capacity as working group Chair, Lybarger set the tone of standards meetings for years to come in the S3-48 working group as well as other working groups concerned with hearing aids. Accurate and complete minutes of working group meetings are critical for continuity of working group activities between meetings. The S3-48 working group has also been, indeed, fortunate to have Wayne Olsen as Secretary for an excess of 20 years. He has set a high standard for the functioning of a working group Secretary by taking very complete minutes at each working group meeting and organizing and distributing them to working group members in a timely fashion with the appropriate handouts from the meeting as attachments.

## Working Group S3-80, Standardization of Probe Tube Measurements of Hearing Aid Performance

Although members of the S3-48 working group considered forming a subcommittee to develop a performance measurement standard for assessing the electroacoustic characteristics of hearing aids on real ears, a separate working group, S3-80, was ultimately split off for this purpose. It was felt that the magnitude of this task warranted the formation of a separate working group so that the ongoing work of S3-48 at the time (the development of the S3.42 standard) would not be disrupted. The title of the S3-80 working group is *Probe-Tube Measurements of Hearing Aid Performance.* Its scope is "to develop standards for the determination of the real ear electroacoustic performance of hearing aids *in situ*" (ASA, 1994).

### Working Group S3-37, Standardization of Coupler Calibration of Earphones

The scope for the S3-37 working group on couplers is: "Coordinate ANSI projects with International Electrotechnical Commission (IEC) working groups. Prepare revisions to existing earphone calibration standards, prepare new standards for circumaural earphones, study and prepare standards for simulation of the human ear for measurement purposes" (ASA, 1994). It is this working group that formulated ANSI standard S3.7, which specifies the dimensions and configurations of the various 2-cc couplers, and ANSI standard S3.25, which specifies the characteristics of the modified Zwislocki ear simulator.

### Working Group S3-81, Standardization of Assistive Listening Devices

The scope of the S3-81 working group on *Hearing Assistive Technologies* is: "To provide definitions for various types of assistive listening devices (ALDs). To determine which assistive listening devices can be measured acoustically and to provide standard procedures for such acoustical measurement" (ASA, 1994). One of the initial goals of this group is to develop a definition for ALDs that would clearly distinguish them from hearing aids. The United States Food and Drug Administration (FDA) regulates the introduction, manufacturing, and performance specifications of medical devices. The FDA eagerly awaits the definition of ALDs because it has been closely watching the introduction and widespread marketing without *FDA 510(k) approval* of low-cost hearing aids posing as non-medical assistive listening devices. [510(k) refers to the section in the Federal Food, Drug, and Cosmetic Act that requires medical device manufacturers to request FDA approval to market a new or a modified medical device.] As of this writing, it appears that one feature distinguishing many ALDs from hearing aids is that ALDs have a remote microphone.

Obviously, the scopes of these four working groups are similar and, consequently, many of their members belong to more than one of these working groups. When they have business to discuss, working group meetings for these four groups normally occur twice a year. For convenience, many of the meetings are held "back to back" in 1 or 2 days of highly concentrated standards activity, usually immediately preceding or following a national convention such as the Acoustical Society of America (ASA) or the American Academy of Audiology (AAA).

## *Standards Development and Approval Process*

The term "standard" implies consensus and approval. Procedures for standards development fulfill the requirements of due process and consensus development as outlined in the *Procedures for the Development and Coordination of American National Standards* (ANSI, 1993). A detailed definition of the elements of due process as they apply to voluntary standards development is given in the *Society Bylaws of the American Society of Testing and Materials* (ASTM, 1992). These include timely and adequate notice of a proposed standard to all persons likely to be materially affected by it; opportunity of all affected interests to participate in the deliberations, discussions, and decisions concerned both with procedural and substantive matters; maintenance of adequate records of discussions and decisions; timely publication and distribution of minutes of meetings of both main committees and subcommittees; adequate notice of proposed actions; meticulously maintained records of drafts of a proposed standard, proposed amendments, action on amendments, and final promulgation of the standard; timely and full reports on the results of balloting; and careful attention to minority opinions throughout the process. Under the due process and consensus requirements of ANSI, if the procedures in a standard under development are obviously going to cause an economic hardship for organizations or individuals, this must be brought out early on in the discussions. Then, the standard can be drafted so as to not cause severe economic hardships. However, in general, it is this author's experience that ANSI working groups try to function as much as possible without the influence of political or commercial interests, keeping the discussions to a scientific format. Often, in fact, attendees of working group meetings are treated to purely tutorial and highly technical, informative presentations, resulting from one or more of its members offering to present data on the results of new measurement methods. Such presentations offer the possibilities of standardizing new techniques in the future if they eventually become widely used.

Once a new standard is drafted, or an old standard is revised by a working group, it must be circulated to and approved by the group of organizations and persons within one of the four committees referenced above that are allowed to vote on draft standards. The process of hearing aid standards development involves achieving a consensus among the working group that drafted it, as well as the full S3 Bioacoustics committee. At the time of this writing, the S3 Bioacoustics committee consists of the representatives of organizations as well as the individual experts shown in Figure 1–1. This approval process involves balloting wherein each representative with voting rights casts one vote, accompanied by technical or editorial comments, if appropriate. "No" votes and comments are resolved by the working group that drafted the standard. This is accomplished either by making changes to the contents of the document or by persuading the dissenter to change the vote to affirmative. Once the "No" votes and comments have been resolved, the new standard is given a number and printed. It is then offered for sale in the ANSI standards catalog.

ANSI standards related to hearing aids usually follow a consistent format: an Abstract, Foreword, list of organizations and experts on the full S3-Bioacoustics Committee, a list of the individuals on the working group, a Table of Contents, Introduction, Scope, Explanation of Terms, References, the main body of the document, and the Appendices.

| Organization | Representative |
|---|---|
| S3 Standards Committee | A. Brenig, Secretariat |
| S3 Standards Committee | T. Frank, Chair |
| S3 Standards Committee | R.F. Burkard, Vice Chair |
| American Academy of Otolaryngology | L.A. Michael |
| American Industrial Hygiene Assn | L.H. Royster |
| American Institute of Ultrasound Medicine | J. Zagzebski |
| American College Occupational and Environmental Medicine | P.J. Brownson |
| American Otological Society, Inc. | R.F. Naunton |
| American Speech-Language-Hearing Assn | R.F. Burkhard |
| AT&T | R.M. Sachs |
| Audio Engineering Society, Inc. | R.H. Campbell |
| Bruel & Kjaer Instruments, Inc. | E. Schonthal |
| Compressed Air and Gas Inst | J.H. Addington |
| Hearing Industries Assn (HIA) | C.D. Conger |
| Industrial Safety Equipment Association, Inc. | J. Birkner |
| International Hearing Society (IHS) | P. Mercola |
| National Institute of Standards and Technology | E.D. Burnett |
| Power Tool Institute, Inc. | J.L. Bennett |
| U.S. Air Force | C.W. Nixon |
| U.S. Army Aeromedical Research Laboratory | J.H. Patterson |
| U.S. Army Human Eng Laboratory (HEL) | G. Garinther |
| U.S. Army Walter Reed Army Medical Center | Ltc Rodney M. Atack, Ph.D. |
| U.S. Dept of the Navy Navy Environmental Health Center | J. Page |

Individual Experts

| | |
|---|---|
| J.R. Bareham | K.D. Kryter |
| S.J. Barry | H. Levitt |
| R.W. Benson | R. McKinley |
| A.J. Brammer | J.D. Toyster |
| D.D. Dirks | H.E. vonGierke |
| K.M. Eldred | D.E. Wasserman |
| J.L. Fletcher | L.A. Wilber |
| R.S. Gales | W. Yost |
| W.J. Galloway | R.W. Young |
| R. Guernsey | |
| D.L. Johnson | |

**Figure 1–1.** Organizational members, their representatives, and individual experts of the Acoustical Society of America Accredited S3 Standards Committee on Bioacoustics at the time of this writing.

## Regulatory Aspects of ANSI Standards

Some individuals who are critical of the procedures specified in certain standards may have presumed that ANSI standards have regulatory power on their own. It is important to note that ANSI standards do not mandate anything. They are strictly recommendations that may be followed on a voluntary basis. It is only when ANSI standards are adopted by a regulatory agency that their measurements become required rather than voluntary.

An example of an ANSI standard that was adopted by a regulatory agency is S3.22 Specifications of Hearing Aid Characteristics, which was originally drafted in the mid-1970s at the request of the FDA to help ensure hearing aid quality control. Because of its adoption by the FDA and resulting regulatory status, S3.22 is probably the most well-known and the most used ANSI hearing aid standard. In fact, S3.22 has been called "the ANSI hearing aid standard," implying that there is only one such document. Other ANSI standards that pertain to hearing aids are less well known to those in the hearing health care field and are less frequently used, evidently because there are no regulatory requirements to use them. These include S3.35, Methods of Measurements of Performance

Characteristics of Hearing Aids Under Simulated *In Situ* Working Conditions and S3.42, Testing Hearing Aids With a Broad-Band Noise Signal.

Widespread use of a standard may also occur when other federal agencies adopt the procedures that have been standardized. For example, the Veterans Administration (VA), which is not a regulatory body, periodically qualifies a small group of hearing aid manufacturers to provide custom ITE hearing aids to VA Medical Center audiology clinics. To qualify, hearing aid manufacturers are asked to design and build custom ITE hearing aids from VA-generated specifications. These hearing aids are submitted to the VA for rigorous tests that have long been in the forefront of the state of the art in hearing aid measurements. To facilitate this activity, the VA hearing aid procurement program works closely with experts from within the VA system and outside consultants, as well as personnel from the *National Institute of Standards and Technology* (NIST—formerly the *National Bureau of Standards*) who measure the electroacoustic performance of the submitted hearing aids. For example, as part of the 1994 solicitation, manufacturers submitting products for qualification were informed that only those hearing aids whose *coherence function* exceeded a certain minimum value would be put on contract (VA, 1994). (The coherence function is a single number ranging from 0 to 1 that indicates the amount of noise and distortion produced by a hearing aid at a particular frequency. That is, coherence indicates the fraction of the hearing aid output that is caused by the input signal.) Because the use of the coherence function as a hearing aid measurement has been recommended in the ANSI S3.42-1992 standard, this mandate gives this standard a higher profile and greater use.

Additionally, often procedures provided in ANSI standards make their way into commercially available test equipment. One example is the Frye 6500, a widely distributed hearing aid analyzer that uses a broad-band noise signal and *Fast Fourier Transform* (FFT) analysis. This instrument was developed during the same time as the deliberations of the S3-48 working group that ultimately led to ANSI S3.42-1992.

## *Updating ANSI Standards*

As technology advances, procedures and parameters in standards may become obsolete over time. Many new standards are based on previous standards that cover the same topic but have been made obsolete by changes in parameter definitions or in current measurement practices. However, rather than formulate new standards, often, working groups revise existing standards, when possible, by bringing them up to date with current practices. Those individuals who are not involved with standards development, but who are critical of how "far behind" certain ANSI standards are from their own current measurement practices or beliefs, need to be reminded of the voluntary nature of standards development and the due process for consensus development that each new or revised standard must undergo before being approved and published. The development of new ANSI hearing aid-related standards or revision of existing standards often takes many years to complete. Such long times are not surprising, considering that the working groups meet only twice a year and most of the work is accomplished on a volunteer basis. In fact, due to the busy schedules of working group members, much of their standards work activity has to be done in the evenings and on weekends. For these extra hours, working group members, including their Chairs and Secretaries, receive no compensation for their efforts, other than the support they receive from the organizations they represent. Most working groups have the philosophy that procedures should not be standardized until they are either already widely utilized and proven, or until they are tested in feasibility studies conducted by working group members. Just to reach a consensus about a particular measurement procedure among the members of a working group can be a major undertaking. An important unwritten policy of most working groups is that a new or revised standard should not limit the development of new technology. Often, during the initial stages of standards development, when the rough outlines are being drawn for a new standard, the work goes quickly and is relatively exciting. However, the pace slows considerably when the details are being worked out and the fine points of the language used in the document are being edited.

Unfortunately, weaknesses and oversights are sometimes found after an ANSI standard has been printed and has been in use. If the oversights involve a serious error, an "Erratum" sheet can be inserted into each copy of the standard that contains the error, much as is done with textbooks that have errors. An ANSI standard is a "living" document. Every 5 years, the Acoustical Society allows working groups to reaffirm, update, or obsolete existing standards they have developed to take into account evolution in thinking about the appropriateness of their past recommendations. An example is ANSI S3.22, whose first printing was in 1976, with revisions in 1982 and 1987. Currently, S3.22 is again being revised to make more meaningful measurements and to resolve a few problems that were found with some of its procedures.

One example of an oversight was found early on, just after the 1987 revision of ANSI S3.22 was printed. The original version of S3.22 in 1976 had specified 70 dB SPL input level for the harmonic distortion test at all three test frequencies. In the 1982 revision of S3.22, the input level was specified as 70 dB SPL for 500 Hz and 800 Hz and 65 dB SPL for 1600 Hz. The rationale of the S3-48 working group for not using the same input level for all three test frequencies in the 1982 revision was that many hearing aid receivers in use at that time were thought to possess a maximum sensitivity at approximately 1600 Hz. This sensitivity created a peak in the response at that frequency that might drive the hearing aid into distortion, even at reference test gain setting. [Reference test gain setting is the reduced gain (volume) control setting at which many of the S3.22 tests are performed.] However, in the 1987 revision, the S3-48 working group initially decided that the input level used at all three test frequencies 500, 800, and 1600 Hz for harmonic distortion measurements could revert back to 70 dB SPL. The rationale of the S3-48 working group for this reversal was based on not finding a significant difference in total harmonic distortion measured values after a considerable amount of testing at 1600 Hz and at the third special purpose average (SPA) frequency in the laboratories of several working group members. (SPA frequencies are a set of three 1/3-octave test frequencies, each separated by 2/3-octave, that may be used in place of the standard distortion test frequencies if the hearing aid passband is extremely high pass or extremely low pass.) For these tests, harmonic distortion was measured at 1600 Hz with both 65 dB and 70 dB SPL input levels for many hearing aids having many widely differing circuits and transducers. It was the opinion of members of the working group that (1) with the increased usage of new receivers that shifted the primary peak in the frequency response up to about 3000 Hz, most hearing aids would no longer have receivers with an impedance resonance in the vicinity of 1600 Hz, and (2) use of the SPA frequencies for extreme high pass and extreme low pass hearing aids would cause their gain controls to be turned down enough to achieve reference test position to avoid significant distortion. Unfortunately, neither was always the case as pointed out by Harry Teder, a member of the working group who provided some examples of hearing aids that still exhibited the problem. Shortly thereafter, an Erratum sheet was issued for S3.22-1987, instructing the use of 65 dB input SPL at 1600 Hz or at the third SPA distortion test frequency.

### International Standards

ANSI is the U.S. member of international standards organizations such as the *International Electrotechnical Commission (IEC)*, which has working groups for hearing aid-related standards development whose scopes are similar to those in the United States provided by the Acoustical Society of America. In the past, IEC standards have been adopted by many member countries for "type approval" of hearing aids. (Type approval refers to the process used to characterize and approve hearing aids for distribution in a country.) As such, IEC hearing aid standards may take on a high degree of regulatory power in some of these member countries. With the advent of the *European Community (EC)*, IEC standards will have even more regulatory power because their test procedures will be required for hearing aids distributed in all of the member countries.

One of the main activities of the ANSI S3-48 hearing aid working group is developing and coordinating comments on hearing aid-related documents generated by the IEC hearing aid working groups. Ideally, ANSI and IEC standards would be technically compatible, and differ possibly only in editorial content. At the very least, it would be advantageous for ANSI and IEC standards not to conflict with one another. To this end, there are provisions in the ANSI Procedures for the Development and Coordination of American National Standards for making an international document an ANSI standard (ANSI, 1993).

Unfortunately, up to this time, there have been very few ANSI and IEC hearing aid-related standards that are technically compatible. There are clear examples of ANSI hearing aid standards being formulated before the IEC standards working groups started developing similar documents. Yet, the IEC documents often evolved with significant technical differences relative to their ANSI predecessors. For example, it appears that the ANSI S3.22-1976 hearing aid measurement standard and the ANSI S3.29-1979 ear simulator standard led to the development in the early 1980s of the IEC 118 series of standards and the IEC 711 ear simulator standard. In spite of the objections of the delegates to the IEC from the United States and several other countries, these two sets of standards are technically incompatible. Somehow, the IEC working groups decided not to adopt the S3.22-

1976 and S3.25-1979 ANSI standards. Fortunately, a more concerted effort between the IEC and ANSI hearing aid working groups to develop new standards and to modify existing standards in a spirit of harmonization is currently under way.

## Brief Overview of Selected ANSI Hearing Aid-Related Standards

The scopes of ANSI hearing aid-related standards range from a relatively simple specification of earhook nozzle threads (S3.37-1987) for postauricular hearing aids to extremely detailed procedures for measuring the electroacoustic parameters of hearing aids. The following is a brief elaboration of the contents of several ANSI hearing aid-related standards, a discussion of the working group rationale for some of the revisions, and how these standards compare to their IEC counterparts. For more detail about each standard, the interested reader is referred to the standards themselves.

### Measurement of Hearing Aid Electroacoustical Characteristics, ASA Standard S3.3-1960

The S3.3 standard, published in 1960, is entitled *Methods of Measurement of the Electroacoustical Characteristics of Hearing Aids.* It was based on one of the first hearing aid measurement standards ever developed, ASA Z24.14-1953, entitled *American Standard Method for Measurement of Characteristics of Hearing Aids* (Lybarger, 1994). The S3.3 standard has been reaffirmed repeatedly, first in 1971, and last in 1990.

S3.3 includes detailed sections on accuracy and limits for test equipment including requirements for the sound source, test enclosure, coupler, reference microphone, coupler microphone, sound pressure measurement system, and apparatus for automatic frequency response recording. The document also specifies requirements for environmental test conditions, test point, sound pressure level control means (*substitution and comparison methods*), power supply, and control settings. The main measurements defined in the S3.3 standard are *full-on acoustic gain, saturation sound pressure level, harmonic distortion at three test frequencies, battery current, a basic frequency response, and a family of frequency response curves.* The S3.3 standard was one of the predecessors of the ANSI S3.22-1976 standard, but was not replaced by S3.22. The procedure for setting the gain control for the basic frequency response specified in S3.3 was the forerunner for the *reference test position* concept in S3.22. The saturation sound pressure level was defined in S3.3 as a frequency-by-frequency measurement of the maximum value of the rms coupler SPL with input level varying as needed rather than with a constant 90 dB input SPL as in S3.22. S3.3 also specifies use of the *HA-1, HA-2,* and *HA-3* type 2-cc couplers for accommodating various styles of hearing aids. (A discussion of these couplers follows in a later section of this chapter.)

Also included in the main body of the S3.3 standard were recommended procedures for obtaining the effect of tone control position on frequency response and optional procedures for determining the effects of power supply voltage variation and gain control rotation on acoustic gain. Future plans by the S3-48 working group call for incorporating these S3.3 tests into the next revision of the S3.22 standard and then making the S3.3 standard obsolete. The interested reader is referred to Staab (1978) for further details on S3.3.

## Specification of Hearing Aid Characteristics, ANSI Standard S3.22-1976 (rev. 1982, 1987)

As mentioned previously, ANSI standard S3.22 entitled *Specification of Hearing Aid Characteristics,* was developed specifically at the request of the FDA. Under the *Medical Device Amendments of 1976* (Federal Register, 1977), hearing aids were categorized by the FDA as a medical device. The intent of the FDA was to regulate hearing aids with a performance standard that would ensure their quality via conformance to specified tolerances. In 1974, the FDA informed the hearing aid industry that the FDA would write a hearing aid performance standard if the S3-48 working group could not develop one in a short time. Michael Gluck, an Engineer with the FDA, actually produced several drafts of a hearing aid performance standard before the S3-48 working group was able to complete what ultimately became ANSI standard S3.22, first published in 1976 (Kasten and Franks, 1986). This document was actually developed in conjunction with the FDA because Michael Gluck was invited by the working group Chair, Sam Lybarger, to become a member of S3-48. To this day, one or two representatives of the FDA continue to attend S3-48 working group meetings on a regular basis. However, in general, their presence has been more relaxed than that in the 1970s, with their current role being mainly supportive and advisory in nature. Due to the FDA action of classifying hearing aids as a medical device, the S3-48 working group must keep in mind that any of the procedures it standardizes might someday be adopted as required tests by the FDA. Many individuals have pointed out how poorly the electroacoustic performance measurements in S3.22 represent the actual performance of hearing aids while being worn. These individuals are reminded that the original purpose of this standard was to ensure quality control, not to depict real-world performance (Kasten and Franks, 1986).

### EARLY EXPERIENCES USING A BROAD-BAND NOISE SIGNAL

Prior to the FDA mandate to develop a hearing aid performance test standard, in the early 1970s, the S3-48 working group investigated whether a noise input signal could be used in place of a pure tone input signal. Such a noise input signal, shaped approximately to the short term speech spectrum, has been used for many years by Edwin Burnett at the National Bureau of Standards (NBS) for testing hearing aids submitted for qualification to the Veterans Administration hearing aid program (Burnett, 1967). The idea for standardizing on noise for an input signal in conjunction with spectral analysis was suggested in the 1970s by Gerald Studebaker, then a member of the S3-48 working group, on hearing aid measurement standards. The essence of his proposal to the working group, and some examples of measurements on hearing aids, can be found in the proceedings of the Wyoming hearing aid conference (Studebaker, 1979).

To determine whether using a broad-band noise input signal was viable, tests were performed in a round robin at the laboratories of working group members on several specifically selected hearing aids. (A round robin, as used here, refers to a series of the same tests conducted on the same hearing aid or hearing aids by different individuals and laboratories. An example of a round robin with a broad-band noise input signal is given in the section of this chapter that discusses the S3.42-1992 standard.) The data showed considerable variations in the *noise gain* and *noise saturation sound pressure level* measurements for the same hearing aids across different laboratories. [The terms noise gain and noise sound pressure level with 90 dB SPL input (NSPL90) are both single figure numbers that were later standardized in ANSI S3.42-1992 Testing Hearing Aids With a Broad-Band Noise Input Signal. They represent the overall root mean square (rms) gain and noise output SPL across frequency with 60 and 90 dB noise input SPL, respectively.] This large variability was thought to be caused by differences in the acoustic spectrum of the noise input signals generated at the various laboratories. Some of the laboratories participating had excellent equalization equipment for shaping the noise input spectrum; others did not. Repeatability of noise gain measurements across laboratories using the noise input signal was poor due to the inability of all laboratories to equalize the spectrum of the noise input signal accurately in different test chambers.

In the mid-1970s, after the results of the round robin with noise input were analyzed, the FDA was pressing the S3-48 working group to develop a quality control standard quickly. Therefore, the idea of using the broad-band noise input signal had to be abandoned in favor of a three frequency average. Averaging at three frequencies to express gain was similar to the procedure of averaging at 500, 1000, and 2000 Hz recommended in United States of America Standards Institute standard S3.8 (USASI, 1967). The selection of the three test frequencies was the result of some eleventh hour measurements made by Sam Lybarger with a number of hearing aids using the laboratory-grade test equipment in his home. His results showed that averaging measurements at 1000, 1600, and 2500 Hz yielded average gain and average saturation sound pressure levels very similar to those obtained by the NBS with their noise input signal. The working group ultimately recommended standardizing these three frequencies for gain and saturation sound pressure level measurements; they became known as the "high frequency average" or HFA gain and HFA SSPL90.

S3.22 defines a *reference test position* (RTP—the gain control position at which reference test gain is obtained) of the hearing aid gain control for conducting most of the tests and a three-frequency average for expressing gain (HFA full-on gain and gain at RTP) and saturation sound pressure level (HFA SSPL90). Additionally, the method for frequency range determination specified in S3.22 is very similar to that recommended in the S3.8 standard (USASI, 1967) in which frequency range was derived from the two intersections of the basic frequency response with a horizontal line drawn 15 dB down from the three-frequency average gain.

HOW TOLERANCES IN S3.22 ARE APPLIED

A primary goal of the S3.22 standard, and one that the FDA especially insisted on, is that any facility having a hearing aid analyzer that meets the performance requirements for measuring equipment specified in S3.22 could test hearing aids in accordance with the standard. This goal was deemed very useful because often dispensers (or governmental facilities) might wish to check hearing aids to determine whether they were within the manufacturer's published specifications. S3.22 was originally conceived to apply mainly to noncustom, postauricular hearing aids that were the most prevalent type distributed in the early 1970s. For such instruments, it is possible to make performance measurements on many samples of the same hearing aid model from which means and standard deviations can be determined for such parameters as HFA SSPL90 and HFA full-on gain. The tolerances specified in the S3.22 standard are then applied around the mean data values (for S3.22 tolerances, see Fig. 1–2).

However, test equipment inaccuracies were not included in the tolerances provided in S3.22 for each parameter being measured. Instead, it was the responsibility of the facility checking the hearing aid to account for the estimated inaccuracies of their test equipment. This procedure, as recommended in section 6.16 of the S3.22 standard, at first may be somewhat difficult to understand. The *Interpretation of Tolerances section* in the S3.22 standard is perhaps best illustrated by an example. The tolerances specified in S3.22 for HFA SSPL90 and HFA full-on gain of ±4 dB and ±5 dB, respectively, are applied by the manufacturer's quality control department for hearing aids being delivered to dispensers. Let us assume that the inaccuracies of the manufacturer's test equipment are hypothetically estimated to be ±2 dB for SSPL90 and ±1 dB for gain. To check a group of postauricular hearing aids against their published specifications, the manufacturer *subtracts* these estimated equipment inaccuracies from the ±4 dB and ±5 dB tolerances for HFA SSPL90 and HFA full-on gain, respectively, that are specified in the standard. Thus, only those hearing aids that fall within ±2 dB for HFA SSPL90 and within ±4 dB for HFA full-on gain could be passed by the manufacturer as meeting specifications. This procedure ensures that any hearing aid of a given model will be shipped from the manufacturer's facility meeting the tolerances given in the S3.22 standard.

If another facility electroacoustically analyzes a hearing aid of the same model, the total allowable tolerances for each parameter are the same tolerances specified in the standard *plus* the estimated test equipment inaccuracies of that facility, centered around the nominal values on the specifications provided for that model by the hearing aid manufacturer. For example, if a dispenser's hearing aid analyzer inaccuracy was hypothetically estimated to be ±3 dB for SSPL90 and ±2 dB for gain, the dispenser would check hearing aids to ±7 dB for HFA SSPL90 and also ±7 dB for HFA full-on gain.

| Maximum SSPL 90 | HF Average SSPL 90 | HF Average Full-on Gain | Reference Test Gain | Frequency Range | Total Harmonic Distortion | | | Equivalent Input Noise Level | Telephone Pickup Coil Sensitivity at 1 KHz | Battery Drain |
|---|---|---|---|---|---|---|---|---|---|---|
| | | | | | 500 Hz | 800 Hz | 1600 Hz | | | |
| Maximum 140 dB | 130 dB | 55 dB | 53 dB | 180 – 5050 Hz | 10% | Maximum 5% | 5% | Maximum 28 dB | 100 dB | Maximum 2 6 mA |
| Typical 138 dB | ±4 dB | ±5 dB | | | 5% | Typical 2% | 1% | Typical 23 dB | ±6 dB | Typical 2.1 mA |

**Figure 1–2.** Published nominal and maximum specifications per ANSI S3.22-1987 for a postauricular hearing aid. Reprinted with permission from Preves, 1988.

For *maximum SSPL90, current drain, equivalent input noise, and harmonic distortion,* hearing aid manufacturers were instructed by the original version of S3.22 (and the FDA) to publish maximum values that no example of a particular model would ever exceed. As with the other toleranced values, these specified maximum values do not include an allowance for measuring equipment inaccuracies. Therefore, when checking a group of postauricular hearing aids, the manufacturer's quality control department subtracts their estimated equipment inaccuracies from the published maximum values as shown by the example in Figure 1–2. If the hypothetical estimated inaccuracy of a manufacturer's test equipment is ±2 dB for SSPL90 measurements, the manufacturer's quality control department would check outgoing hearing aids to 2 dB less than the 140 dB published maximum SSPL90 value. Similarly, estimates of the inaccuracies of measuring equipment at another facility used to check the hearing aid against published specifications must be *added* to these specified maximum values to predict the actual allowable maximum values to test against. If the estimated equipment inaccuracy of the test equipment at an audiological clinic, for example, is hypothetically ±3 dB for SSPL90, when checking a hearing aid of that type against published specifications, to establish a valid upper limit to check against, the clinic would have to add 3 dB to the manufacturer's published maximum SSPL90 value (e.g., 140 dB in Fig. 1–2) for that hearing aid model.

The procedure outlined above cannot be applied very well to one-of-a-kind custom hearing aids, for which the individual measurements obtained on each hearing aid serve as the published specifications for that particular instrument (Preves, 1988). These individual measurements are sent out, as required by the FDA, on a data sheet accompanying each custom hearing aid. Consequently, in 1987, S3.22 was revised to take into account the prevalence of custom-designed ITE hearing aids. For this revision, the S3-48 working group proposed that the actual data, rather than estimated maximum values, could be reported for maximum SSPL90, current drain, equivalent input noise, and harmonic distortion for custom-designed hearing aids. Also included in the 1987 revision of the S3.22 standard were one set of estimated equipment inaccuracies that applied to the hearing aid manufacturer or to an off-site test facility, saving everyone the trouble of having to estimate the equipment inaccuracies. These are: ±3 dB for Maximum SSPL90 and equivalent input noise, ±20% for current drain, and ±3% for harmonic distortion measurements.

With the 1987 revision of the standard, therefore, when checking custom-designed hearing aids, the manufacturer's quality control department simply reports the values actually measured on each custom hearing aid and sends a hard copy along with the hearing aid. As far as the FDA is concerned, these values serve as the published specifications for that hearing aid. Measurements obtained at another facility checking the hearing aid would have to fall within the above-published tolerances, added to the manufacturer's reported values for maximum SSPL90, current drain, equivalent input noise, and harmonic distortion that accompanied the hearing aid. For example, if an audiological clinic wanted to check the equivalent input noise of a custom ITE hearing aid against the 30 dB SPL measurement (specification) reported by the hearing aid manufacturer, the clinic would test the hearing aid for a maximum equivalent input noise of 30 dB SPL + the 3 dB tolerance = 33 dB SPL.

APPLYING S3.22 TO EXTREME HIGH-PASS AND LOW-PASS HEARING AIDS

S3.22 was also revised in 1987 to accommodate those hearing aids with extreme high-pass or extreme low-pass frequency responses. An example of the problem was brought to the attention of the S3-48 work group by Mead Killion who manufactures an accessory earhook that results in hearing aids with extreme low-frequency emphasis. Subsequent testing by S3-48 working group members revealed that hearing aids having passbands that were outside the frequency range of the three HFA test frequencies (1000 to 2500 Hz) usually would not result in their gain controls being turned down very far to achieve the reference test position. In fact, many of these hearing aids would have the reference test position at full-on, because of not having sufficient gain in comparison to SSPL90 to require turning the gain control down at all. Obtaining the performance of hearing aids at full-on is contradictory to the original intention of S3.22, which was to test hearing aid performance at a reduced gain control setting. The working group felt that hearing aids tested at full-on might be penalized due to possible instability, resulting in greater peaks and troughs in the frequency response. Additionally, at full-on, higher equivalent input noise, higher harmonic distortion, and higher current drain may also occur.

USE OF SPECIAL-PURPOSE FREQUENCIES

In the 1987 revision of S3.22, for these extreme high-pass or low-pass hearing aids, the hearing aid manufacturer is allowed to select "special purpose frequencies" with which to form a special purpose average *(SPA) full-on gain* and a *SPA SSPL90* that more closely represented the passband of the hearing aid than the set (1000, 1600, and 2500 Hz) that are used for the HFA full-on gain and HFA SSPL90 tests. For example, for the hearing aid whose frequency response and SSPL90 curves are shown in Figure 1–3, because the calculated gain at reference test position is 103.6 dB SPL–77 dB = 26.6 dB, and the HFA full-on gain of the hearing aid is only 23.3 dB, the gain control is at full-on to achieve reference test position using the set of HFA test frequencies (1000, 1600, and 2500 Hz) (Preves, 1988). Note the high value of harmonic distortion at 500 Hz (11.5%). To determine whether this hearing aid is a candidate for testing with three SPA test frequencies, the criterion specified in S3.22-1987 is whether the full-on gain at one of the HFA test frequencies is more than 15 dB less than the peak full-on gain. In this example, the full-on gain (lower curve) at 1000 Hz is more than 15 dB less than the peak gain (at 1800 Hz) so the criterion for using SPA test frequencies is met. To choose the SPA test frequencies, the reader is referred to Figure 1–4. Figure 1–4 shows the output SPL by frequency with 60 dB input SPL (left panel— representing gain) and 90 dB input SPL (right panel—representing SSPL90) in both graphic and tabular form for the hearing aid used for Figure 1–3. S3.22 specifies that the SPA test frequencies can be a combination of three preferred one-third octave frequencies, each separated by two-thirds octave (ANSI, 1967). From Figure 1–4, the set (2000, 3150, and 5000 Hz) would produce an SPA full-on

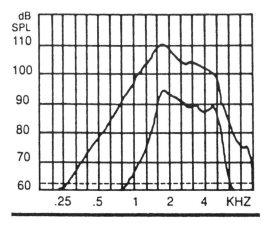

SSPL90 CURVE RUN AT 90 dB SPL INPUT
PEAK SSPL=110.6 dB SPL @ 1.800 KHZ

HFA SSPL90=103.6 dB SPL

REF TEST GAIN= 22.3 dB
HFA FULL ON GAIN= 23.3 dB @ 50 dB INPUT SPL

FREQ RESPONSE RUN AT 60 dB SPL INPUT
F1(LF)= .870 KHZ ; F2(HF)=6.530 KHZ

TOTAL HARMONIC DIST
.500 KHZ: 11.5% @ 70 dB SPL INPUT
.800 KHZ: N/A
1.600 KHZ: 1.5% @ 65 dB SPL INPUT

EQ INPUT NOISE LEVEL= 28.1 dB SPL
BATTERY I= 0.60 MA @ 1 KHZ, 65 dB INPUT SPL
BATTERY TYPE= ZINC-AIR, V=1.30 V

**Figure 1–3.**  Electroacoustic data per ANSI S3.22-1987 using high-frequency average (HFA) test frequencies for a custom ITE hearing aid with high-pass frequency response. Upper curve: SSPL90. Lower curve: frequency response. Reprinted with permission from Preves, 1988.

gain of 29.8 dB (6.5 dB higher than that with the HFA test frequencies in Fig. 1–3) and an SPA SSPL90 of 103.6 dB SPL, the same as with the HFA test frequencies (Fig. 1–3). From the left panel in Fig. 1–4, this is 2.2 dB higher total output SPL with a 60 dB input SPL at the three frequencies than would have been produced if the set (1600, 2500, and 4000 Hz) had been used. Thus, the SPA gain at reference test position is calculated as 103.6 dB–77 dB = 26.6 dB. Using these frequencies for SPA test frequencies for the hearing aid would, therefore, cause a 3.2 dB gain control setback (SPA full-on gain of 29.8 dB–calculated gain at RTP of 26.6 dB). For this lower reference test position setting, the harmonic distortion at 1000 Hz (1/2 of the lowest SPA test frequency) was 3%.

With the exception of the change in input level mentioned previously for the harmonic distortion test at 1600 Hz (65 dB SPL instead of 70 dB SPL), the 1982

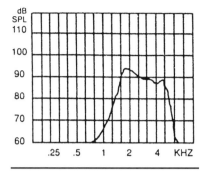

| Freq (KHZ) | dB SPL | Freq (KHZ) | dB SPL |
|---|---|---|---|
| .200 | 60.0 | 2.500 | 91.0 |
| .250 | 60.0 | 2.650 | 90.4 |
| .315 | 60.0 | 2.800 | 89.8 |
| .400 | 60.0 | 3.000 | 89.4 |
| .500 | 60.0 | 3.150 | 89.4 |
| .560 | 60.0 | 3.350 | 89.4 |
| .630 | 60.0 | 3.550 | 88.6 |
| .710 | 60.0 | 3.750 | 87.8 |
| .800 | 60.6 | 4.000 | 87.0 |
| .900 | 63.4 | 4.250 | 87.0 |
| 1.000 | 66.6 | 4.500 | 88.2 |
| 1.060 | 68.0 | 4.750 | 89.4 |
| 1.120 | 70.0 | 5.000 | 86.2 |
| 1.180 | 72.0 | 5.300 | 82.6 |
| 1.250 | 74.4 | 5.600 | 77.2 |
| 1.320 | 78.2 | 6.000 | 70.2 |
| 1.400 | 81 0 | 6.300 | 65.0 |
| 1.500 | 84.6 | 6.700 | 60.4 |
| 1.600 | 89.2 | 7.100 | 60.0 |
| 1.700 | 92.8 | 7.500 | 60.0 |
| 1.800 | 94.2 | 8.000 | 60.0 |
| 1.900 | 93.8 | 8.500 | 60.0 |
| 2.000 | 93.8 | 9.000 | 60.0 |
| 2.120 | 93.2 | 9.500 | 60.0 |
| 2.240 | 92.4 | 9.999 | 60.0 |
| 2.360 | 91.8 | | |

| Freq (KHZ) | dB SPL | Freq (KHZ) | dB SPL |
|---|---|---|---|
| .200 | 60.0 | 2.500 | 104.4 |
| .250 | 60.8 | 2.650 | 103.8 |
| .315 | 66.8 | 2.800 | 103.4 |
| .400 | 72.4 | 3.000 | 103.6 |
| .500 | 77.8 | 3.150 | 103.8 |
| .560 | 81.0 | 3.350 | 103.6 |
| .630 | 84.6 | 3.550 | 103.2 |
| .710 | 87.2 | 3.750 | 103.0 |
| .800 | 90.8 | 4.000 | 102.0 |
| .900 | 93.6 | 4.250 | 101.6 |
| 1.000 | 97.0 | 4.500 | 101.4 |
| 1.060 | 99.4 | 4.750 | 100.8 |
| 1.120 | 100.8 | 5.000 | 98.4 |
| 1.180 | 102.0 | 5.300 | 94.6 |
| 1.250 | 103.0 | 5.600 | 90.0 |
| 1.320 | 104.4 | 6.000 | 86.8 |
| 1.400 | 105.6 | 6.300 | 84.0 |
| 1.500 | 107.4 | 6.700 | 80.8 |
| 1.600 | 109.6 | 7.100 | 78.4 |
| 1.700 | 110.4 | 7.500 | 76.6 |
| 1.800 | 110.6 | 8.000 | 75.4 |
| 1.900 | 109.8 | 8.500 | 75.4 |
| 2.000 | 108.8 | 9.000 | 76.2 |
| 2.120 | 107.4 | 9.500 | 70.8 |
| 2.240 | 106.2 | 9.999 | 63.6 |
| 2.360 | 105.2 | | |

**Figure 1–4.** Graphical and tabular frequency responses at a full-on gain control setting for the hearing aid used for Figure 1–3. Swept pure tone at 60 dB input SPL (Left) and 90 dB input SPL (Right). Reprinted with permission from Preves, 1988.

revision of the S3.22 standard consisted mainly of editorial changes to the original version of 1976. Interested readers are referred to Lybarger (1985) and to Kasten and Franks (1986) for more information on the ANSI S3.22 standard.

### INCOMPATIBILITY OF IEC STANDARDS AND ANSI STANDARDS

In the early 1980s, shortly after the formulation and subsequent publication of ANSI S3.22-1976, the IEC hearing aid standards working group developed the 118 series of hearing aid measurement standards. These standards followed the general intent of the ANSI S3.22 standard, but not the specific details. Among these standards was 118-7, *Measurement of Performance Characteristics of Hearing Aids for Quality Inspection for Delivery Purposes.* Because IEC 118-7 uses the same 2-cc couplers as ANSI S3.22, the IEC 118-7 standard is unlike the IEC 118-0 type characterization hearing aid standard (*Measurement of Electroacoustic Characteristics*), which uses the *IEC 711 ear simulator.* (The IEC 118-0 standard is a type characterization standard because it is used to characterize the electroacoustic performance specifications of hearing aids rather than to check quality control of hearing aids.) Another significant difference is that the IEC hearing aid working group decided to use a single frequency to set the gain control to reference test position (rather than the three frequency average as in ANSI S3.22) and a 15 dB gain control setback (rather than the 17 dB setback specified in S3.22). The reader is referred to Table 1–1 for more information on the differences between the tests in ANSI S3.22 and IEC 118-7.

The formulation of technically incompatible ANSI and IEC hearing aid quality control standards is representative of the difficulty ANSI and IEC have had in developing compatible standards for measuring hearing aid performance. These differences present an economic penalty for those hearing aid manufacturers that export their products internationally; as a result of the procedural differences between ANSI and IEC hearing aid standards, these manufacturers must provide two sets of data, one set in accordance with ANSI S3.22 for use in the United States and Canada, and the other set for use in countries requiring the IEC 118 series of hearing aid standards.

To promote a spirit of harmonization between IEC and ANSI, Ole Dyrlund, the current Chair of IEC working groups 13 and 14 on hearing aid standards, attended the April, 1992, meetings of the ANSI S3-37, S3-48, and S3-80 working groups during the American Academy of Audiology convention in Nashville. During his visit, an "ad hoc" meeting was arranged for interested members of these three ANSI working groups to meet with Dyrlund and any other interested members of IEC hearing aid working groups also in Nashville at that time. At the ad hoc meeting, differences between comparable ANSI and IEC standards were discussed, but there was considerable doubt as to whether greater harmonization in hearing aid measurement standards could be obtained. The IEC working group

**Table 1–1.**  Comparison of Main Test Methods and Conditions Specified in ANSI S3.22-1987 to those in IEC 118-7

| Subject | IEC | ANSI |
| --- | --- | --- |
| RTGCP | Single frequency, 15 dB gain control setback | HFA (SPA), 17 dB gain control setback |
| Battery current | 60 dB SPL input | 65 dB SPL input |
| Input, full-on gain | 50 dB SPL if OSPL90-SPL60 is <5 dB | 50 dB SPL if OSPL90-SPL60 is <4 dB |
| Distortion | 1 frequency | 3 frequencies |
| Frequency range | No | Yes |
| Tolerances | No | Yes |
| AGC measurements | No | Yes |
| Directional mic. | No | Yes |
| Ambient condition | | Small differences |

RTGCP is reference test gain control position. Reprinted with permission from Dyrlund, 1992.

is committed to utilizing the 711 ear simulator as per IEC in 118-0 to determine hearing aid performance for specification sheets. Their contention is that the IEC 711 ear simulator represents the real ear gain, SSPL90, and frequency response of a hearing aid better than a 2-cc coupler does. In contrast, the ANSI working group is committed to utilizing the 2-cc coupler because it has been proven in round-robin measurements to provide repeatable measurements on the same hearing aid across multiple laboratories and because its frequency response approximates real ear insertion gain frequency responses more closely than those responses obtained with the IEC 711 ear simulator.

Dyrlund suggested at the ad hoc meeting that if ANSI could consider using an ear simulator rather than a 2-cc coupler, IEC would consider using the three-frequency average (rather than a single frequency) and a 17 dB gain control setback (rather than 15 dB) for reference test position. Dyrlund also proposed considering the Madsen ear simulator for this purpose, but it has not as yet been completely characterized. Also, there is some concern about the stability of the Madsen ear simulator in varying environments because it uses an electret rather than a condenser microphone. Further, preliminary data obtained in Dyrlund's laboratory shows that the Madsen ear simulator does not meet all of the tolerances of the IEC 711 ear simulator standard. (Figure 1–5 shows that the IEC 711 tolerances would have to be doubled for an example of a Madsen ear simulator to conform). The National Institute of Standards and Technology (NIST, formerly NBS), has been asked by the S3-48 working group and the Veterans Administration

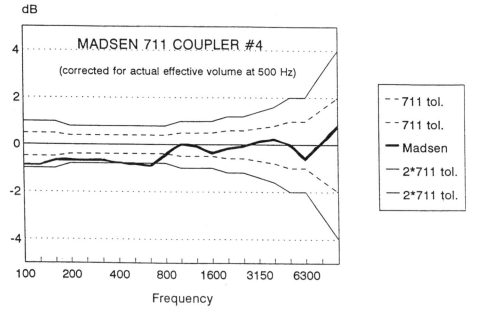

**Figure 1–5.** Normalized SPL produced in one example of a Madsen ear simulator with Bruel & Kjaer 4136 1/4 inch microphone as the sound source. Overlaid are the allowable upper and lower limits of SPL variation specified in the IEC 711 ear simulator standard (711 tol.—dashed curves) and two times this allowable SPL variation (2*711 tol.—top and bottom curves). Reprinted with permission from Dyrlund, 1993.

(as part of their hearing aid testing program) to assist in characterizing the Madsen ear simulator. NIST has long been an advocate of standards development and has done much to support hearing aid standards activities (NIST, 1986). Use of the IEC 711 and modified Zwislocki ear simulators for hearing aid testing has been discussed by the S3-48 working group during the formulation of the IEC 118-0 standard. A change from the 2-cc coupler to an ear simulator for determining the performance specifications of hearing aids would result in an immediate increase in gain and SSPL90 for existing hearing aids (Lybarger, 1981). Likewise, a change from ear simulator to 2-cc coupler for IEC would produce an immediate decrease in gain and SSPL90 for existing hearing aids now specified by IEC 118-0. Both situations pose a serious problem for currently produced hearing aids because their specifications would have to be republished. (Like a real ear canal/eardrum/middle ear, an ear simulator produces higher gain and SSPL90 than a 2cc coupler. However, it is questionable how important this is for purely quality control purposes.) There is the issue of which ear simulator to use because there are two different ear simulator standards. The modified Zwislocki ear simulator specified in ANSI S3.25-1979 is in wide use in the United States, but is not accepted by the IEC. Also, the Zwislocki ear simulator is probably not sufficiently rugged for use in high volume production. There was some discussion about the possibility of standardizing a Type 2–711 ear simulator with Barbara Kruger, a member of the S3-48 working group, Chair of the ANSI S3-37 working group on couplers, and former chair of the IEC working group on couplers. (For example, a Type 2–711 ear simulator might have wider tolerances as depicted by the 2*711 lines in Fig. 1–5.) The purpose would be to specify the tolerances for a Type 2–711 ear simulator so that both the modified Zwislocki ear simulator and the Madsen ear simulator would meet its specifications. Those at the ad hoc meeting finally decided that one of the best chances for future harmonization between ANSI and IEC standards lay in compromise of the entrenched positions held by ANSI and IEC regarding the S3.22 and 118-7 standards. At least the 711 ear simulator/2-cc coupler issues would not be involved with these two standards. Differences between the ANSI Standard S3.22 and IEC Publication 118-7 as shown in Table 1–1 were discussed (Arndt, 1992; Dyrlund, 1992). However, 3 years have passed since the Nashville ANSI/IEC ad hoc meeting, and so far there have been no compromises from either side. The ANSI and IEC hearing aid standards continue to remain technically incompatible.

## Coupler Calibration of Earphones (ANSI Standard S3.7-1973)

ANSI S3.7-1973, *Method for Coupler Calibration of Earphones,* provides specifications for several couplers and guidance for their use in calibrating hearing aid and audiometric earphones. (Note: a hearing aid earphone pertains to the receiver). The original 1973 version of S3.7 was a revision and extension of American National Standard Z24.9-1949 that had the same title. The S3.7 standard was reaffirmed in 1986 and has been revised by the S3-37 working group since then. "No" votes have been resolved for the latest revision of S3.7 and the document is being printed at the time of this writing. The following discussion applies to this latest revision of S3.7.

The Purpose section of the S3.7 standard states that no single coupler exists that can be used with all types of earphones, and can produce stable and repeatable results while adequately representing the real ear over a wide-frequency range. Thus, the document covers several different types of couplers that are used for earphone calibration for hearing aids (HA types) and audiometers. The IEC 126-1973 standard on 2-cc couplers is compatible with the 1973 version of S3.7.

All of the HA series couplers except the HA-1 type incorporate an internal earmold simulator. Among the 2-cc couplers used for hearing aid testing are:

HA-1 COUPLER

This coupler allows direct coupling of an earmold of a postauricular hearing aid, a molded insert with an internal earphone or a shell of an ITE hearing aid without additional tubing. Modeling clay or putty is used to seal the earmold or shell into the coupler. When this coupler began to be heavily used in the late 1970s resulting from the growth of ITE hearing aid sales, some effort was made to replace the clay or sealing putty with rubber "O" rings of various sizes. However, this was to no avail, because canals of ITE hearing aids vary widely in diameter and shape. Frequently, it took more time to find the appropriate size rubber "O" ring that would seal completely the earmold or shell to the coupler than to use the clay or putty.

One common problem in using the HA-1 coupler occurred when the vent in an ITE hearing aid or earmold remained open. This created an artifactual resonance, as shown by the top curve in Figure 1–6, rather than the smoother lower curve obtained with the vent closed by placing clay or putty over the vent opening. (The S3.22 standard recommends testing with the vent closed.) Similar effects can occur if the areas around the shell or earmold are not completely sealed around the coupler.

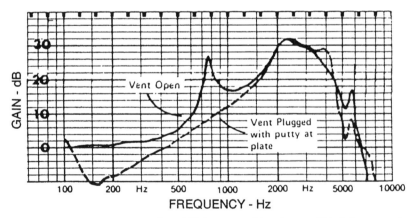

**Figure 1–6.** Frequency response of an ITE hearing aid using an HA-1 2-cc coupler with vent open and vent closed at the faceplate. Spike in upper-frequency response is caused by the vent opening resonating with the 2-cc cavity.

HA-2 COUPLER

This coupler is used for earphones with nubs (e.g., an external receiver from a body aid). Also, the HA-2 coupler has been extensively used for many years for tests with an external entrance tubing connecting an earphone in a hearing aid to an earmold or an ear insert. The earmold simulator in the HA-2 coupler has a 3 mm bore diameter, which may produce a high frequency boost compared to an actual earmold with 2 mm bore diameter tubing (Lybarger, 1985). The reader is referred to Chapter 6 for more details.

For high volume testing, the external tubing may be rigid for longer wear. The length and diameter, as specified by the manufacturer, simulates the actual tubing used in practice. Unless otherwise stated, the connecting tubing outside of the coupler has a length of 25 mm and an inner diameter of 1.93 mm (#13 tubing).

HA-3 COUPLER

This coupler is used for testing modular ITE hearing aids as well as earphones and insert type receivers that do not have nubs. The entrance tubing may be flexible or rigid and has a length of 10 mm and a diameter of 1.93 mm (i.e., #13 tubing) unless otherwise stated by the manufacturer.

HA-4 COUPLER

This coupler is a modification of the HA-2 coupler using entrance tubing. It is intended for postauricular or eyeglass hearing aids in which the sound path bore from the hearing aid output through the earmold is assumed to have a uniform diameter of 1.93 mm. The interested reader is referred to Lybarger (1985) for further information on couplers.

**Occluded Ear Simulator (ANSI Standard S3.25-1979)**

Unlike the various hearing aid couplers discussed above, ear simulators have been specifically designed to represent the characteristics of a normal real ear over a wide frequency range. The occluded ear simulator standard specifies the physical configuration and acoustical performance of the four-branch modified Zwislocki ear simulator. This ear simulator is used in the Knowles Electronics Manikin for Acoustic Research or KEMAR (Burkhard and Sachs, 1975). It simulates the acoustical behavior of an ear canal between the tip of an earmold and the eardrum. It also simulates the median acoustic impedance at the eardrum of persons with normal middle ear function (see Chapter 2 for more detail on this).

In the early 1980s, rather than use the specifications for the well-documented and widely used modified Zwislocki coupler, as described in the published ANSI S3.25-1979 ear simulator standard, the IEC ear simulator working group, led by Per Bruel, decided to make their standard slightly different. The IEC 711 ear simulator ultimately conformed to the specifications of a Bruel and Kjaer ear simulator that was not yet commercially available at that time. Because of slight differences in measurement data, unfortunately, the tolerances of the acoustical performance in the IEC 711 ear simulator standard barely missed conforming to the tolerances of the four-branch modified Zwislocki ear simulator provided in ANSI S3.25-1979. Mahlon Burkhard of Knowles Electronics, the "father of KEMAR," was Chair of the ANSI S3-37 working group at that time. He and his working group were incredulous that the IEC 711 standard contained tolerances that caused the four-branch modified Zwislocki ear simulator to miss the allowable acoustical impedance at a few frequencies by less than 1 dB. The Zwislocki ear simulator already had been widely used in many countries besides the United States. However, formulation of the IEC 711 ear simulator standard rendered the use of the Knowles Zwislocki ear simulator unacceptable in any country that adopted the IEC 711 ear simulator standard. The formulation of separate ANSI and IEC ear simulator standards is another representative example of the difficulty ANSI and IEC have had in developing compatible standards for measuring hearing aid performance. It would seem that politics and commercial interests may have out-ranked practicality and pure science in this standardization case.

The S3.25 standard was reaffirmed in 1989. Future plans by the S3-37 working group call for possibly merging the ANSI S3.25 Occluded Ear Simulator Standard with the S3.7 Coupler Calibration of Earphone Standard. The interested reader is referred to Lybarger (1985) for further information on differences between couplers and ear simulators.

### Manikin Measurements (ANSI Standard S3.35-1985)

ANSI standard S3.35-1985, entitled *Methods of Measurement of Performance Characteristics of Hearing Aids Under Simulated In Situ Working Conditions*, is intended to provide guidance on how to use a manikin such as KEMAR for esti-mating hearing aid performance on a typical wearer. Measurements performed in accordance with this standard are to be obtained in a near-reflectionless test space with low ambient noise levels such as the acoustical environment pro-duced in an anechoic chamber.

The document provides acoustical requirements for the test space and a coor-dinate system to reference loudspeaker position and direction of sound incidence to the manikin. Among the measurements defined in the standard are: *manikin frequency response, simulated in situ gain, simulated insertion gain frequency response,* and *simulated in situ SSPL90 frequency response.*

In the early 1980s, members of the S3-48 working group conducted a round robin series of measurements with one postauricular hearing aid in accordance with the procedures outlined in the S3.35 standard. The goals of the round robin were to determine the repeatability of measurements on KEMAR between labo-ratories using one hearing aid and to isolate possible causes for any inconsis-tencies across laboratories. Repeatability achieved in the high frequencies of simulated insertion gain frequency responses across laboratories was somewhat disappointing, and the measurements were repeated after the initial results were analyzed. The interested reader is referred to Teder (1984) for a detailed report on the outcome of this round robin.

The S3.35 standard was reaffirmed in 1990. The ANSI manikin standard is very similar to IEC 118-8, which is categorized as a report rather than a standard. The contents of these documents have formed valuable input to the working group that is currently drafting a standard for real ear measurements with probe microphones. The interested reader is referred to the Manikin Measurements Conference Proceedings (Burkhard, 1978).

## Correction Factors to Convert Between Coupler Gain and Insertion Gain

Although not incorporated into a standard, correction factors have been used widely to estimate insertion gain frequency response on KEMAR as well as on real ears from 2-cc coupler frequency response data. For example, some hearing aid manufacturers use correction factors to provide on their hearing aid specification sheets estimated insertion gain frequency response, derived from the 2-cc frequency response.

Technically, the abbreviation CORFIG stands for Coupler Response for Flat Insertion Gain (Killion and Monser, 1980). CORFIG refers to a set of transformations that converts a required insertion gain frequency response to a target 2-cc coupler frequency response. Therefore, the inverse of CORFIG would be used to convert coupler frequency response to insertion gain frequency response. This inverse of CORFIG has been termed somewhat jokingly "GIFROC" (the reverse of CORFIG) by Killion and Revit (1993) and has been used by others (e.g., Meskan, 1994) for converting 2-cc gain values to insertion gain values.

The S3-48 working group initially became involved with CORFIGs in the early 1980s when its Chair, Sam Lybarger, calculated the insertion gain that should result from a 2-cc coupler frequency response and from a frequency response on the Zwislocki ear simulator for ITE, BTE, and ITC hearing aids (Lybarger and Teder, 1986). The S3-48 working group wished to evaluate these calculations against actual measurements for ITE hearing aids, so another "*in situ*" round robin was created. This time, the round robin consisted of the same six laboratories [that were in the previous round robin reported on by Teder (1984)] making 2-cc coupler and simulated insertion gain frequency response measurements on KEMAR for one ITE hearing aid. The calculated GIFROC and the mean measured GIFROC for the six laboratories, reproduced from Lybarger and Teder (1986), is shown in Figure 1–7. These correction values would have to be added to the 2-cc frequency response to obtain the predicted insertion gain. Up to 4000 Hz, the calculated and mean measured inverse CORFIG curves agreed to within approximately 2 dB. The reader is reminded that the correction values shown in Figure 1–7 would be different for BTE, ITC, and CIC hearing aids and also that insertion gain obtained with KEMAR may not be a good predictor of insertion gains on individuals. (See Chapter 2 for more details.)

One mandated requirement for estimating insertion gain comes from the Veterans Administration hearing aid distribution program. That is, any hearing aid that is distributed to a VA audiology clinic must be accompanied by either the actual measured insertion gain on KEMAR or an estimated insertion gain. Because it is difficult to get custom ITE hearing aids having earmolds of various shapes and sizes to fit into the available KEMAR ears, an estimate of insertion gain becomes mandatory for a production situation. For this purpose, a frequently used set of correction factors to predict insertion gain is one recommended by

| Frequency, Hz | ITE Aid Calculated | Measured Mean | S |
|---|---|---|---|
| 200 | 3.6 | 4.8 | 2.5 |
| 300 | 3.2 | 3.5 | 1.1 |
| 400 | 3.7 | 3.3 | 0.9 |
| 500 | 4.0 | 2.7 | 0.9 |
| 600 | 4.1 | 2.2 | 0.9 |
| 700 | 3.8 | 1.9 | 1.2 |
| 800 | 3.7 | 2.0 | 0.9 |
| 900 | 3.8 | 2.8 | 1.2 |
| 1000 | 4.2 | 2.8 | 0.5 |
| 1200 | 3.7 | 2.6 | 0.5 |
| 1400 | 1.1 | 3.2 | 1.0 |
| 1600 | 0.7 | 3.4 | 1.3 |
| 1800 | 0.4 | 1.8 | 0.7 |
| 2000 | −0.6 | 1.5 | 1.3 |
| 2200 | −1.8 | 0.6 | 1.8 |
| 2400 | −2.4 | −1.8 | 2.1 |
| 2600 | −2.4 | −3.7 | 2.4 |
| 2800 | −2.1 | −3.4 | 1.8 |
| 3000 | −1.6 | −1.2 | 2.5 |
| 3200 | −1.0 | −0.9 | 1.9 |
| 3400 | −0.4 | 2.4 | 1.0 |
| 3600 | 0.5 | 3.5 | 1.8 |
| 3800 | 1.3 | 4.5 | 2.5 |
| 4000 | 2.5 | 6.7 | 1.7 |
| 4500 | 5.2 | 10.0 | 4.2 |
| 5000 | 6.9 | 8.6 | 3.0 |
| 5500 | 7.7 | 10.2 | 1.6 |
| 6000 | 7.6 | 12.6 | 2.1 |
| 6500 | 8.5 | 15.3 | 4.0 |
| 7000 | 13.3 | 18.2 | 3.7 |
| 7500 | | 16.7 | 3.2 |
| 8000 | 14.1 | 15.2 | 1.9 |

**Figure 1–7.** Column 2: calculated values to be added to coupler gain to predict insertion gain (GIFROC) on KEMAR. Column 3: means of measurement differences at six laboratories between insertion gain for one ITE hearing aid on KEMAR and its 2-cc coupler gain. Column 4: standard deviations (S) of the insertion gain/coupler gain measurement differences at the six laboratories. Reprinted with permission from Lybarger and Teder, 1986.

Burnett and Beck (1987). These correction factors are a result of the S3-48 working group round robin mentioned above (Lybarger and Teder, 1986).

Although the Burnett and Beck (1987) correction factors predict insertion gain on KEMAR for custom ITE hearing aids with their vents closed, these predicted insertion gain responses can be indicative of the actual insertion gain responses obtained by some, but not all, hearing aid wearers. As an example, comparisons between the predicted insertion gain on KEMAR using the Burnett and Beck (1987) correction factors and actual real ear measurements of insertion gain with the ITE instruments fitted on the persons for whom they were designed were made at a Veterans Administration hospital on 10 ears. Data for one of the well-predicted examples in this study is shown in Figure 1–8; the 0.177-inch diameter vent in the ITE hearing aid was left unoccluded. In this example, to normalize for differences in gain control positions (reference test for coupler measures versus MCL for real ear measures), the predicted and actual insertion gain frequency responses were adjusted for the same gain at 1000 Hz. The interested reader is referred to Lybarger (1985) for further information on CORFIG.

### Noise Test Standard (S3.42-1992)

ANSI S3.42–*Testing Hearing Aids With a Broad-Band Noise Signal* was developed specifically to provide measurements that depict the steady-state electroacoustic behavior of compression hearing aids and hearing aids with level-dependent frequency response. ANSI S3.22-1987 specifies a 50 dB SPL swept pure tone input level for obtaining the frequency response of hearing aids with compression or automatic gain control (AGC) circuitry. The reasoning behind such a low input signal level was to obtain the frequency response of AGC hearing aids while they were operating in linear mode, at a level below the *compression kneepoint.* However, newer AGC hearing aids, with lower compression kneepoints, have been recently developed. (The reader is referred to Chapters 4 and 5 for more detail on these hearing aids.) Some of these hearing aids have AGC kneepoints below 50 dB SPL input, and their operation cannot be completely characterized by pure tones (Kates, 1991).

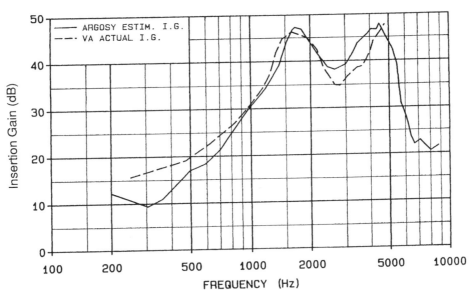

**Figure 1–8.** Real Ear Insertion Response (REIR—dashed line) measured with a probe microphone for an ITE hearing aid on the wearer and the predicted Simulated Insertion Gain Frequency Response on KEMAR (SIGFR per ANSI S3.35-1985—solid line) estimated from the 2-cc frequency response using correction figures from Burnett and Beck, 1987. Curves were normalized at 1000 Hz for comparison purposes.

SINGLE- AND MULTIPLE-BAND COMPRESSION HEARING AIDS
AND THE PROBLEM OF BLOOMING

The term "Automatic Signal Processing" *(ASP)*, as applied to hearing aids, theoretically includes single and multiple band compression hearing aids (Killion et al., 1990). Also, some of these so-called ASP hearing aids operate so that their frequency responses change from moment to moment, depending on changes in input sound pressure level. For these hearing aids with frequency response shaping dependent on input level, the gain in different frequency regions changes with different input levels. For multiple-band compression hearing aids, level-dependent frequency response shaping may occur because the kneepoints may be different in the different frequency regions. With the development of such complex signal processing algorithms, standardized measurement methods were needed that could characterize the performance of these hearing aids at input levels for which compression occurs. A swept sinusoid tests at one frequency at a time. As a result, the frequency responses for hearing aids with nonlinear signal processing such as single or multiple-band compression, obtained with a swept pure tone signal at high input levels (e.g., 70, 80, and 90 dB SPL), may have an artifactually high low frequency gain ("blooming"), or a discontinuity in their frequency responses, if the hearing aid begins to compress part way through during the time of the sweep (Preves et al., 1989). An example of the *blooming phenomenon* is shown in Figure 1–9 for a single-band compression hearing aid using an HA-2 2cc coupler. Note how the low-frequency output SPL increases relative to the high-frequency output SPL, particularly for the 70 dB and 80 dB SPL input levels. These response curves indicate that compression has begun to occur approximately midway through these pure tone sweeps.

BIAS TONE METHOD

A bias tone method has been advocated by the IEC hearing aid working group to determine the frequency response as a function of input level for AGC hearing aids. With this method, one or more fixed frequency bias tones are presented while another tone is swept across the frequency range of interest. The resulting measurements may have artifacts in the frequency response caused by inclusion or elimination of the bias tone. For example, Figure 1–10 shows a family of frequency responses using the HA-2 2-cc coupler for the same hearing aid as in Figure 1–9, but obtained with a 3000 Hz bias tone. It is evident from the sharp dip at 3000 Hz that the bias tone was eliminated from the output of the hearing aid with a sharply tuned notch filter (Preves et al., 1989). With this method, if the fine details of the hearing aid circuit algorithm are not known, the tester must experiment first to find the appropriate bias tone frequency. Thus, the frequency responses obtained with the bias tone method will be heavily dependent on the bias tone frequency and input level selected. For multiple-band AGC hearing aids, one bias tone must be used for each band having a separate compression circuit. In this complicated test setup, the frequencies and input levels of these bias tones must be selected appropriately to reveal the performance characteristics of the multiple band circuit. Despite the objections of the U.S. conveyed to the IEC working group about the complexity of the instrumentation and proce-

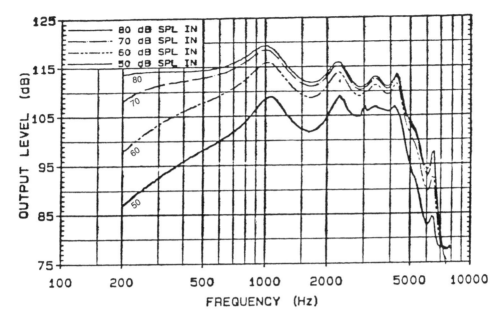

**Figure 1–9.** Illustration of "blooming" effect in family of frequency response curves at high input levels (70–80 dB SPL) of a swept pure tone for a single band postauricular compression hearing aid.

dures, the bias tone method has been adopted as a supplement to the IEC 118-2 hearing aid standard *(Hearing Aids With Automatic Gain Control Circuits).*

BROAD-BAND NOISE METHOD

As an attractive alternative to the bias tone method, spectrum analyzers can be used to measure hearing aid performance, using frequency shaping of a broad-band noise to produce a speech spectrum noise input signal (Burnett, 1967). These measurements are based on conventional *Fast Fourier Transform (FFT)* and *cross spectrum* techniques. One advantage of using a steady-state noise input signal to obtain frequency responses of hearing aids with nonlinear processing, such as multiple-band compression, is that at all frequencies are tested simultaneously, thereby eliminating the artifact caused by the compression circuit activation during the frequency response measurement with a pure tone sweep. Thus, in the mid 1980s, after almost a 10-year hiatus, the S3-48 working group once again took up the task of developing a standard for testing hearing aids using a broad-band noise input signal.

As a reminder, ANSI S3.22 expresses the overall gain and overall saturation sound pressure level of hearing aids by averaging at three frequencies (normally 1000, 1600, and 2500 Hz). As mentioned earlier, these three frequencies were selected so the HFA full-on gain and the HFA SSPL90 were comparable to the NIST measurements for gain and SSPL90 using a shaped broad-band noise input (Staab, 1978). Also, as mentioned previously, ANSI S3.22-1987 allows the manufacturer to select the three frequencies for the average gain and SSPL90 for special

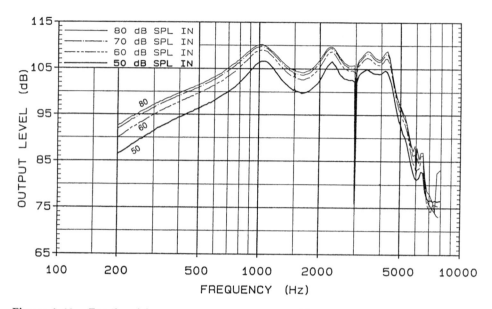

**Figure 1–10.**   Family of frequency–response curves of hearing aid used for Figure 1–9 with a 3000 Hz bias tone summed with the swept pure tone at the same input level. Spike at 3000 Hz is caused by a notch filter removing bias tone from hearing aid output.

purpose hearing aids. Measurements using a broad-band noise signal would have the advantage of averaging at more than three frequencies, and special frequencies would not be needed for measurements on extreme high-pass or low-pass hearing aids. The spectrum of this noise input signal is defined in Figure 1–11, and must lie between the upper and lower smooth lines in Figure 1–11. The jagged middle line in Figure 1–11 shows the actual spectrum measured using a Bruel & Kjaer 4212 hearing aid analyzer test chamber with 1/3 octave equalization and random noise generated by a Bruel & Kjaer 2032 FFT spectrum analyzer having 16 Hz FFT resolution (an FFT analysis bin every 16 Hz).

SEVERAL TESTS SPECIFIED BY ANSI S3.42-1992

Several new tests are defined in the S3.42-1992 standard *"Testing Hearing Aids With a Broad-Band Noise Signal."* These tests employ the steady-state, speech-shaped noise discussed above. The new measurements include *overall gain and saturation sound pressure level (NSPL90) with the noise input* as well as *a family of frequency response curves* and an *input/output (I/O) characteristic* as the input sound pressure level of the shaped noise is varied. NSPL90 is a single number rms output sound pressure level in a 200 to 5000 Hz bandwidth produced by a hearing aid with its gain control set at maximum using a 90 dB rms noise input SPL. *Full-on noise gain* is a single number gain value expressed in decibels calculated by subtracting the overall rms noise input SPL to the hearing aid from the rms noise output SPL from the hearing aid over a 200 to 5000 Hz bandwidth. The input sound pressure level for the full-on noise gain measurement is 60 dB.

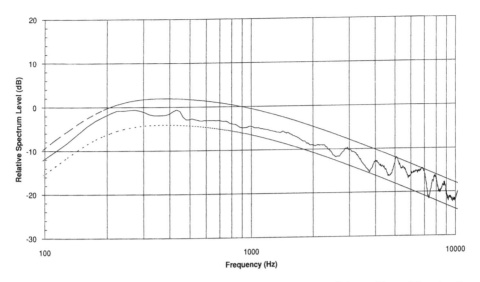

**Figure 1–11.** Upper and lower allowable limits for spectrum of shaped broad-band noise input specified in ANSI S3.42-1992. Middle curve is actual spectrum obtained in a Bruel & Kjaer 4212 test chamber using a 1/3 octave equalizer to shape the noise signal generated by a Bruel & Kjaer 2032 spectrum analyzer.

Recall that the S3-48 working group had conducted round-robin tests in the early 1970s to determine whether or not testing with such a noise input was viable. These round-robin tests with noise input were conducted before the widespread availability of many FFT-based spectrum analyzers. These devices generate their own complex signals that are easily equalized and are automatically time-synchronized with the analysis period. The development and availability of these analyzers allow for the generation of the desired input noise spectrum and repeatable measurements of input and output noise spectra across test facilities. Consequently, to determine whether modern spectrum analysis equipment would produce acceptable repeatability of hearing aid measurements using broad-band noise input signals, in 1987 the S3-48 working group conducted another round robin among five laboratories with a single postauricular AGC hearing aid. Table 1–2 summarizes some of the data obtained on HA-2 2-cc couplers with tube extensions during these round-robin tests. The table shows data from the five laboratories that participated in the measurements. The noise gain at full-on gain control setting at the five laboratories ranged from 51.5 dB to 53.5 dB, resulting in a standard deviation of 0.8 dB. NSPL90 measures at the five laboratories ranged from 111.5 to 113.4 dB SPL, resulting in a standard deviation of 0.8 dB. Thus, the agreement for these measures with the noise input signal among the five laboratories was quite good. By comparison, for this post auricular instrument, the hearing aid manufacturer specified HFA full-on gain per ANSI S3.22-1976 of 53 dB and HFA SSPL90 as 111 dB SPL. Therefore, for this hearing aid the single number full-on noise gain correlates well with the three-frequency average HFA full-on gain and the NSPL90 correlates well with HFA SSPL90 as Lybarger found in the mid 1970s.

**Table 1–2.**   Round-Robin Data Obtained at Five Laboratories for a Single Compression Hearing Aid Whose Frequency Responses Are Shown in Figure 1–12.

| Laboratory | NSPL90 (dB SPL) | Noise Gain (dB) |
|---|---|---|
| 1 | 111.5 | 52 |
| 2 | 113.3 | 53.5 |
| 3 | 113 | 52 |
| 4 | 113.4 | 52.6 |
| 5 | 112.5 | 51.5 |
| Mean | 112.7 | 52.3 |
| Standard deviation | 0.8 | 0.8 |

Measurements are full-on noise gain and output SOL with a 90 dB SPL noise input (NSPL90) on five HA-2 2 cc couplers.

The frequency–response curves obtained at the five laboratories using 5 HA-2 2-cc couplers for this hearing aid with a noise input of 50 dB SPL are shown in Figure 1–12. The frequency response is measured over a 200 to 6500 Hz bandwidth. For comparison purposes, the curves have been shifted vertically to have the same gain at 1000 Hz. With this normalization, the agreement among laboratories is within 3 dB over the frequency range 400 Hz to 4000 Hz, indicating that shaping the noise input spectrum satisfactorily at the five laboratories was not a problem.

After much experimenting and deliberation to determine the method of setting reference test position using the noise input signal, the S3-48 working group concluded that the procedure for gain control setback recommended by Richard

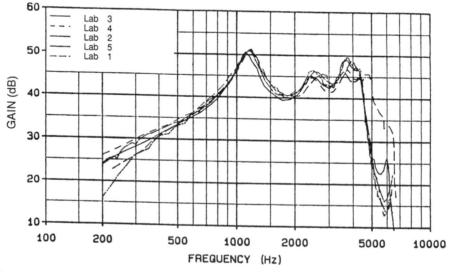

**Figure 1–12.**   Frequency-response curves for the hearing aid used for Table 1–2 obtained at five laboratories using HA-2 2-cc couplers with a 50 dB noise input SPL per ANSI S3.42-1992. Curves normalized to have equal gain at 1000 Hz.

Brander, a member of the working group, should be like that in S3.22. (The gain control is turned down until the output SPL from a hearing aid with a 60 dB noise input SPL is 17 dB below the NSPL90.) A 60 dB noise input SPL was selected to help ensure that the input level would be above the environmental noise level in most test enclosures, but not so high as to overload most hearing aids.

A family of frequency–response curves with a noise input signal indicates how the frequency response of a hearing aid changes as the noise input level is changed. The family of curves as a function of noise input SPL at full-on gain obtained at one laboratory for the hearing aid used in the 1987 round-robin tests is shown in Figure 1–13. The response curves for this single-band AGC hearing aid remain essentially parallel for shaped noise inputs ranging in 10 dB steps from 50 dB to 80 dB SPL. This was the same hearing aid used for the data in Figures 1–9, 1–10, and 1–12 and Table 1–2. Recall that, for this hearing aid, Figure 1–9 had shown that similar curves developed with a swept pure tone input exhibited a "blooming" phenomenon, i.e., increased low frequency response at higher input levels.

The units on the ordinate of a family of frequency response curves can be shown in output SPL or in gain. However, if output SPL is chosen for the ordinate, the shape of the noise input spectrum will be included in the frequency–response curve unless it is first subtracted out (e.g., the output SPL ordinate in Figure 1–13 indicates that the noise input spectrum has been subtracted out). Consequently, the S3.42 standard specifies that gain in decibels should be used to label the ordinate scale for frequency–response curves. The increments in noise input levels for a family of curves is usually a multiple of 5 dB.

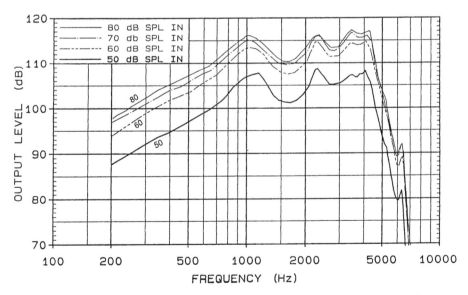

**Figure 1–13.** Family of frequency–response curves obtained with shaped random noise input per ANSI S3.42-1992 of hearing aid used for Figures 1–9, 1–10, and 1–12 and Table 1–2.

## LEVEL-DEPENDENT FREQUENCY RESPONSE

The shaped noise input signal is useful for determining whether an "ASP" hearing aid has a level-dependent frequency response. For example, Figure 1–14 from Killion, Staab, and Preves (1990) shows a family of curves obtained with a noise input for a "BILL" (Bass Increases at Low Levels)-type hearing aid (Argosy Manhattan II) in which the low-frequency gain is reduced as noise input SPL increases. Figure 1–15 from the same paper shows a family of curves for a "TILL" (Treble Increases at Low Levels)-type hearing aid (K-AMP) in which the high-frequency gain is reduced as noise input SPL increases.

## INPUT/OUTPUT CHARACTERISTIC

The input/output characteristic obtained with a noise input is a plot of noise output SPL over a range of noise input SPLs. This characteristic is useful in determining over what range(s) of input SPLs a hearing aid performs linearly and nonlinearly. Examples of families of frequency responses and their associated input/output characteristics are provided in Figures 1–16 and 1–17. These figures were obtained with the shaped noise signal using a linear hearing aid and using a two-band hearing aid with AGC in the lower band, respectively. The response curves in Figure 1–16 for the linear hearing aid remain relatively unchanged as the noise input SPL increases until saturation begins to occur (at

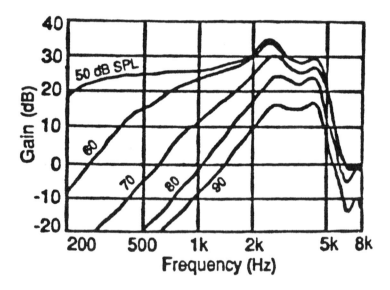

**Figure 1–14.** Family of frequency response curves using an HA-1 2-cc coupler for an ITE hearing aid with *Bass Increases at Low Levels* (BILL)-type level-dependent frequency response (Argosy Manhattan II). Measurements were obtained with speech-shaped random noise at input levels ranging from 50 to 90 dB SPL in 10 dB steps per ANSI S3.42-1992. Reprinted with permission from Killion et al., 1990.

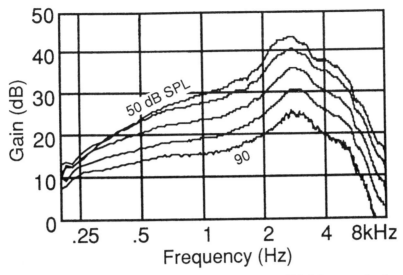

**Figure 1–15.**  Family of frequency response curves using an HA-1 2-cc coupler for an ITE hearing aid with *Treble Increases at Low Levels* (TILL)-type level-dependent frequency response. Measurements were obtained with speech-shaped random noise input at input levels ranging from 50 to 90 dB SPL in 10 dB steps per ANSI S3.42-1992.

about 70 dB noise input SPL). For example, at 80 dB noise input SPL, gain across the frequency range has been significantly reduced due to increased saturation. In Figure 1–17, compression in the lower band of the two-band hearing aid reduces predominately low-frequency gain as the input SPL increases, while the high-frequency gain is relatively unchanged. This family of level-dependent frequency response is similar to that shown in Figure 1–14.

Other examples of frequency responses, families of response curves, and input/output characteristics using the shaped noise input signal and the protocols outlined in the standard may be found in Walker and Dillon (1982), Frye (1987), Preves and Newton (1989), Bareham (1990a, 1990b), Stelmachowicz, Lewis, Seewald, and Hawkins (1990), and Preves (1990).

AMBIENT NOISE RESTRICTIONS

The procedures specified in S3.42-1992 are intended for measurements made with 2-cc couplers in acoustic test chambers as well as measures made on a manikin such as KEMAR in anechoic chambers. (The procedures in this standard also apply to real ear probe tube microphone measurements if the requirements for test conditions and equipment are met. However, ANSI working group S3-80 is producing a separate document for these real ear measurements.) In any of these environments, the residual noise level (ambient noise) in the enclosure must be low enough to not affect the measurements significantly. The standard specifies that the overall residual noise SPL in the enclosure be less than 40 dB SPL over the frequency range 200 to 5000 Hz and less than 50 dB SPL over the

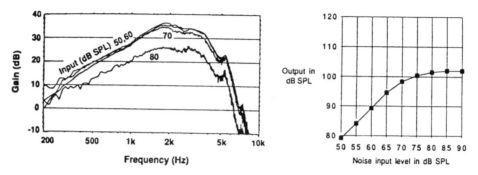

**Figure 1–16.**  Measurements per ANSI S3.42-1992 using speech-shaped random noise to develop: (left) family of frequency–response curves at input levels ranging from 50 to 80 dB SPL in 10 dB steps and (right) the Input/Output characteristic. Measurements were made using an HA-1 2-cc coupler for an ITE hearing aid with "linear" processing. Reprinted with permission from Preves and Woodruff, 1990.

frequency range 100 to 5000 Hz. Additionally, it requires that the signal-to-noise ratio in each analysis band must be greater than 10 dB. Testing in environments not meeting these requirements may result in measurements that have been contaminated by environmental noise. The symptom of such a problem is a jagged frequency response curve. Increasing the number of measurement averages can help to minimize this problem and smooth the frequency response.

COHERENCE FUNCTION MEASUREMENTS

Spectral analysis procedures also offer other new tests for characterizing hearing aid performance using a noise input signal. For example, the *coherence function*, which compares input and output signals, provides an indication of the validity of the frequency response measurement (Reddy and Kirlin, 1979; Burnett et al., 1982). The intent of this application of coherence is to consider as valid only that portion of a frequency–response curve for a hearing aid for which the coherence is at least 0.5 (Fig. 1–18). The darkened portions of the curves in Figure 1–18 indicate the frequency range for which the coherence is greater than 0.5. A coherence

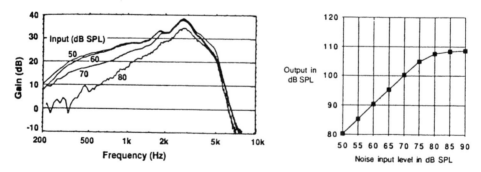

**Figure 1–17.**  Same as Figure 1–16 for a two-band AGC ITE hearing aid with compression in the low frequency band. Reprinted with permission from Preves and Woodruff, 1990.

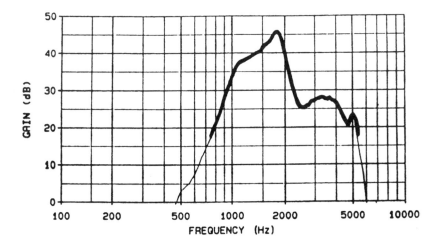

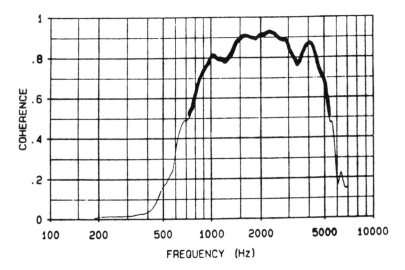

**Figure 1–18.** Example of insertion gain frequency response (upper panel) and coherence function (lower panel) for a hearing aid on KEMAR. To indicate the frequency range over which the frequency response measurement is valid on the basis of coherence, the frequency–response and coherence curves are darkened for those portions of the curves at which coherence ≥ 0.5.

less than 0.5 indicates that the output from the hearing aid is composed of more noise and/or distortion than input signal. (At higher input levels, coherence of 0.5 represents equal amounts of distortion and input signal, thus representing a 100% distortion condition). For this hearing aid, the insertion gain frequency response shown in the upper panel would be considered valid from approximately 750 Hz to about 5500 Hz. For some hearing aids, coherence is reduced at low input levels because of circuit noise, thus rendering the transfer function questionable. An example of such a condition is shown in Figure 1–19 for a low-gain completely-in-the-canal (CIC) hearing aid with a "linear" circuit. Figure 1–19a shows data in accordance with ANSI S3.22. Note that the equivalent input noise is high–38.5 dB SPL. Figure 1–19b depicts the family of frequency–response curves obtained with the speech-shaped noise input signal increasing in 10 dB steps over a range of 50 to 90 dB SPL. Because of the high circuit noise in the hearing aid, the frequency response with a 50 dB input SPL has considerable jaggedness. Figure 1–19c shows the coherence functions for this hearing aid at the same input levels used for Figure 1–19b. Because the coherence with a 50 dB noise input SPL is less than 0.5 over much of the high frequency range, the jagged frequency response in Figure 1–19b with a 50 dB noise input SPL has questionable validity. Coherence values in Figure 19c improve for this hearing aid as the noise input level is raised. Unfortunately, at this time, the coherence measurement is not yet widely available in commercial hearing aid analyzers. The data per ANSI S3.42 in Figures 1–19b and 1–19c were obtained with a Bruel & Kjaer 2032 spectrum analyzer using speech-shaped random noise as the input signal with 50 averages for the analysis.

ANSI VERSUS IEC

Recently, the IEC hearing aid working group has also been interested in formulating a new standard using a noise input signal. In the spirit of harmonization of ANSI and IEC standards, the Chair of the IEC hearing aid working groups 13 and 14 requested a copy of ANSI S3.42 on a computer disk. At the time of this writing, however, the IEC working group is recommending that the spectrum of the noise input signal be specified in third octave bands rather than by spectrum level, as it is in S3.42. This is occurring in spite of negative comments from the United States pointing out potential problems with the third octave method. These differences in specifying the noise signal could, in effect, allow the spectrum of the noise input signals specified by the ANSI and IEC standards to be significantly different.

NEW TYPES OF NOISE SIGNALS FOR THE FUTURE

The steady-state shaped broad-band noise, as described in the standard, is an appropriate test signal for hearing aids that automatically change gain as a function of input level (e.g., amplitude-compression hearing aids) or for those hearing aids that have filters that adaptively change frequency response as a function of input level. However, because these hearing aids also react to temporal fluctuations in the input signal, a temporally varying test signal is needed to characterize their behavior more completely. For such hearing aids, an input signal having a pulsing speech-spectrum noise may be appropriate (Bareham, 1990b). Steady-state narrow band noise or continuous pure tone signals could be added to the pulsing speech-spectrum noise to simulate speech in a continuous background noise. Alternatively, speech itself might be used (Burnett, 1991; Dyrlund, Ludvigsen, Olofsson, and Poulsen, 1994).

Thus, future revisions of the standard might include use of pulsing signals or speech itself. Also, the discussion of the use of maximum length sequences (MLS)

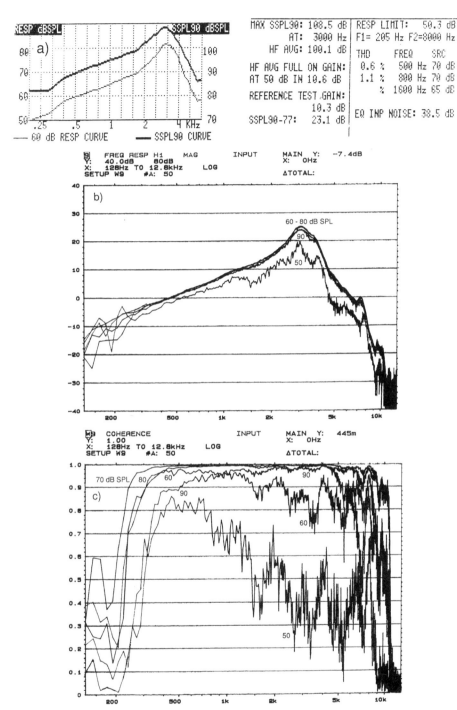

**Figure 1–19.** (a) Data per ANSI S3.22-1987 of a low-gain completely-in-the-canal hearing aid; (b) family of frequency–response curves using speech-shaped noise at input levels ranging from 50 to 90 dB SPL in 10 dB steps per ANSI S3.42-1992; (c) coherence functions for same noise input levels used in Figure 1–19b.

for input signal generation might be expanded in future revisions. This method for generating the noise input signal is mentioned only briefly in S3.42. Among the personal computer-based, commercially available implementations using MLS are the *Maximum Length Sequence System Analyzer* (MLSSA) and a system from Audio Precision, although neither was developed specifically for hearing aid testing. Because the signal generated by MLSSA is pseudorandom, it is deterministic and well-defined, and therefore, full two-channel analysis is not needed (Burnett, 1992). However, the MLS signal also retains some of the benefits of two-channel analysis with a random test signal in that it has a Gaussian probability density function (Burnett, 1992) and so cross-spectral analysis can be performed. Also, the MLS signal can be designed to meet the requirements for a crest factor of 12 dB, as specified in S3.42. Thus, MLS analysis appears to have the advantages of a pseudorandom test signal, in that it produces results very quickly while retaining the advantages of two-channel analysis with a random test signal, in being able to obtain the coherence function (Campbell, 1991). Since the time of publication of S3.42, a number of studies have demonstrated that the MLS is a viable method of generating the broad-band signal specified in the standard and for testing hearing aids in accordance with the standard (Schneider and Jamieson, 1993a, 1993b).

## *Appendices in ANSI Hearing Aid-Related Standards*

Procedures in the appendix of an ANSI standard are not considered to be included in the main body of the standard and, thus, are not required procedures if the standard is adopted by a regulatory agency. For example, while the procedures and other material in the appendices of ANSI S3.22 have considerable technical and informational value, they are regarded as optional because they are not required by the FDA. Thus, appendices give working groups the opportunity to include informational material or to suggest additional procedures that the working group wishes to be optional, either because they add too much testing time for production line use, or because they have not been sufficiently tested and proven at the time of publication of the standard.

Among the additional tests that can be completed on hearing aids for informational purposes are those that have been formulated previously in ANSI S3.3-1960 (R-1971) and in the IEC 118-0 standard. Methods in the proposed appendix of the next revision of S3.22 taken from ANSI S3.3-1971 and IEC 118-0 include: *Characteristic of the Gain Control (volume control taper), Effect of Tone-Control Positions on Frequency Response,* and *the Effect of Power-Supply Voltage and Impedance Variation on Acoustic Gain and SSPL90.* At the time of this writing, additional optional measurements that may be recommended as appendices in the next revision of S3.22 are: expressing battery drain current as a function of quiescent current and maximum current, effect of the output limiting control on SSPL90 and frequency response, hearing aid output noise spectrum, total harmonic distortion as a function of input sound pressure level, compression ratio and its inverse, compression factor, Test Loop Sensitivity, and maximum sensitivity of induction coil pickup.

## Standardizing Real Ear Probe Microphone Measurements

The S3-80 working group on *Probe Tube Measurements of Hearing Aid Performance* has been in the process of developing a standard for several years. Due to the considerable diversity of the strong opinions of some working group members, it has been quite difficult to reach a consensus on the basic framework and contents of the standard. Efforts of the working group have been impeded somewhat because severe time constraints of regular work schedules have led to three changes in the Chair of the working group. After several years of discussions without much writing being accomplished, William Cole, the current Chair of the working group, wrote a document that has served as a good basis for discussion and that has been modified mostly in editorial content. Members of the working group have tried to ensure that some of the terms defined in the draft document become standardized in articles and presentations. Included are such familiar terms as *Real Ear Unaided Response (REUR)*, *Real Ear Insertion Response (REIR)*, *Real Ear Aided Response (REAR)*, and *Real Ear Occluded Response (REOR)* as well as comparable terms for gain at one frequency. At this time, the IEC working group on real ear measurements appears to be preparing a document that is generally compatible to that being formulated by the ANSI S3-80 working group.

## Future Directions of the ANSI S3-48 Working Group on Hearing Aid Standards

At the time of this writing, the next revision of S3.22 has been evolving within the S3-48 working group for almost 7 years. Without compromising the original quality control purpose of the standard, in the next revision, the S3-48 working group is trying to make the measurements in the standard more predictive of hearing aid performance in real-world situations. To accomplish this goal, persons with behavioral testing background have been encouraged to augment the predominately electroacoustical background of current working group members. For example, in the future, the working group may be considering a procedure for relating the spectrum of the noise output of a hearing aid to the threshold of a hearing impaired person so as to be able to predict whether the hearing aid circuit noise will be audible and, if so, over what frequency range. In all likelihood, because the primary intent of S3.22 is still to ensure quality control, predicting the audibility of hearing aid circuit noise will probably form the basis for another standard that will be directed at tests related primarily to hearing aid performance in actual use conditions. For further information, the reader is referred to the discussion in the section on Possible Future Measurements of Hearing Aid Circuit Noise for S3.22.

The working group has been in search of other types of distortion measurements that might be more predictive of the sound quality of hearing aid-processed signals. Some work has been done in this area by Bell Northern Research (1986) and by Kubichek, Atkinson, and Webster (1991) in correlating subjective opinions of sound quality to the coherence function and pattern recognition results to identify the amount of distortion. The interested reader is referred to the section on Possible New Measurements of Hearing Aid Distortion.

Following the format of the IEC 118 series of standards, officers of the S3-Bioacoustics committee have expressed the desire to have one standard that would cover all aspects of hearing aids and assistive listening devices. This would involve merging the standards already produced by the S3-48 working group (S3.3, S3.22, S3.35, S3.37, and S3.42) with the standards that will be produced by the S3-80 and S3-81 working groups.

The following is a brief description of several new measurement techniques the working group has been studying in the hope of making the resulting measurements more meaningful to those fitting hearing aids.

## Possible New Methods for Measuring the Performance of Induction Coils for S3.22

The 1987 revision of S3.22 was published after a "No" vote was resolved conditionally by the S3-48 working group. The individual voting "No" for his organization agreed to give conditional approval with the proviso that the next revision of the standard would contain more thorough and more representative measurement procedures for characterizing induction coil performance in hearing aids. The existing induction coil test procedure in S3.22 specifies that the hearing aid is to be positioned relative to the magnetic field input for maximum sensitivity at one test frequency. S3.22-1987 states that as an option, the maximum induction pickup sensitivity at other frequencies also can be provided. The comments that accompanied the "No" vote pointed out that such a procedure does not distinguish how well a hearing aid picks up inductive signals emanating from different directions. This is an important consideration because in the actual application of induction coil pickup with hearing aids, there are at least three different inductive signal sources that must be considered: signals from a telephone handset, signals from a loop provided in a room designed for assistive listening, and signals from a neck loop on a hearing aid wearer that is connected to an assistive listening device such as an FM receiver.

### INDUCTION COIL PICKUP OF TELEPHONE VERSUS LOOP

The three inductive sources cited above have different orientations and magnetic field strengths, making the amount of inductive energy transduced by a hearing aid heavily dependent on the orientation of the induction pickup coil inside the hearing aid. (The reader is referred to Chapter 3 for more details on telecoil design.) As shown in Figure 1–20, hearing aid-compatible telephones have both radial (to the sides) and axial (straight out on axis)-radiated inductive energy. The radial component is usually about 6 dB weaker than the axial component (EIA, 1983). Thus, the induction coil in the hearing aid shown in Figure 1–20 is aligned for maximum pickup of the axial magnetic component radiated from the telephone receiver, but only if the telephone handset is held in the unnatural position behind the hearing aid shown. A result of this induction coil orientation problem was illustrated at an S3-48 working group meeting with pictures supplied by W. F. Hopmeier, a hearing aid dispenser and member of the working group. The photographs showed hearing aid wearers holding telephone handsets at awkward angles, presumably in order to obtain maximum signal strength

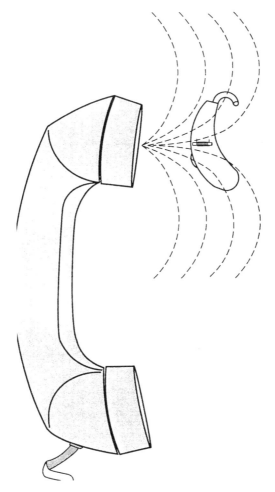

**Figure 1–20.** Schematic illustration of axial and radial magnetic fields emanating from a telephone receiver and sensed by a hearing aid having an induction coil aligned for maximum pickup when the telephone handset is held behind the hearing aid.

from the telephone via the induction coil pickup in their hearing aids. In Figure 1–20, if the telephone handset is held in a more normal telephone use position, the induction coil would be aligned to pick up one of the weaker radial induction components. To have optimal pickup of the induction field from telephones, as shown in Figure 1–21a, hearing aids must have their induction coils mounted *horizontally* and perpendicular to the surface of the receiver in the telephone handset. In this position, there will be relatively poor pickup of the induction field from neck loops and almost no pickup from room loops. Hearing aids with induction coils mounted *vertically* when worn will have good pickup from room loops and neck loops and about 6 dB less than optimal pickup from telephones (Fig. 1–21b). Some members of the S3-48 working group felt strongly that the hearing aid dispenser and the consumer should be able to determine how well a

**a.** Good for telephone pickup.

(Induction coil horizontal)

**b.** Good for room loop and neck loop pickup.

(Induction coil vertical)

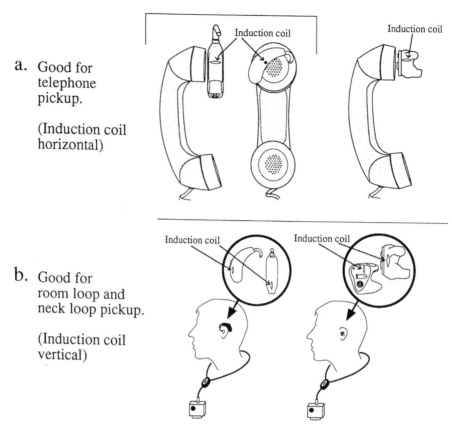

**Figure 1–21.** Illustration showing that directional sensitivity of magnetic pickup depends on the orientation of the induction coil in a hearing aid. Recommended telecoil orientation for good inductive pickup of: (a) telephones and (b) room loops and neck loops.

hearing aid with induction coil picks up signals from different directions by the results of the induction coil tests performed. To this end, measuring induction coil pickup from three directions is a procedure that has been followed for several years by NIST for testing hearing aids submitted for qualification in the VA hearing aid program (VA Handbook of Hearing Aid Measurement, 1991). Such knowledge is especially important in view of the Americans With Disabilities Act (ADA, 1991), which requires means of effective communication be provided for hearing impaired persons in public facilities. One result of this act is a recent proliferation of loop systems being installed in theaters, museums, airports, and many other places.

TELEPHONE MAGNETIC FIELD SIMULATOR

Soon after the 1987 revision of S3.22 was completed, the S3-48 working group embarked on a new measurement procedure for testing induction coil pickup that was recommended by William Cole, a member of the S3-48 working group.

In his protocol, several new measurements were defined based on a new test fixture called the *Telephone Magnetic Field Simulator (TMFS)*. This fixture is of comparable shape and size to the receiver portion of a telephone handset and simulated the axial and radial magnetic fields radiated by a typical hearing aid-compatible telephone (EIA, 1983). The magnetic field strength produced in the axial direction by the TMFS is about 31.6 milli-Ampere/meter (mA/m) at 1 kHz at a distance of 1 cm from the test surface of the TMFS. This magnetic field strength is considerably greater than the 10 mA/m field strength currently specified in S3.22-1987. Measurements with the TMFS are labeled coupler *Sound Pressure Level In a Telephone Magnetic Field Simulator (SPLITS)*.

The TMFS fixture currently being evaluated by the S3-48 working group is shown in Figure 1–22. Postauricular hearing aids are laid on their side and ITE hearing aids are laid faceplate down on the TMFS. In Cole's proposal, measurements with the TMFS fixture are used to predict the induction coil pickup performance of a hearing aid with a telephone. Hearing aid output SPL in the 2-cc coupler with a 60 dB SPL input (i.e., the acoustic mode using microphone input) is compared to the hearing aid output when switched to induction coil mode (i.e., using the telecoil input) and driven by the magnetic field produced by the TMFS. The hearing aid gain control is maintained at the same setting (reference

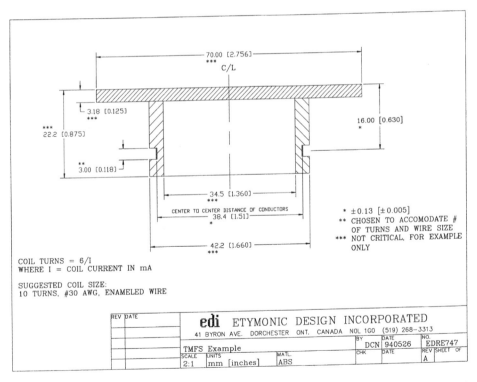

**Figure 1–22.** Dimensional drawing of the current version of the Telephone Magnetic Field Simulator (TMFS) and specification for drive current. Reprinted with permission from William Cole.

test position) for both tests. Following a recommendation some years ago by S3-48 working group member, Harry Teder, the difference between the two measurements is an estimate of how much a hearing aid wearer would have to adjust the gain control on the hearing aid when switching from normal microphone use to the induction coil mode.

NEW METHODS FOR EXPRESSING TELECOIL SENSITIVITY

In his recommended protocol, Cole proposed that the difference between the acoustic mode and induction coil mode HFA output SPL using the TMFS (HFA SPLITS) be called the *Simulated Telephone Sensitivity (STS)*. When the STS is negative, the HFA output SPL with induction coil is less than the HFA output SPL with microphone input using a 60 dB input SPL, a condition typically found with older hearing aids not having an induction coil preamplifier. When the STS is positive, the HFA SPLITS with induction coil pickup is greater than the HFA output SPL with microphone input. The ideal hearing aid would obviously provide an STS of 0 dB. At the time of this writing, the working group is conducting another round robin to evaluate a lighter weight version of the TMFS designed by Sam Lybarger and constructed by William Cole.

Because hearing aids with an induction coil can perform differently with *room loops* and *neck loops* than with telephones, Cole also recommended testing the hearing aids positioned vertically within a larger loop to simulate use conditions with room loops and neck loops. For this test, an imaginary vertical axis is defined to reference the vertical positioning of postauricular and in-the-ear hearing aids. Cole proposed that the hearing aid output SPL in induction coil mode with vertical orientation be called coupler *Sound Pressure Level In a Vertically-oriented magnetic field (SPLIV)*. Similar to the protocol proposed for telephone pickup, the difference between the HFA hearing aid output SPL in acoustic mode with 60 dB input SPL and the HFA SPLIV is called the *Test Loop Sensitivity (TLS)*. When the TLS is negative, the HFA output SPL with induction coil in a vertically oriented magnetic field (HFA SPLIV) is less than the HFA output SPL with microphone input using a 60 dB input SPL. When the TLS is positive, the HFA SPLIV is greater than the HFA output SPL with microphone input. The ideal hearing aid would provide a TLS of 0 dB.

Using the protocol suggested by Cole, several round-robin studies were conducted by interested working group members with the same telephone and five hearing aids at six different laboratories. Three of the hearing aids were postauricular and two were in-the-ear. Because postauricular hearing aids worn on the right ears and left ears may cause an asymmetrical location of the induction pickup coil, measurements were taken for both sides of the hearing aid. One of the ITE hearing aids had the telecoil mounted perpendicular to the faceplate or approximately horizontal as worn. The other ITE hearing aid had the same circuit and the same telecoil, but the telecoil was mounted parallel to the faceplate or approximately vertical as worn. The working group also wished to determine whether a monotonic relationship existed between STS in the coupler and in the real ear. Therefore, the round-robin tests included acoustic and inductive mode tests with the same hearing aids using 2-cc couplers and real ears. For this purpose, a telephone line simulator was constructed in accordance with EIA standard RS-504, 1983. The purpose of the telephone line simulator was to simulate the effects of the telephone network and a representative length of telephone line. For the induction-mode real ear measurements, the real ear measurement system output was connected to the input of the telephone line simulator and the telephone was connected to the output of the telephone line simulator.

A summary sheet for the results of the last round robin determining the STS for the same hearing aids at several laboratories is shown in Table 1–3. The STS values in column 4 of Table 1–3 indicate that the HFA output SPL for microphone (column 2) was greater than that for telecoil (HFA SPLITS—column 3) for the Avanti hearing aid and about the same for the Suprimo hearing aid, whereas the HFA output SPL for microphone was less than that for telecoil for the E25 hearing aid and the two ITE hearing aids. The effect of rotating the telecoil within a hearing aid by 90 degrees to achieve optimal induction coil pickup of signals from the telephone can be seen by comparing the HFA SPLITS data for the two ITE hearing aids. As expected, on average, the induction pickup (HFA SPLITS) is about 6 dB greater with the telecoil mounted perpendicular to the faceplate (ITE PERP—coil approximately horizontal as worn) than with it mounted parallel to the faceplate (ITE PARA—coil approximately vertical as worn). From this data, the working group concluded that the relatively small amount of variation in the 2-cc coupler induction coil pickup data (i.e., HFA SPLITS data in column 3) obtained with the TMFS fixture was quite encouraging. For right ear mounting, for example, the maximum variation between the six laboratories (Beltone is listed twice because two different telephone receivers were used for their real ear measurements) was 5.5 dB for HFA SPLITS for four of the five different hearing aids mounted on the TMFS. (There was an 8.1 dB maximum variation in HFA SPLITS measurements between laboratories for the fifth hearing aid, the ITE hearing aid with the telecoil mounted parallel to the faceplate). The grand means of the maximum variations between the six labs for HFA output SPL in the 2-cc coupler from the five hearing aids was 5.5 dB variation in induction mode (for all the data in column 3) for right ear mounting and 3.3 dB variation in acoustic mode (for all data in column 2). Thus, for this small sample size, the induction mode measurements made with the TMFS had only a 2.2 dB higher grand mean (5.5–3.3 dB) of the maximum variations across the six laboratories for the five hearing aids than that for the acoustic measurements. It was also encouraging to find that the relative STS values between hearing aids in the 2-cc coupler (column 4) were similar to the relative differences between hearing aids in comparing the inductive and acoustic output SPLs in the real ear measurements.

A similar procedure was followed for the same five hearing aids used for the STS calculations, but this time positioning the hearing aids *vertically* relative to a large test loop, as they would be used for inductive pickup of room loops. The results are shown in Table 1–4. The TLS data for each hearing aid in column 4 of Table 1–4 are different from the STS results in Table 1–3 and indicate that the HFA output SPL for microphone was significantly greater than that for telecoil for all of the hearing aids, except the E25 for which the HFA output SPL for microphone was about the same or a little higher than that for telecoil. The TLS values in Table 1–4 are much lower than the STS values in Table 1–3, in part, because the

**Table 1–3.**   HFA Output SPL via Acoustic Input and via Inductive Inputs Using the Telephone Magnetic Field Simulator (TMFS) in a Round Robin with Six Laboratories Testing the Same Five Hearing Aids

| Lab | Acoustic 60 dB SPL input HFA out (dB SPL) | Inductive SPLITS HFA out (dB SPL) | STS (dB)* |
|---|---|---|---|
| **Hearing Aid: Avanti (right ear)** | | | |
| Argosy | 90.8 | 87.6 | –3.2 |
| Beltone MR | 92.8 | 83.2 | –9.7 |
| Beltone U1 | 92.8 | 83.2 | –9.7 |
| Mayo | 92.7 | 86.3 | –6.4 |
| Etymonic | 93.7 | 88.7 | –5.0 |
| 3M | 89.8 | 84.3 | –5.6 |
| VA-WASH., DC | 93.1 | 85.0 | –8.1 |
| **Hearing Aid: Suprimo (right ear)** | | | |
| Argosy | 94.7 | 95.4 | +0.7 |
| Beltone MR | 95.0 | 92.9 | –2.1 |
| Beltone U1 | 95.0 | 92.9 | –2.1 |
| Mayo | 94.0 | 95.3 | +1.3 |
| Etymonic | 95.1 | 96.3 | +1.2 |
| 3M | 92.2 | 95.0 | +2.9 |
| VA-WASH., DC | 93.1 | 92.4 | –0.7 |
| **Hearing Aid: E25 (right ear)** | | | |
| Argosy | 91.4 | 100.0 | +8.6 |
| Beltone MR | 93.4 | 99.2 | +5.8 |
| Beltone U1 | 93.4 | 99.2 | +5.8 |
| Mayo | 93.3 | 103.7 | +10.4 |
| Etymonic | 93.6 | 100.8 | +7.2 |
| 3M | 90.2 | 101.2 | +11.0 |
| VA-WASH., DC | 93.9 | 101.3 | +7.4 |
| **Hearing Aid: ITE Para coil** | | | |
| Argosy | 98.6 | 103.3 | +4.7 |
| Beltone MR | 98.7 | 95.2 | –3.5 |
| Beltone U1 | 98.7 | 95.2 | –3.5 |
| Mayo | 97.3 | 98.7 | +1.4 |
| Etymonic | 99.6 | 103.0 | +3.4 |
| 3M | 98.8 | 96.3 | –2.5 |
| VA-WASH., DC | 94.8 | 100.5 | +5.7 |
| **Hearing Aid: ITE Perp coil** | | | |
| Argosy | 97.6 | 106.4 | +8.8 |
| Beltone MR | 97.4 | 102.5 | +5.1 |
| Beltone U1 | 97.4 | 102.5 | +5.1 |
| Mayo | 97.7 | 106.3 | +8.6 |
| Etymonic | 98.6 | 107.2 | +8.5 |
| 3M | 98.2 | 108.0 | +9.8 |
| VA-WASH., DC | 98.8 | 104.3 | +9.2 |

*The difference between HFA output SPL with inductive and acoustic inputs is the Simulated Telephone Sensitivity (STS) or the estimated gain needed to equalize the output SPL when switching from microphone mode to induction coil mode for telephone pickup.

**Table 1–4.**  HFA Output SPL via Acoustic Input and via Inductive Input
Using a Large Test Loop in a Round Robin with Six Laboratories Testing
the Same Five Hearing Aids Used for Table 1–3

| Lab | Acoustic 60 dB SPL input HFA out (dB SPL) | Inductive SPLIV HFA out (dB SPL) | TLS (dB)* |
|---|---|---|---|
| **Hearing Aid: Avanti** | | | |
| Argosy | 90.8 | 82.9 | –7.9 |
| Beltone | 92.8 | 79.1 | –13.7 |
| Mayo | 92.7 | 82.3 | –10.4 |
| Etymonic | 93.7 | 79.7 | –14.0 |
| 3M | 89.8 | 80.2 | –9.6 |
| VA-WASH., DC | 93.1 | 80.7 | –12.4 |
| **Hearing Aid: Suprimo** | | | |
| Argosy | 94.7 | 88.1 | –6.6 |
| Beltone | 95.0 | 83.7 | –11.3 |
| Mayo | 94.0 | 88.7 | –5.3 |
| Etymonic | 95.1 | 81.3 | –13.8 |
| 3M | 92.2 | 78.7 | –13.5 |
| VA-WASH., DC | 93.1 | 86.0 | –7.1 |
| **Hearing Aid: E25** | | | |
| Argosy | 91.4 | 92.1 | +0.7 |
| Beltone | 93.4 | 90.7 | –2.7 |
| Mayo | 93.3 | 93.7 | +0.4 |
| Etymonic | 93.6 | 89.8 | –3.8 |
| 3M | 90.2 | 90.5 | +0.4 |
| VA-WASH., DC | 93.9 | 90.2 | –3.7 |
| **Hearing Aid: ITE para coil** | | | |
| Argosy | 98.6 | 92.4 | –6.2 |
| Beltone | 98.7 | 88.3 | –10.4 |
| Mayo | 97.3 | 92.3 | –5.0 |
| Etymonic | 99.6 | 87.2 | –12.4 |
| 3M | 98.8 | 93.8 | –5.0 |
| VA-WASH., DC | 94.8 | 89.7 | –5.1 |
| **Hearing Aid: ITE perp coil** | | | |
| Argosy | 97.6 | 88.4 | –9.2 |
| Beltone | 97.4 | 74.3 | –23.1 |
| Mayo | 97.7 | 79.3 | –18.4 |
| Etymonic | 98.6 | 74.9 | –23.7 |
| 3M | 98.2 | 74.8 | –23.4 |
| VA-WASH., DC | 96.3 | 91.5 | –4.8 |

*The difference between HFA output SPL with inductive and acoustic inputs is the Test Loop Sensitivity (TLS) or the estimated gain needed to equalize the output SPL when switching from microphone mode to induction coil mode for room loop pickup.

loop used for the SPLIV measurements and TLS calculations produced only a 10 mA/m magnetic field strength. Additionally, however, some of these results are not surprising, because a telecoil mounted within a hearing aid horizontally as worn (e.g., the ITE PERP hearing aid with coil mounted perpendicular to the faceplate) is expected to have poor inductive pickup from loops. The maximum variation between SPLIV measurements (column 3) across the six laboratories produced by three of the five different hearing aids (Avanti, E25, ITE with tele-coil mounted parallel to faceplate or approximately vertical as worn) was 6.6 dB. For the other two hearing aids, the maximum variation between laboratories in HFA SPLIV measurements was 17.2 dB for the ITE hearing aid with the telecoil mounted perpendicular to the faceplate (approximately horizontal as worn) and 10.0 dB for the Suprimo hearing aid. These large spreads suggest that the various laboratories were having difficulty in positioning the hearing aids at the same imaginary vertical axis. Currently, the S3-48 writing group is recommending a 31.6 mA/m inductive field strength for SPLIV tests and is attempting to provide a better definition of a vertical reference axis for this measurement.

As of this date, the procedure specified for determining STS is in the main body of the current draft of the next revision of the S3.22 standard. The currently used procedure described in S3.22-1987 to position the hearing aid for maximum induction pickup sensitivity and the method for determining TLS are in the appendix of the next draft revision of S3.22.

It is gratifying to note that, as the performance tradeoffs of induction coil pick-up have become better understood, integrated circuit technology has been applied to solve the low induction coil sensitivity problem; hearing aid manufac-turers have begun to include an induction coil preamplifier as a standard feature in many current hearing aids. Also, more attention is being paid to the orienta-tion of the telephone coil within the hearing aid for its intended application. The STS and the TLS indicate how well a particular hearing aid with telecoil picks up inductive signals from the telephone and from loops, respectively. Having this information should provide considerable help in the selection of the best hearing aid, depending on the individual needs of the hearing aid wearer. If the hearing aid wearer has equal need for induction pickup of telephones and loops, a hear-ing aid with high values of STS and TLS should be fitted. To this end, a single, vertically mounted telecoil or, if physical space allows, two telecoils, orthogonally positioned, seem to be the best solutions (Compton, 1994; Preves, 1994).

ELECTROMAGNETIC INTERFERENCE

Although inclusion of a telecoil preamplifier and appropriate orientation of the telecoil within the hearing aid generally resolved the issue of low induction coil sensitivity, it may have created another problem. That is, the more sensitive induction coils in current hearing aids now may pick up greater interference from other sources of electromagnetic energy that may be close by. These include fluorescent lights, computer monitors, printers, and even hearing aid analyzers. One would hope that the *electromagnetic interference (EMI)* of these devices could be removed relatively easily by adding high-pass and low-pass filters to the front-end amplifier stages of hearing aids with induction pickup coils. However, this problem may not be solved so easily because preliminary study of the spec-tra radiated by these devices reveals broad-band EMI signals. For example, the spectra of the electromagnetic fields radiated by a computer monitor and a dot matrix printer are shown in Figures 1–23a and 1–23b, respectively. These spectra are too broad band to be filtered out in a hearing aid with induction coil by simple

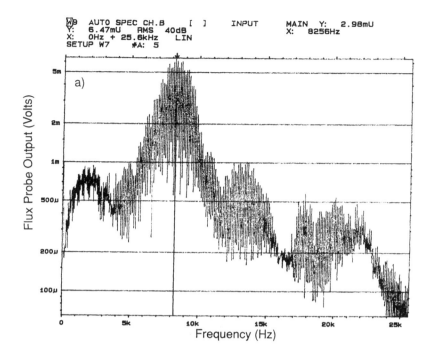

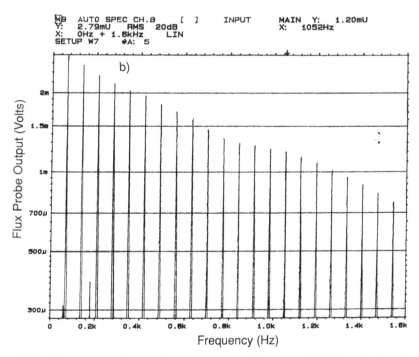

**Figure 1–23.** Electromagnetic spectra sensed by a Magnetek 1846 Flux Probe at a distance of four inches that were radiated from (a) an Acer 330 SVGA computer monitor and (b) an Epson FX-185 dot matrix printer (not while printing).

high-pass or low-pass filters. (A related discussion follows in the section on Digital Cordless Telephone Interference.)

IEC VERSUS ANSI TELECOIL TEST PROCEDURES

The IEC 118-1 standard, entitled Part 1: *Hearing Aids With Induction Pick-up Coil,* has recently been modified to obtain induction coil sensitivity and frequency response with a magnetic field strength of 31.6 mA/m. However, the standard still specifies that the hearing aid be oriented for the maximum induction coil sensitivity, and that this orientation is to be stated, but it does not specify the reference coordinates that should be used. The revised document also includes a distortion test with a 100 mA/m magnetic field strength input, which is the typical magnetic field emanating from a room loop.

## Possible New Methods for Measuring the Performance of AGC Hearing Aids for S3.22

INPUT LEVEL AND GAIN CONTROL POSITION

ANSI standard S3.22-1987 specifies a 50 dB SPL swept pure tone input for obtaining the frequency response curve of an AGC hearing aid. This relatively low input level was deliberately selected by the S3-48 working group in the early 1970s to obtain the frequency response of AGC hearing aids operating linearly. An input of 50 dB SPL was below the AGC kneepoint for most hearing aids at that time. Since that date, however, it is more common for AGC hearing aids to have kneepoints below 50 dB SPL. Also, it is desirable to determine the frequency response of AGC hearing aids while they are in compression. Another difference in current test methods between AGC and linear hearing aids is that reference test gain control position is defined as full-on. Testing at a full-on position may penalize some AGC hearing aids that have Class B or Class D amplifier output stages because their current drains are dependent on output signal level. Testing at a full-on gain control position also is in contradiction to the concept of determining reference test position from HFA SSPL90. Testing at full-on may result in AGC hearing aids being penalized by higher harmonic distortion and frequency response curves that have large peaks and troughs. Consequently, to eliminate these problems, the S3-48 working group is presently advocating that S3.22 be modified so that the gain controls of AGC hearing aids are adjusted with the same procedure used for linear hearing aids. That is, the current draft of the revised S3.22 standard recommends testing AGC hearing aids with a 60 dB input SPL and with their gain controls set to the reference test position, as determined by the HFA SSPL90 measurement.

ATTACK AND RELEASE TIMES

Another problem that has arisen after years of using S3.22 is the measurement of attack and release times of AGC hearing aids. To determine attack and release times, the currently used procedure is to abruptly change the input level between 55 dB and 80 dB SPL and count the time for the hearing aid output to decay or rise, respectively, to within 2 dB of its final value. There are few problems with this 2 dB settling "window" for older-generation, single time constant AGC hearing aids. However, with the widespread proliferation of hearing aids with compression circuits having variable time constants, the 2 dB settling window, in combination with hearing aids that may have very long AGC time constants (i.e., greater than a few hundred milliseconds), can lead to erratic values and poor repeatability in measurements of attack time. For example, a plot of output SPL versus time of the attack time for a K-AMP hearing aid shown is in Figure 1–24a. For this measurement, as specified in S3.22, the input was a 2000 Hz sinusoid abruptly changed from 55 dB SPL to 80 dB SPL. Note the extremely long, nearly horizontal portion of the waveform as it decays. The time taken for the envelope of the hearing aid output to settle to its final value of 88.2 dB SPL is nearly 2 seconds. Per S3.22, the time taken for the output to be within 2 dB of 88.2 dB SPL is 85 milliseconds. The initial portion of this attack time is expanded in Figure 1–24b to see the dual time constant of the K-AMP more clearly. At first, a brief spike occurs, followed by a much longer time constant with gradual decay. The current test procedure for the attack time specified in S3.22 requires using the longer, nearly horizontal portion of the attack time waveform to get within 2 dB of the final value. Applying this procedure to K-AMP hearing aids often produces poor repeatability and wide tolerances for attack time. Repeatable measurements are hard to achieve because the output SPL during the longer decay portion only changes by a few tenths of a dB over many milliseconds.

This variable time constant situation raises a philosophical question: in Figure 1–24b, which time constant best represents the attack time of the hearing aid? The more dominant attack time seems to be the shorter portion, because the output SPL of the hearing aid during the short decay changes by many dB in a very few milliseconds. Note from Figure 1–24b that if either a 3-dB or a 4-dB settling window had been used, the attack time would have been 1.5 milliseconds (at full-on gain control setting). On other hearing aids, however, further testing has revealed that a 4 dB settling level might cause the attack time to be missed altogether. Consequently, taking all of this into consideration, the S3-48 working group is recommending that the settling level for the attack time measurement be changed from 2 dB to 3 dB in the next revision of S3.22.

Because a similar problem was found with the release time measurement, a change in the settling level from 2 dB to 4 dB for the release time measurement is being recommended in the next revision of S3.22. For an output compression hearing aid whose electroacoustic performance per ANSI S3.22 is illustrated in Figure 1–25a, the effect of this change on the release time is illustrated in Figure 1–25b. This figure indicates, that with an abrupt change in 2000 Hz input from 80 to 55 dB SPL, the release time is reduced from 1.35 seconds for a 2 dB settling level to 0.725 seconds for a 4 dB settling level.

TEST FREQUENCIES

Currently, the AGC input/output curve and attack and release times are obtained at 2000 Hz. More information is needed at other frequencies to more completely characterize hearing aids with level-dependent frequency response (Killion et al., 1990), such as those with multiple-band compression. Conse-

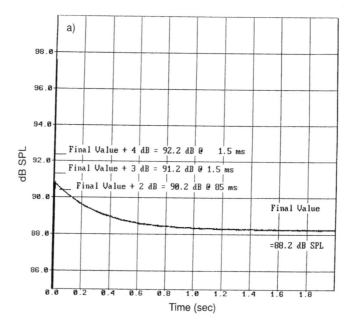

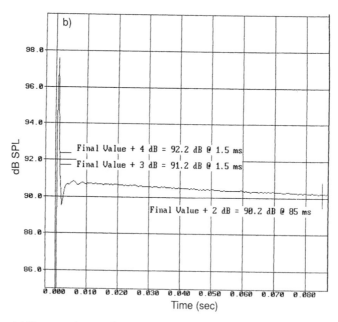

**Figure 1–24.** (a) Temporal waveform envelope of the output of an ITE hearing aid on a 2-cc coupler resulting from K-AMP compression in response to an abrupt change in a 2000 Hz input from 55 to 80 dB SPL. Attack time is 85 milliseconds per ANSI S3.22-1987 with 2 dB settling window and 1.5 milliseconds with either a 3 or a 4 dB settling window. (b) Enlarged view of first 80 milliseconds in Figure 1–24 (a) showing dual attack time constant of K-AMP circuit.

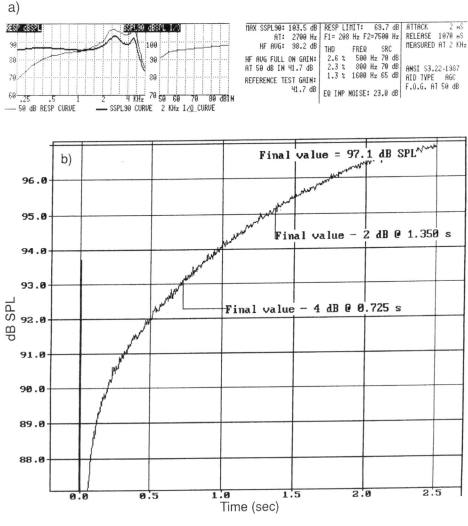

**Figure 1–25.** (a) Data per ANSI S3.22-1987 for an output compression hearing aid. (b) Temporal waveform envelope for hearing aid used in (a) in a 2-cc coupler resulting from compression in response to an abrupt change in 2000 Hz input from 80 to 55 dB SPL. Release time would be 1.350 seconds per ANSI S3.22-1987 with 2 dB settling window and 0.725 seconds with a 4 dB settling window.

quently, the next revision of S3.22 will specify that 250, 500, 1000, and 4000 Hz could be used optionally at the discretion of the manufacturer as additional test frequencies for measurement of input/output function and the attack and release times. Even without specific mention in the standard, hearing aid manufacturers always have had the option of reporting the results of measurements at any test frequency for additional information.

KNEEPOINT AND COMPRESSION RATIO

There has been considerable discussion within the S3-48 working group regarding the advantages and disadvantages of including a definition of AGC kneepoint in the next revision of S3.22. The main problem is developing a singular definition of kneepoint that accurately describes the input/output (I/O) characteristic for all types of compression hearing aids, including those with curvilinear and logarithmic I/O characteristics, multiple kneepoints, and nonmonotonic kneepoints. After considerable time over many months was spent by members of the S3-48 working group in trying to define kneepoint, no agreement could be reached on a unambiguous definition that would cover the behavior of all known compression hearing aids. Thus, at the time of this writing, the S3-48 working group plans not to include a definition of kneepoint in the next revision of S3.22.

A possible future change in S3.22 is the measurement of the "effective" compression ratio of AGC hearing aids (Stone and Moore, 1992). Currently, the input/output characteristic and compression ratio for AGC hearing aids is determined for steady-state conditions. Stone and Moore (1992) have demonstrated that the compression ratio for normally encountered temporally modulating signals, such as speech or pulsatile noises, is smaller than for steady-state signals. They point out that this phenomenon can occur when part, but not all, of the modulating waveform is below the AGC kneepoint or when the compression release time is similar to the temporal modulation period of the input signal.

### Battery Current Drain With Noise Input or as an Average at Three Pure Tone Frequencies

S3.22-1987 specifies that the current drain of hearing aids be obtained at the reference test position with a 1000 Hz input signal of 65 dB SPL. However, many current hearing aids use class B and Class D amplifier output stages in which current drain varies with input level and gain control setting rather than remaining fixed as in a class A output stage. Although the selection of 65 dB SPL input at 1000 Hz for the S3.22 current drain test in the 1970s was designed to represent current drain for a wide range of hearing aids containing class B as well as class A output stages, after so much time has passed a more representative procedure is being sought. Because hearing aids rarely amplify fixed input level sinusoids, Jeremy Agnew, a member of the working group, suggested that an investigation be conducted regarding the possibility of using broad-band noise or a three-frequency average to measure hearing aid current drain. Also to be assessed in this study were the effects of different input levels on current drain. A subgroup within the S3-48 working group was formed to conduct the investigation. The subgroup, chaired by William Cole, concluded that there was good correlation between the current drain measurement at 1000 Hz per S3.22-1987 and current drain obtained using the broad-band noise input signal specified in S3.42-1992 or with a high-frequency average using the three HFA test frequencies as input signals. Their data are summarized in the worksheet shown in Table 1–5. The first column "INST. ID" identifies the designation of the amplifier used in the hearing aids. The second column "CLASS" identifies whether each hearing aid had a Class A, AB, B, or D output stage. The third column "RECEIVER" provides the Knowles

Table 1–5.  Current Drain Measurements Obtained with Various Methods for Different Hearing Aids

| Inst. ID | Class | Receiver | HF Avg SSPL90 | A Idle | B Per s3.22 | C HF Avg Per s3.22 | D 90 dB Hf Avg @ FOG | E 60 dB Noise −17 dB | F 90 dB Noise @ Fog | G A/E | H B/E | I C/E | J D/F | K A/B | L 80% Iq + 20% Ipk |
|---|---|---|---|---|---|---|---|---|---|---|---|---|---|---|---|
| 91A0280 | B | Dual BK | 122.9 | 0.41 | 1.58 | 1.40 | 5.29 | 0.99 | 6.26 | 0.41 | 1.60 | 1.41 | 0.85 | 0.26 | 1.39 |
| 90M0683 | B | ? | 116.4 | 0.34 | 1.02 | 0.98 | 4.30 | 0.67 | 4.94 | 0.51 | 1.52 | 1.46 | 0.87 | 0.33 | 1.13 |
| 90M1288 | D | EP | 109.2 | 0.31 | 0.32 | 0.34 | 0.61 | 0.33 | 0.59 | 0.94 | 0.97 | 1.03 | 1.03 | 0.97 | 0.37 |
| 90M1573 | D | EP | 111.4 | 0.32 | 0.32 | 0.33 | 1.13 | 0.33 | 1.07 | 0.97 | 0.97 | 1.00 | 1.06 | 1.00 | 0.48 |
| ULTIMA III | AB | EF | | 0.32 | 1.30 | 1.30 | 5.40 | 0.96 | 5.40 | 0.33 | 1.35 | 1.35 | 1.00 | 0.25 | 1.34 |
| ULTIMA III | AB | ED | | 0.32 | 0.90 | 0.87 | 3.20 | 0.67 | 3.30 | 0.48 | 1.34 | 1.30 | 0.97 | 0.36 | 0.90 |
| ULTIMA II | D | EP | | 0.56 | 0.70 | 0.70 | 5.10 | 0.65 | 5.30 | 0.86 | 1.08 | 1.08 | 0.96 | 0.80 | 1.47 |
| GENNUM 531 | AB | BK | 119 | 0.55 | 1.28 | 0.77 | 3.20 | 0.70 | 5.40 | 0.79 | 1.83 | 1.10 | 0.59 | 0.43 | 1.08 |
| PP7 | AB? | BK | 118 | 0.57 | 1.21 | 1.00 | 3.40 | 0.84 | 3.50 | 0.68 | 1.44 | 1.19 | 0.97 | 0.47 | 1.14 |
| 3073 | D | EP | 104.2 | 0.30 | 0.31 | 0.30 | 0.57 | 0.31 | 0.58 | 0.97 | 1.00 | 0.97 | 0.98 | 0.97 | 0.35 |
| 3074 | D | EP | 108.9 | 0.40 | 0.46 | 0.42 | 1.30 | 0.42 | 1.44 | 0.95 | 1.10 | 1.00 | 0.90 | 0.87 | 0.58 |
| 3075 | D | EP | | 0.71 | 0.75 | 0.74 | 3.30 | 0.72 | 3.00 | 0.99 | 1.04 | 1.03 | 1.10 | 0.95 | 1.23 |
| 3106 | D | EP | | 0.32 | 0.32 | 0.32 | 0.57 | 0.32 | 0.52 | 1.00 | 1.00 | 1.00 | 1.10 | 1.00 | 0.37 |
| 3107 | D | EP | | 0.37 | 0.38 | 0.38 | 1.30 | 0.37 | 1.12 | 1.00 | 1.03 | 1.03 | 1.16 | 0.97 | 0.56 |
| 3108 | D | EP | | 0.65 | 0.67 | 0.67 | 3.40 | 0.65 | 2.90 | 1.00 | 1.03 | 1.03 | 1.17 | 0.97 | 1.20 |
| E28P | AB | CI | 130.1 | 1.14 | 2.99 | 3.29 | 10.1 | 1.83 | 9.99 | 0.62 | 1.63 | 1.80 | 1.01 | 0.38 | 2.93 |
| A2000-AFMP | B | CI | 133.1 | 0.56 | 3.11 | 2.67 | 10.12 | 1.38 | 13.98 | 0.41 | 2.25 | 1.93 | 0.72 | 0.18 | 2.47 |
| | | | | | | | | | AVG = | 0.76 | 1.30 | 1.22 | 0.97 | 0.66 | |
| | | | | | | | | | SD = | 0.24 | 0.36 | 0.28 | 0.14 | 0.32 | |
| | | | | | | | | | SD/AVG = | 0.32 | 0.27 | 0.23 | 0.15 | 0.48 | |

Column A: quiescent or idle current; B: current drain per S3.22; C: average current drain at 1000, 1600, 2500 Hz with 65 dB input SPL at reference test position; D: same as C with a 90 dB input SPL at reference test position; E: current drain with 60 dB SPL speech-shaped noise input at reference test gain per S3.42; F: same noise input signal as E at 90 dB SPL and full-on gain. From Cole, 1991.

Electronics receiver model type used in the hearing aid. Column A reports the idle current drain (that at minimum gain control setting with no input signal). Column B reports the current drain using the existing S3.22 procedure; column C reports the current drain using an HFA average current drain; and columns E and F report current drain using a 60 dB SPL and 90 dB SPL, respectively, speech-shaped broad-band noise input. For ease in interpreting these data, Cole computed ratios to compare these measurements. A ratio close to 1.0 indicates that the two techniques being compared result in about the same measured current drain. The averages and standard deviations across all hearing aids tested with the various methods are shown at the bottom of the table. For example, the AVG ratio of 0.97 in column J indicates that, on the average, measuring current drain with a 90 dB input SPL using the three-frequency average (Column D) or the speech-shaped noise (Column F) results in about the same current drain. These two measurements are estimates of the maximum current drain. The average ratio of 1.30 in Column H indicates that current drain, as measured by S3.22 (at reference test gain control position with a 1000 Hz sinusoid at 65 dB input SPL—Column B), is about the same as that measured with the speech-shaped noise input signal at 60 dB SPL (Column E) when the hearing aid gain control is set at reference test position as specified in S3.42.

Because only small differences in current drain were observed across these different procedures, no change in the S3.22 drain current procedure is being recommended in the main body of the standard. The last column (L) of Table 1–5 shows the current drain using a weighted sum of 80% of the idle current (column A) plus 20% of the maximum or peak current (Column D). Using this procedure to express current drain is being included as an optional method in the appendix of the next draft revision of S3.22.

## Possible New Measurements of Hearing Aid Distortion

For several years, the S3-48 working group has been investigating new methods of characterizing distortion in hearing aids to represent better their performance in real-world listening situations. The harmonic distortion measurements specified in S3.22 are intended to ensure quality control, and not necessarily to provide an indication of the sound quality of sounds processed by a hearing aid. The amount of intermodulation distortion has been shown to relate more closely to degradation of sound quality and speech intelligibility than harmonic distortion (Harris et al., 1961; Schweitzer et al., 1977; Jirsa and Norris, 1982; Pryce, 1989). Consequently, a long-standing suggestion has been for ANSI to recommend measuring the intermodulation distortion produced by hearing aids. A measurement procedure for determining intermodulation distortion in hearing aids is included in IEC 118-0.

As mentioned previously, coherence measurements described in the appendix of the S3.42 noise test standard are used as an indication of the validity of the frequency response measurement. There is some indication that coherence may also be a good indicator of the distortion produced in a hearing aid, and how it might affect sound quality. Several investigators have suggested that coherence can be used to measure the nonlinear distortion of hearing aid circuitry (Dyrlund, 1989;

Preves, 1990; Schweitzer et al., 1991; Hawkins and Naidoo, 1993; Kates and Kozma-Spytek, 1994). For example, Kates and Kozma-Spytek (1994) found extremely close correlation between a distortion index, as measured by the coherence function, and sound quality ratings of processed sentences as the level of peak clipping and frequency response were varied (see Table 1–6). Three different frequency responses were used: (a) flat, (b) 20 dB low-frequency emphasis, and (c) 20 dB high-frequency emphasis. Symmetric hard clipping was used at four clipping levels 0, 4, 8, and 12 dB above the sentence rms power level. These clipping levels resulted in the speech waveform being clipped about 20% of the time for the 0 dB clipping level and less than 0.5% of the time for the 12 dB clipping level. The subjective rating values reported in Table 1–6, column 3, and distortion index values reported in Table 1–6, column 4 were first normalized by their highest raw rating values, respectively, to provide rating scales between 0 and 1. Subjective ratings of sound quality (column 3) are generally lower for the low-frequency (LF) boost condition than for the flat and high-frequency (HF) emphasis conditions, presumably because the more intense low-frequency energy of the voiced sounds in the sentences were clipped more than the weaker high frequency energy of the unvoiced sounds. The correlation coefficient between the subjective ratings and the distortion index was 0.998.

In another study, Schweitzer, Grim, Preves, Kubichek, and Woodruff (1991) found a high correlation between hearing aid-processed speech quality and coherence using five different types of hearing aid signal processing, as shown in Figure 1–26. Their study included a linear amplifier having a class A output stage with no peak clipping (H.A. L) and with symmetrical peak clipping (H.A. B). Nonlinear processing amplifiers having a class D output stage included in the study were input compression (H.A. C), Argosy Manhattan II with "BILL" processing (H.A. M), a high-pass filter followed by an infinite amplitude clipping at

**Table 1–6.** Mean Sound Quality Ratings of Eight Normal Hearing Subjects versus Distortion Index Computed from Coherence Measurements for Three Simulated Hearing Aid Frequency Responses and Four Symmetric Clipping Conditions

| Frequency Response | Clipping Threshold, dB | Normal Subject Rating | Distortion Index |
|---|---|---|---|
| 20-dB LF Boost | 0 | 0.239 | 0.239 |
| | 4 | 0.355 | 0.426 |
| | 8 | 0.633 | 0.736 |
| | 12 | 0.981 | 1.000 |
| Flat | 0 | 0.442 | 0.483 |
| | 4 | 0.652 | 0.664 |
| | 8 | 0.873 | 0.976 |
| | 12 | 1.000 | 1.000 |
| 20-dB HF Boost | 0 | 0.477 | 0.548 |
| | 4 | 0.665 | 0.727 |
| | 8 | 0.831 | 0.984 |
| | 12 | 0.939 | 1.000 |

Reprinted with permission from Kates and Kozma-Spytek, 1994.

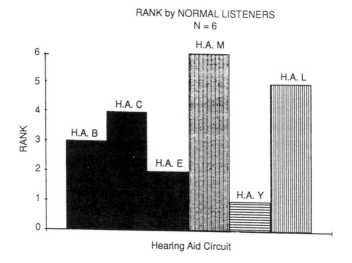

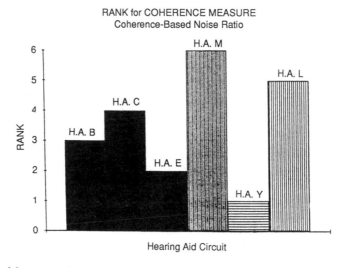

**Figure 1–26.** Mean sound quality ranking by six normal listeners (upper panel) and rank by coherence measurements (lower panel) for hearing-aid processed 10-second male voice segments of the "Rainbow Passage" presented at 65 dB input SPL. Digital recordings were made with all hearing aids adjusted to 30 dB HFA gain on a HA-1 2-cc coupler in a Bruel & Kjaer 4212 sound chamber. Hearing aid circuits: (B) class A linear circuit with 10 dB symmetrical peak clipping; (C) input compression with class D output stage; (E) class D output stage with high-pass filter followed by linear amplification at low input levels and infinite amplitude clipping at high input levels; (M) "BILL" circuit with adaptive high-pass filter and class D output stage; (Y) same as hearing aid E with infinite amplitude clipping occurring at all input levels; (L) same as B with no peak clipping. Reprinted with permission from Schweitzer et al., 1991.

higher input levels only (H.A. E), and at all input levels (H.A. Y). In the upper panel, speech processed by each hearing aid was rank ordered by six normal listeners for sound quality with 6 being the best ranking and 1 being the worst ranking. In the lower panel, the coherence values shown for each hearing aid were first converted to a 1 to 6 scale for comparison to the upper panel sound quality rankings. Visual inspection of the top and bottom panels in Figure 1–26 shows almost identical ranking values among the 6 hearing aids by sound quality and by coherence.

## Possible Future Measurements of Hearing Aid Circuit Noise for S3.22

PROBLEMS WITH THE CURRENT METHOD

The *equivalent input noise measurement* specified in ANSI S3.22 has been one of the most difficult measurements in the standard to perform. The major problems with the equivalent input noise measurement method specified in S3.22 are its sensitivity to: (1) the hearing aid gain, (2) the low-frequency response slope of the hearing aid, (3) the environmental noise present in the test chamber of the hearing aid analyzer, and (4) test equipment system noise. These problems were brought to the attention of the S3-48 working group by William Johnson, a member of the working group. Measurements of equivalent input noise made in accordance with the existing method in S3.22 result in hearing aids with low gain and those with steeply sloping frequency responses exhibiting higher equivalent input noise than hearing aids having a flatter frequency response. Johnson theorized that the peak noise energy is the primary factor in determining the overall amount of circuit noise output SPL from the hearing aid.

An example produced by Johnson of equivalent input noise being indirectly proportional to gain is shown in the top panels of Figures 1–27a, 1–27b, and 1–27c. These panels report data per ANSI S3.22 obtained on a Frye 6500 hearing aid analyzer for the same hearing aid at three different gain control settings. This hearing aid was especially created for these tests with an instrumentation quality operational amplifier (Analog Devices AD 560). The equivalent input noise was 19.4, 30.2, and 42.0 dB SPL for peak gains of approximately 50, 25, and 15 dB, respectively. The intent of these tests was to demonstrate the effect on equivalent input noise when three different hearing aids were created by varying the gain of a single hearing aid circuit. If the equivalent input noise measurement is independent of the hearing aid gain, it should not change when the gain control is adjusted. In this case, part of the cause of the high equivalent input noise in Figures 1–27b and 1–27c appeared to be relatively high levels of ambient noise in the test chamber and/or the analyzer system noise. This problem can be seen in the lower panels of Figures 1–27a, 1–27b, and 1–27c. For the three gain control settings, these three lower panels show the noise output spectra of the hearing aid (and amplified system noise and ambient noise in the test chamber) with no input and the overall noise output SPL (labelled RMS OUT). Note by comparing the lower panels in Figures 1–27a and 1–27b that the overall hearing aid output SPL with no input decreases by only 15 dB (60.3 dB SPL to 45.1 dB SPL) as a result of a 25 dB gain reduction (from 50 dB to 25 dB peak gain). The overall hearing aid noise output SPL actually increases by almost 2 dB (45.1 to 46.9 dB SPL) when the peak gain is

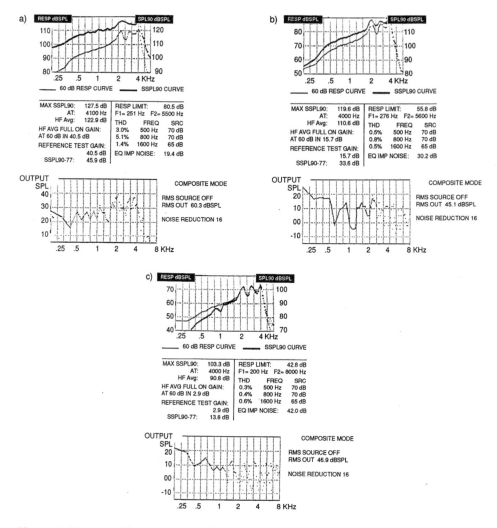

**Figure 1–27.** (a-c) Upper panels—data per ANSI S3.22-1987 obtained with Frye 6500 hearing aid analyzer for the same hearing aid adjusted to three peak gains. Lower panels—total rms output noise SPL from the hearing aid and its spectrum with no input signal. Peak gains were approximately 50 dB (a), 25 dB (b), and 15 dB (c). Reprinted with permission from Johnson, 1992.

reduced by 10 dB from 25 dB to 15 dB (Figs. 1–27b and 1–27c). The noise output SPL with no input indicated by RMS OUT in the bottom panels of Figures 1–27b and 1–27c should differ by 10 dB if the hearing aid output noise level is not being affected by ambient noise in the test chamber noise or by analyzer system noise. Because 10 dB difference was not achieved, the high value of 42.0 dB SPL equivalent input noise in Figure 1–27c is probably artifactual because it appears that the actual hearing aid noise is being masked by the ambient noise in the test chamber and/or the system analyzer noise.

EFFECT OF FREQUENCY RESPONSE ON EQUIVALENT INPUT NOISE

An example of equivalent input noise being indirectly proportional to the slope of the low-frequency response is shown in Figures 1–28a and 1–28b. In this example, the intent was to demonstrate what would happen when two different hearing aids were created by varying the low-frequency response of a single hearing aid circuit. If the equivalent input noise measurement was independent of low-frequency response slope, the equivalent input noise should not change by adjusting the low-frequency tone control. These data were obtained with a Bruel & Kjaer 2032 spectrum analyzer for the same hearing aid used for Figure 1–27 at two different low-frequency tone control settings. For each condition, the gain control was adjusted to maintain the peak gain at about 45.5 dB. In the flatter response configuration shown in Figure 1–28a, HFA full-on gain was 38.5 dB and equivalent input noise per S3.22 was 29.3 dB SPL (neither is shown in Figure

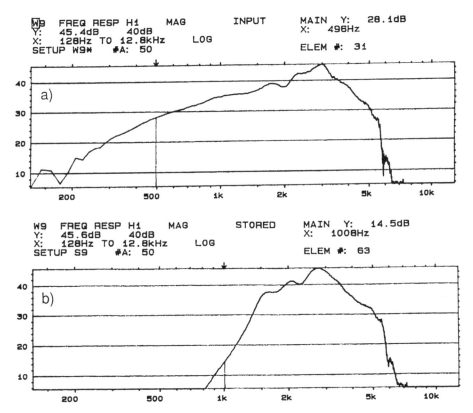

**Figure 1–28.** Frequency responses obtained with a Bruel & Kjaer 2032 spectrum analyzer for two tone control settings of same hearing aid used for Figure 1–27. (a) Flat response condition produced HFA gain of *38.5 dB and equivalent input noise of *29.3 dB SPL; (b) High-frequency emphasis condition produced HFA gain of *31.8 dB and an equivalent input noise of *33.4 dB SPL. If 1600, 2500, and 4000 Hz was used for condition (b), SPA gain was *38.9 dB and equivalent input noise was *26.3 dB SPL. *These data are not shown in the figures.

1–28a). Thus, the hearing aid noise output SPL with no input was 67.8 dB SPL (38.5 dB + 29.3 dB SPL) over a bandwidth of 200–5000 Hz. When the low-frequency tone control was adjusted for the high-pass frequency response shown in Figure 1–28b, HFA full-on gain decreased about 6 dB to 31.8 dB, but the equivalent input noise rose about 4 dB to 33.4 dB SPL (neither is shown in Fig. 1–29b). The equivalent input noise increased for the high-pass frequency response because the hearing aid noise output with no input was 65.2 dB SPL (31.8 dB + 33.4 dB SPL), a decrease of only about 3 dB from that in Figure 1–28a, while the HFA gain decreased by 6 dB. In Figure 1–28b, because there was a 31.1 dB difference in the frequency response between the peak gain and the gain at 1000 Hz, this hearing aid qualifies for use of SPA frequencies rather than HFA frequencies. Choosing 1600, 2500, and 4000 Hz as the SPA frequencies, the full-on SPA gain for the hearing aid in Figure 1–28b was 38.9 dB and the equivalent input noise was 26.3 dB SPL rather than the 33.4 dB SPL value obtained when the HFA frequencies were used. Thus, with SPA frequencies, in this example, when the low-frequency tone control was adjusted, equivalent input noise actually decreased by 3 dB (29.3 dB SPL for Fig. 1–28a versus 26.3 dB SPL with SPA frequencies for Fig. 1–29b) because gain stayed about the same while noise output SPL decreased by 3 dB. This—and other examples—led the working group to conclude that hearing aids with extreme high-frequency emphasis are not penalized by artifactually high equivalent input noise measurements if SPA frequencies are used.

ANOTHER METHOD OF EXPRESSING EQUIVALENT INPUT NOISE

However, because low-gain hearing aids can be penalized by artifactually high equivalent input noise measurements, the S3-48 working group has been investigating other ways of measuring and expressing the circuit noise of hearing aids.

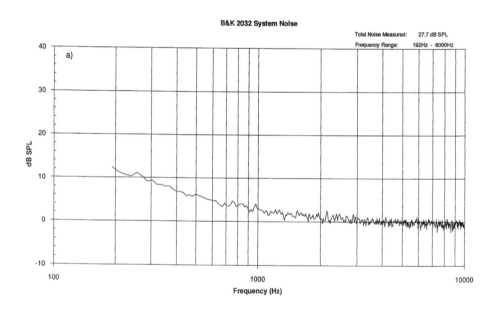

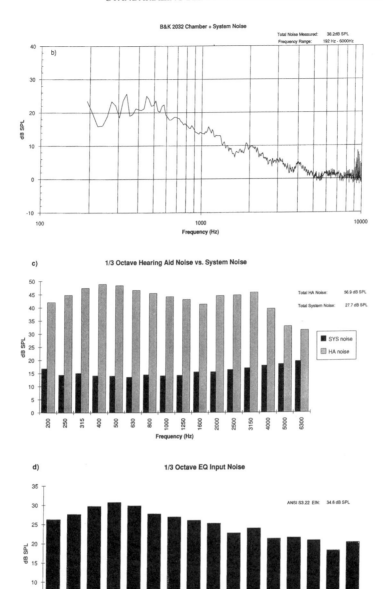

**Figure 1–29.**  Spectrum of the: (a) system noise of Bruel & Kjaer 2032 spectrum analyzer using a 1/2 inch coupler microphone and the opening to the HA-1 coupler occluded; (b) system noise shown in (a) plus ambient noise in a Bruel & Kjaer 4212 test chamber. (c) Noise output with no input of a hearing aid having 23.3 dB HFA gain (taller bars) and system noise of spectrum analyzer with 1/2 inch microphone (shorter bars), both with 1/3 octave analysis. (d) Equivalent input noise in 1/3 octave bands for hearing aid used for (c).

One consideration is the possibility of reporting the spectrum of the hearing aid noise output in 1/3 octave bands as is specified in IEC standard 118-0. This procedure would help to circumvent the problems shown in Figure 1–27 of high system noise and ambient noise in the test chamber contaminating the measurements. In response to Johnson's comments, George Frye, a member of the S3-48 working group, suggested a modification of the method specified in IEC 118-0. According to Frye's proposal, the equivalent noise measurement is judged invalid in any 1/3 octave band in which the system noise SPL is within 6 dB of the hearing aid output noise SPL. Frye noted that the IEC 118-0 requirement for system noise to be 10 dB below hearing aid output noise is too difficult for production or commercial testing environments and that a requirement for system noise SPL being 6 dB below hearing aid output noise SPL would produce a maximum error of only about 1 dB.

An example of this method of analyzing hearing aid circuit noise is shown in Figure 1–29. The spectrum for the system noise of a Bruel & Kjaer 2032 spectrum analyzer is shown in Figure 1–29a. As reported in the upper right corner of the figure, the total rms system noise over the frequency range from 192 to 6000 Hz was 27.7 dB SPL. These system noise data were obtained with the input signal turned off and the output SPL measured with the 1/2 inch condenser coupler microphone while occluding the opening into the HA-1 2-cc coupler. Figure 1–29b depicts the spectrum of the ambient noise in a Bruel & Kjaer 4212 test chamber used with the spectrum analyzer added to the system noise spectrum shown in Figure 1–29a. This measurement was made by removing the 2-cc coupler from the coupler microphone and leaving the sound source off in the test chamber. As shown in the upper right corner of Figure 1–29b, the total rms system plus the ambient test chamber noise from 192 Hz to 6000 Hz was 38.2 dB SPL. Figure 1–29c shows the result of applying Frye's proposal of 1/3 octave hearing aid output noise analysis to an ITE hearing aid having 23.3 dB HFA full-on gain. The shorter group of bars is the system noise spectrum from Figure 1–29a, converted to 1/3 octave bands. The taller group of bars is the spectrum of the hearing aid noise output in 1/3 octave bands with no input signal. The total system noise and hearing aid noise output with no input signal over a bandwidth of 192 to 6000 Hz were 27.7 dB SPL and 57.9 dB SPL, respectively. The two sets of bars in Figure 1–29c are more than 6 dB apart across the entire frequency range, so, according to Frye's proposal, the resulting 1/3 octave spectrum of the equivalent input noise shown in Figure 1–29d is valid in all the 1/3 octave bands. The equivalent input noise for this hearing aid obtained per ANSI S3.22 was 34.6 dB SPL (57.9 dB SPL noise output—23.3 dB HFA gain).

To emulate a low-gain hearing aid, the same measurements were performed using the same equipment on the hearing aid used for Figure 1–29 with its gain control adjusted to an HFA gain of 9.8 dB. The taller set of bars in Figure 1–30a shows the spectrum in 1/3 octave bands of the hearing aid output with no input, and the shorter set of bars in Figure 1–30a is the same system noise spectrum using 1/3 octave analysis shown in Figure 1–29c. The total hearing aid noise output with no input over the frequency range 192 to 6000 Hz was 45.3 dB SPL. Because the shorter set of bars is within 6 dB of the taller set of bars at the highest 1/3 octave band (6300 Hz), the calculated equivalent input noise in 1/3 octave

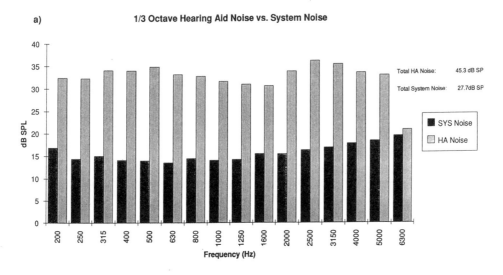

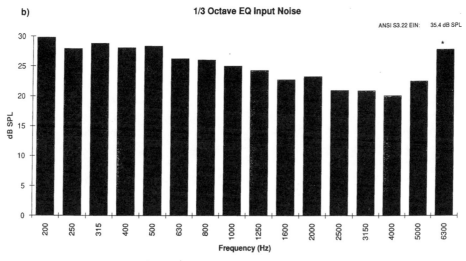

**Figure 1–30.** (a) Noise output with no input of same hearing aid used for Figure 1–29 with its gain adjusted to 9.8 dB HFA gain (taller bars) and system noise of Bruel & Kjaer 2032 spectrum analyzer with 1/2 inch microphone (shorter bars), both with 1/3 octave analysis. (b) Equivalent input noise in 1/3 octave bands for the hearing aid used for (a).

bands shown in Figure 1–30b is valid per Frye's proposal for all but the 6300 Hz 1/3 octave band. (Consequently, there is an asterisk above the equivalent input noise bar for this band). For this hearing aid, the equivalent input noise was 35.4 dB SPL per ANSI S3.22, essentially unchanged from that for the higher gain condition with this same hearing aid.

At the time of this writing, the S3-48 working group is recommending that the 1/3 octave analysis method for hearing aid circuit noise be included in the Appendix of the next revision of the S3.22 standard. To make the equivalent input noise measurement independent of ambient noise, the working group is also considering a recommendation that the 1/3 octave test chamber noise be subtracted from the 1/3 octave hearing aid output noise with no input. This subtraction can be done in real time with a two-channel hearing aid analyzer, and thereby account for variations in environmental noise outside the test chamber.

### Future Possibilities for More Realistic Hearing Aid Battery Simulators

Appendix B of ANSI S3.22-1987 contains a table with recommended battery simulator characteristics. The working group generally considers these values still appropriate for the steady-state values of open circuit battery voltage and series internal impedance if values for new batteries such as the 10A/230 and 5A are added. However, as shown by several members of the S3-48 working group members, beginning with Elmer Carlson, hearing aid batteries have loaded *steady-state voltages* and *voltage time constants* that are dependent, respectively, on the amount of steady-state current and pulsed current drawn (Carlson, 1992). Thus, the dynamic behavior as well as the steady-state behavior of batteries used in hearing aids needs to be considered, for example, as input levels and gain control settings change. In essence, because of its internal impedance, the loaded voltage of a hearing aid battery can change continuously and has attack and release times as a result of changes in input level and the resulting current drawn. For example, Figure 1–31a shows the effect on the loaded battery voltage of a 10 second, 0.8 mA current pulse drawn from a typical fresh #13 battery. Note the exponential "attack" and "release" times, respectively, in the voltage at the terminals of the loaded battery as the current pulse is applied at time 0 and removed at 10 seconds. Furthermore, the amount of steady-state voltage drop created by the combination of the steady-state current drawn from the battery and the internal impedance appears not to be a simple linear function. For example, Figure 1–31b shows that the best piece-wise linear fit for the mean steady-state voltage drop as a function of steady-state load current drawn from 15 fresh #13 batteries might consist of two straight lines intersecting at approximately 0.5 mA. Creating a battery simulator to simulate these effects is not a simple task because the behavior shown in Figures 1–31a and 1–31b varies for other battery types and for batteries that are partially discharged rather than fresh.

### Digital Cordless Telephone Interference

There has been considerable attention generated in Canada (Northern Telecom, 1993; Arndt, 1993), in Australia (Joyner et al., 1993), and in some member countries of the IEC (EHIMA, 1993) concerning electromagnetic interference (EMI) in hearing aids caused by the use of digital cordless telephones in those countries. Although inevitable, at the time of this writing, digital cordless telephones have not as yet been marketed in the United States. In Europe and Australia, the *CT2+* and *Personal Communication System (PCS)* both belong to the family of the *Digital Cordless Telephone (DCT)* system and are described as a *Global System for Mobile Communication (GSM)*. IEC working group 13 on hearing aid standards has an open work item at the request of the British delegate to investigate methods for measuring the amount of EMI generated in hearing aids by digital cordless tele-

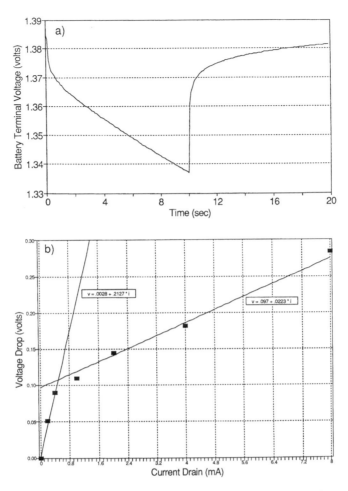

**Figure 1–31.** (a) "Attack" and "release" times of the voltage drop at the terminals of a fresh #13 battery resulting from a 10-second 0.8 milliampere current pulse being drawn from the battery from 0 to 10 seconds. (b) Best piecewise linear curve fit for the mean steady-state voltage drop at the terminals of 15 fresh #13 batteries as a function of steady-state current drain delivered by the battery.

phones (IEC, 1994). The ANSI S3-48 working group will monitor the progress of this IEC committee in this endeavor of characterizing of EMI in hearing aids to be prepared with a course of action when digital cordless telephones are marketed in the United States.

## Conclusions

The ANSI S3-48 working group has a strong tradition in developing hearing aid-related standards over the last 35 years. This is principally due to the leadership provided by Samuel Lybarger and the efforts of many highly competent working group members who have contributed much of their time and expertise. Some of these ANSI standards have preceded similar documents that have been formulated by IEC hearing aid standards working groups. These include ANSI S3.7-1960 and S3.22-1976 on electroacoustic hearing aid measurements, S3.35-1985 on measurements of hearing aids on a manikin, and S3.42-1992 on use of a broad-band noise input signal. Although effort has been made to harmonize ANSI and IEC hearing aid-related standards, often they are different and not technically compatible.

Near-term future developments of ANSI hearing aid-related standards will attempt to focus on how well hearing aids function in real-world listening situations, as well as on ensuring quality control. This will be done by attempting to relate measurements such as internal circuit noise and distortion produced by hearing aids to the wearer's performance, perception, and ratings of these devices.

### Acknowledgements

The author thanks Jay Jendersee, Brian Woodruff, and Dr. Todd Fortune at Argosy Electronics and members of the ANSI S3-48 working group for obtaining some of the data reported in this chapter. Sincere appreciation is also extended to Samuel Lybarger, Wayne Olsen, and Michael Valente for their valuable suggestions in reviewing an earlier version of this chapter.

### *References*

Acoustical Society of America. (1953). *American Standard Method for Measurement of Characteristics of Hearing Aids (ASA Z24.14-1953).* New York.
Acoustical Society of America. (1994). *Minutes of Accredited Standards Committee on Bioacoustics, S3.* Cambridge, MA.
ADA. (1991). Americans With Disabilities Act in brief, focus on employment, public accommodations, transportation, telecommunications. *Fed Reg* (Parts I, II, III, IV, and V). Friday, July 26, 1991.
American National Standards Institute. (1967). *Preferred Frequencies, Frequency Levels and Band Numbers for Acoustical Measurements (ANSI S1.6-1967, R1976).* New York: Acoustical Society of America.
American National Standards Institute. (1987). *Specification of Hearing Aid Characteristics (ANSI S3.22-1987).* New York: Acoustical Society of America.
American National Standards Institute. (1987). *Preferred Earhook Nozzle Thread for Postauricular Hearing Aids (ANSI S3.37-1987).* New York: Acoustical Society of America.
American National Standards Institute. (1992). *Testing Hearing Aids With a Broad-Band Noise Signal (ANSI S3-42-1992).* New York: Acoustical Society of America.
American National Standards Institute. (1979). *Occluded Ear Simulator (ANSI S3.25-1979, R1989).* New York: Acoustical Society of America.
American National Standards Institute. (1973). *Method for Coupler Calibration of Earphones (ANSI S3.7-1973, R1986).* New York: Acoustical Society of America.
American National Standards Institute. (1984). *Preferred Frequencies, Frequency Levels, and Band Numbers for Acoustical Measurements (ANSI S1.6-1984).* New York: Acoustical Society of America.
American National Standards Institute. (1985). *Methods of Measurement of Performance Characteristics of Hearing Aids Under Simulated In Situ Working Conditions (ANSI S3.35-1985).* New York: Acoustical Society of America.
American National Standards Institute. (1960). *Methods of Measurement of the Electroacoustical Characteristics of Hearing Aids (ANSI S3.3-1960, R1990).* New York: Acoustical Society of America.
American National Standards Institute. (1993). *Procedures for the Development and Coordination of American National Standards.* New York: Acoustical Society of America.
American Society for Testing and Materials. (1992). *Regulations Governing ASTM Technical Committees.* Philadelphia, PA.
Arndt H. (1992). IEC 118-7, 1983 Summary of Test Conditions & Limits ANSI S3.22-1987. Unitron Industries, Ltd., Kitchener, Ontario, Canada.
Arndt H. (1993). EMI Interaction Between the CT2 Digital Handset and Hearing Aids, February 16, 1993. Unitron Industries, Ltd., Kitchener, Ontario, Canada.

Bareham J. (1990a). Part 2: Hearing instrument measurements using dual channel signal analysis. *Hear Instrum* 41(1):32.

Bareham J. (1990b). Part 3: Hearing instrument measurements using dual channel signal analysis. *Hear Instrum* 41(3):34–35.

Bell Northern Research. (1991). Objective evaluation of non-linear distortion effects on voice transmission quality, Contribution to CCITT, COM XII-46-E.

Burkhard M. (1978). *Manikin Measurements.* Elk Grove Village, IL: Knowles Electronics.

Burkhard M, Sachs R. (1975). Anthropometric manikin for acoustic research. *J Acoust Soc Am* 58(1):214–222.

Burnett E. (1967). A new method for the measurement of non-linear distortion using a random noise test signal. *Bull Prosth Res.*

Burnett E. (1991). Complex signal testing of hearing aids limitations and improvements. In: Studebaker G, Bess F, Beck L, eds. *The Vanderbilt Hearing Aid Report II,* Chapt. 14. Parkton, MD: York Press, pp. 175–182.

Burnett E. (1992). Notes about MLS analysis, S3-48 working group minutes from Nashville meeting dated 4-8-92.

Burnett E, Beck L. (1987). A correction for converting 2 cm$^3$ coupler responses to insertion responses for custom in-the-ear nondirectional hearing aids. *Ear Hear Suppl* 8:89S–94S.

Burnett E, Corliss E, Nedzelnitsky V. (1982). Research problems in coupler and in situ measurements on hearing aids. In: Studebaker G, Bess F., eds. *The Vanderbilt Hearing Aid Report I.* Upper Darby, PA: Monographs in Contemporary Audiology, pp. 67–77.

Campbell R. (1991). Letter dated 7-12-91 about the MLSSA system accompanying "No" vote on S3.42 draft standard.

Carlson E. (1992). Some comments on the source impedance provided by batteries, Knowles Electronics memo dated 4-6-92, Itasca, IL.

Cole W. (1991). Memo entitled Battery Drain to ANSI S3-48 working group battery life subcommittee dated April 22, 1991.

Compton C. (1994). Providing effective telecoil performance with in-the-ear hearing instruments. *Hear J* 47(4):23–33.

Dyrlund O. (1989). Characterization of non-linear distortion in hearing aids using coherence analysis, a pilot study. *Scand Audiol* 18:143–148.

Dyrlund O. (1992). IEC, ANSI Co-operation IEC 118-7, ANSI S3.22 Comparison. ANSI S3-48 working group minutes for Nashville meeting.

Dyrlund O. (1993). Performance test of "Madsen 711 couplers," Technical-Audiological Laboratory Project report 3911-62, Odense, Denmark.

Dyrlund O, Ludvigsen C, Olofsson A, Poulsen T. (1994). Hearing aid measurements with speech and noise signals. *Scand Audiol* 23(3):153–157.

Electronic Industries Association. (1983). Magnetic field intensity criteria for telephone compatibility with hearing aids (EIA RS-504). Washington, DC.

European Hearing Instrument Manufacturers Assn. (1993). EHIMA GSM Project Development Phase, DELTA Acoustics & Vibration Technical-Audiological Laboratory—TAL Project Report (Rev. A), carried out for EHIMA, October, 1993, Wemmel, Belgium.

Federal Register (1977). Medical device amendments of 1976. Pub. L. 94-295, May 28, 1976.

Frye G. (1987). Crest factor and composite signals for hearing aid testing. *Hear J* 40(10):15–18.

Harris J, Haines H, Kelsey P, Clack T. (1961). The relation between speech intelligibility and the electroacoustic characteristics of low fidelity circuitry. *J Aud Res* 1:357–381.

Hawkins D, Naidoo S. (1993). Comparison of sound quality and clarity with asymmetrical peak clipping and output limiting compression. *J Am Acad Audiol* 4:221–228.

International Electrotechnical Commission. (1973). IEC reference coupler for the measurement of hearing aids using earphones coupled to the ear by means of ear inserts. *IEC Publication 126.* New York.

International Electrotechnical Commission. (1981). Occluded-ear simulator for the measurement of earphones coupled to the ear by ear inserts. *IEC Publication 711.* New York.

International Electrotechnical Commission. (1983). Measurement of electroacoustic characteristics. *Hearing Aids (IEC Publication 118-0).* New York.

International Electrotechnical Commission. (1983). Hearing aids with induction pick-up coil input. *Hearing Aids (IEC Publication 118-1).* New York.

International Electrotechnical Commission. (1983). Hearing aids with automatic gain control circuits. *Hearing Aids (IEC Publication 118-2).* New York.

International Electrotechnical Commission. (1983). Measurement of performance characteristics of hearing aids for quality inspection for delivery purposes. *Hearing Aids (IEC Publication 118-7).* New York.

International Electrotechnical Commission. (1983). Measurement of hearing aids under simulated in-situ working conditions. *Hearing Aids (IEC Publication 118-8).* New York.

International Electrotechnical Commission. (1994). Electromagnetic compatibility for hearing aids—Immunity to radio frequency fields. *29/77B(Secretariat)281/138 First IEC/CD 118.*

Jirsa R, Norris T. (1982). Effects of intermodulation distortion on speech intelligibility. *Ear Hear* 3(5):251–256.

Johnson W. (1992). Letter to George Frye and ANSI S3-48 working group dated October 23, 1992 regarding problems in measuring equivalent input noise.

Joyner K, Wood M, Burwood E, Allison D, Strange R. (1993). Interference to Hearing Aids by the new Digital Mobile Telephone System, Global System for Mobile (GSM) Communications Standard, National Acoustic Laboratories, March 30, 1993, Sydney, Australia.

Kasten R, Franks J. (1986). Electroacoustic characteristics of hearing aids. In: Hodgson W, ed. *Hearing Aid Assessment and Audiologic Habilitation.* Baltimore, MD: Williams & Wilkins, pp. 38–70.

Kates J. (1991). New developments in hearing aid measurements. In: Studebaker G, Bess F, Beck L, eds. *The Vanderbilt Hearing Aid Report II.* Parkton, MD: York Press, pp. 149–163.

Kates J, Kozma-Spytek L. (1994). Quality ratings for frequency-shaped peak-clipped speech. *J Acoust Soc Am* 95(6):3586–3594.

Killion M, Monser E. (1980). CORFIG: Coupler response for flat insertion gain. In: Studebaker G, Hochberg I, eds. *Acoustical Factors Affecting Hearing Aid Performance.* Baltimore, MD: University Park Press, pp. 147–168.

Killion M, Staab W, Preves D. (1990). Classifying automatic signal processors. *Hear Instrum* 41(8): 24.

Killion M, Revit L. (1993). CORFIG and GIFROC: Real ear to coupler and back. In: Studebaker G, Hochberg I, eds. *Acoustical Factors Affecting Hearing Aid Performance.* Boston, MA: Allyn and Bacon, pp. 65–85.

Kubichek R, Atkinson D, Webster A. (1991). *Advances in Objective Voice Quality Assessment.* Paper presented at IEEE Global Telecommunications Conference, IEEE Communications Society, New York.

Lybarger S. (1981). Should an ear simulator be used to directly replace a 2-cc coupler in hearing aid measurements? Memo dated 9-13-81.

Lybarger S. (1985). The physical and electroacoustic characteristics of hearing aids. In: Katz J, ed. *Handbook of Audiology.* Baltimore, MD: Williams & Wilkins, pp. 849–884.

Lybarger S, Teder H. (1986). 2-cc coupler curves to insertion gain curves: Calculated and experimental results. *Hear Instrum* 37(11):36–40.

Lybarger S. (1994). Hearing aid related standards published by American Standards Association, United States of America Standards Institute and American National Standards Institute. Personal communication.

Meskan M. (1994). Fitting completely-in-the-canal instruments. *Hear Res* 1(7):25–28.

National Institute of Standards & Technology. (1986). Standards Management Program, Office of Standards Services, Procedures for the Development of Voluntary Product Standards. *Fed Reg* 51(119):22497–22503.

Northern Telecom. (1993). Draft recommendations of Ad-Hoc Committee on DCT Hearing Aid Compatibility, February 16, 1993, Bell Northern Research, Ottawa, Ontario, Canada.

Preves D. (1988). Revised ANSI Std. S3.22 for hearing instrument performance measurement. *Hear Instrum* 39(3):26–34.

Preves D, Beck L, Burnett E, Teder H. (1989). Input stimuli for obtaining frequency responses of automatic gain control hearing aids. *J Speech Hear Res* 32:189–194.

Preves D, Newton J. (1989). The headroom problem and hearing aid performance. *Hear J* 42(10):21.

Preves D, Woodruff B. (1990). Some methods of improving and assessing hearing aid headroom. *Audecibel* 39(3):8–13.

Preves D. (1990). Expressing hearing aid noise and distortion with coherence measurements. *ASHA* 32:56–59.

Preves D. (1994). A look at the telecoil—Its development and potential. *Self Help for the Hard of Hearing People (SHHH)* 15(5):7–10.

Pryce D. (1989). Audio DACS push CD players to higher performance. *EDN* 34(25):116.

Reddy S, Kirlin R. (1979). Evaluation of hearing aid and auditory response using pseudorandom noise. In: Larson V, Egolf D, Kirlin R, Stiles T, eds. *Auditory and Hearing Prosthetics Research.* Proceedings of Conference of Auditory and Hearing Prosthetics Research. New York: Grune and Straton, pp. 377–409.

Schneider T, Jamieson D. (1993a). A dual-channel MLS-based test system for hearing-aid characterization. *J Audio Eng Soc* 41(7/8):583–593.

Schneider T, Jamieson D. (1993b). Signal-biased MLS-based hearing-aid frequency response measurement. *J Audio Eng Soc* 41(12):987–997.

Schweitzer H, Causey D, Tolton M. (1977). Nonlinear distortion in hearing aids: The need for reevaluation of measurement philosophy and technique. *J Am Audiol Soc* 2(4):132.

Schweitzer H, Grim M, Preves D, Kubichek R, Woodruff B. (1991). *Qualitative Assessment of Hearing*

*Aid Performance by an Expert Pattern Recognition System.* Poster presentation at American Academy of Audiology Convention, Denver, CO.

Skafte M. (1994). A "Living Legend": Samuel F. Lybarger. *Hear Res* 1(7):6–9.

Staab W. (1978). *Hearing Aid Handbook.* Blue Ridge Summit, PA: Tab Books, pp. 107–157.

Stelmachowicz P, Lewis D, Seewald R, Hawkins D. (1990). Complex and pure-tone signals in the evaluation of hearing aid characteristics. *J Speech Hear Res* 33:380–385.

Stone M, Moore B. (1992). Syllabic compression: Effective compression ratios for signals modulated at different rates. *Br J Audiol* 26:351–361.

Studebaker G. (1979). Utilization of real-time spectral analyzers for the electroacoustic evaluation of hearing aids. In: Larson V, Egolf D, Kirlin R, Stile S, eds. *Auditory and Hearing Prosthetics Research.* New York: Grune and Stratton, pp. 347–376.

Teder H. (1984). Repeatability of KEMAR insertion gain measurements. *Hear Instrum* 35(10):16–22.

United States of America Standards Institute. (1967). USASI S3.8-1967. Method of expressing hearing aid performance.

US Department of Veterans Affairs. (1991). *Handbook of Hearing Aid Measurement.* Veterans Health Services and Research Administration, Washington, DC.

US Department of Veterans Affairs. (1994). *Solicitation RFP 791-01-94, Contract for Custom In-The-Ear Hearing Aids.* Denver, CO: VA Denver Distribution Center.

Walker G, Dillon H. (1982). *Compression in Hearing Aids: An Analysis, a Review and Some Recommendations.* NAL Report No. 90. Canberra: Australian Government Publishing Service, 13.

# 2

## Real-Ear Measures: Individual Variation and Measurement Error

### ROBERT DE JONGE

### Introduction

The performance of a hearing aid depends to a great extent upon what is engineered into the device. Characteristics of the microphone, amplification circuitry, and the receiver can be thought of as intrinsic factors. Extrinsic factors can also have a pronounced effect upon the frequency response and saturation level of the aid. For convenience, these extrinsic factors can be divided into two categories, based upon whether the input to the hearing aid is being affected or the output from the aid is being affected. The first, baffle effects occur as a consequence of how the physical presence of the individual disturbs the sound field. Scattering of the sound wave by the head, pinna, and torso influence the sound pressure level (SPL) developed at the microphone of the hearing aid and, therefore, can change the hearing aid output. The physical size and unique pinna contours of individuals vary and is, therefore, likely to have a unique effect upon the diffraction of sound in the field. The second category of extrinsic factor relates to what load the hearing aid is coupled. Characteristics of the ear canal and middle ear determine the load impedance and also vary from individual to individual. The SPL developed at the output of the hearing aid, often referenced to the eardrum, depends upon the load impedance that is being driven by the receiver.

The purpose of this chapter is to investigate the sources of objective, physical variation from person to person. The magnitude of the expected differences from normal will be estimated, and the variables that are likely to produce the greatest effect will be identified. The issue of measurement error will be explored more fully so that the interpretation of individual differences can be made more appropriately. Although this is not a chapter about probe microphone measurements per se, information will be presented that will facilitate the interpretation of these measures. It is assumed that the reader is familiar with the basic methods, procedures, and terminology associated with real-ear probe microphone measurements.

## Baffle Effects

Regarding baffle effects, when a sound wave encounters an obstacle, certain phenomena may occur: the energy in the sound wave can be transmitted to the object, the object may absorb and dissipate some of the sound energy, the wave may reflect off the object, or the wave may bend around the object. In the case of a low-frequency tone, the wavelength of the sound may be large when compared to the physical dimensions of the object (i.e., a person's head, pinna, neck, or torso). The tendency is for the wave to bend around the object, and there is minimal disturbance of the sound field. If the reverse is true, and the frequency is high (short wavelength) and the size of the object is comparatively large, then the wave will reflect off the object. When the object substantially disturbs the sound field, there is a buildup of pressure in the vicinity of the obstacle (Olson, 1957). Because behind-the-ear (BTE) and in-the-ear (ITE) hearing aids are worn on the head, the SPL entering the microphone is affected by the baffle produced by the head and pinna and, to a smaller extent, the neck and torso. Also, because the position occupied by the microphone is different for a BTE as compared to an ITE, the SPL developed at the microphone will be different. There will also be differences for progressively deeper in-the-canal (ITC) and completely-in-the-canal (CIC) microphone locations. Here, the resonant effects of the concha bowl and ear canal become more important. Generally, most of these effects will be restricted to the higher frequencies (above 1000 Hz) where the wavelength becomes small compared to the size of the baffle.

For linear hearing aids, it would be expected that increases (or decreases) in SPL at the hearing aid microphone produced by baffling effects would appear as direct changes in output levels, at least up to the point where the hearing aid would begin to saturate. For nonlinear aids, where gain varies as a function of input level, the situation is more complex. Because compression instruments generally reduce output levels as input levels increase, baffling effects become progressively less important as the input levels to the hearing aid increase.

## Load Impedance Effects and Computer Simulations

Normally, the hearing aid is coupled to an individual's ear, and the output of the instrument is dependent upon the load impedance of that ear. Important considerations involve both the geometry of the ear canal and the impedance of the middle ear. Together, the ear canal and middle ear combine to form a unit with an impedance that varies with frequency. Although it has been demonstrated that there are limitations to considering the output of the hearing aid as a constant-current source, usually the impedance of the ear canal and middle ear are low when compared to the receiver (Egolf et al., 1986). Under these conditions, the SPL developed varies directly with the load impedance. The general principle is that for instruments, especially ITE aids, increases in the impedance of the ear canal/middle system cause increases in the SPL developed within the ear canal (Larson et al., 1991). The distribution of SPL varies in the ear canal. Measurements are greatest when made in close proximity to the eardrum, especially for higher frequencies. For lower frequencies (below approximately 3000 to 4000 Hz) the occluded ear canal SPL does not change much as the distance from the eardrum increases. For frequencies above 8000 Hz, the greatest SPL is only measured for distances close to the eardrum (Dirks and Kincaid, 1987).

It is usually assumed that extrinsic factors do not affect, or only minimally affect, the intrinsic properties of the hearing aid. However, under certain circumstances, changing the load impedance of the individual ear can change the current flowing into the receiver of the hearing aid. This, in turn, can alter the energy flow through both the hearing aid amplifier and even the microphone, causing additional changes in the frequency response of the hearing aid.

The interaction between the hearing aid circuitry and the ear canal/middle ear system has been extensively studied through computer modeling techniques, and excellent summaries are available on the topic (Egolf, 1980; White et al., 1980; Larson et al., 1991). Modeling techniques are attractive alternatives to the expensive and time-consuming process of carefully obtaining experimental data on human subjects. Models may suffer from errors in prediction, but a model that has been experimentally verified and proven valid has two important qualities. First, the predictions of the model are not influenced by measurement error, and secondly, individual elements of the model can be changed while all other features are held constant. For example, it would be possible to study the effect of varying ear canal diameter while holding canal length and middle ear impedance constant. This would be very difficult to do with a conventional experiment using human subjects.

Gardner and Hawley (1972) mathematically modeled the ear canal as an electrical analog transmission line. The model was terminated with an electrical network mimicking the impedance offered by the middle ear. The resistance and reactance of the middle ear simulation accurately predicted experimentally measured values, and the transfer characteristic of the model agreed very well with the ear canal to middle ear transform given by Wiener and Ross (1946). Studebaker and Cox (1977) used electrical analogs to predict the behavior of different types of vents. Egolf (1977), in a more "black box" approach, used a four-pole electrical analog for mathematically modeling the small-diameter capillary tube used in a probe microphone. Experimental verification showed very little error, less than 2 dB, in the prediction over a range of 10 to 10,000 Hz. This is an important finding, because much of the coupling from a hearing aid receiver to the eardrum are right circular cylinders. Egolf has since extended this work and has used the same techniques to show that accurate models can be constructed to investigate many effects. Simulated hearing aid output on real ears was compared to 2-cc couplers. Also investigated were: the effects of changing receiver type, earmold tubing length and diameter, ear canal length and diameter, and the effects of changing vent length and diameter (Egolf, 1980). Model predictions agreed well with experimental results. Gilman, Dirks, and Stern (1981) reported that changing ear coupler impedance to represent the range of normal middle ear impedances had an effect upon the low frequency (less than 2000 Hz) response of a hearing aid. A computer model gave the same predictions.

A mathematical simulation of an electrical analog model of the receiver, earhook, earmold tubing, venting, ear canal, and middle ear was created by de Jonge (1982, 1983). He investigated effects of varying ear canal length and diameter and middle ear impedance on the SPL developed at the eardrum by a hearing aid. The predictions of this model were virtually identical to those obtained by Egolf (1980) and, later, in a model by Kates (1988a, 1988b). The difference between the SPL developed in a normal ear versus that found in a 2-cc coupler (the real-ear coupler difference, RECD) was also accurately predicted. These findings were confirmed by Egolf, Feth, Cooper, and Franks (1985), who suggested that normal variation in eardrum impedance is likely to be a prime source of variation in hearing aid output. They also used modeling techniques to show that the RECD does not seem to be sensitive to differences between high impedance hearing aid receivers (Knowles BI versus a Danavox DA51). Previously, it had been demonstrated that a lower impedance button style receiver (Danavox SM-H) could interact with ear simulators to affect hearing aid frequency response (Gilman et al., 1981). Egolf's modeling efforts have been extended to include the hearing aid microphone (Egolf et al., 1988a) and amplifier (Egolf et al., 1988b) for the purpose of investigating feedback within hearing aids (Egolf et al., 1989).

In general, the results of these and other efforts (Bade et al., 1984) have demonstrated that computer simulation is an accurate and powerful technique for investigating hearing aid performance. In this chapter, an expanded model based on that reported by de Jonge (1983) has been developed for illustrating effects of individual variability in load impedance. This model was used to simulate the effects upon a hearing aid frequency response of changing ear canal dimensions and middle ear impedance. Features of the model are illustrated in Figure 2–1. By varying the parameters of the simple electrical analog of a hearing aid receiver, resonant peak frequency and amplitude can be adjusted to generically match the frequency response and impedance characteristics of a typical receiver (Egolf et al., 1986). The first 3 elements (resistor, inductor, capacitor) represent a series resonant circuit corresponding to the frictional losses (*Rreceiver*), mass (*Lreceiver*), and compliance (*Creceiver*) of the diaphragm of the miniature loudspeaker. This is followed by a parallel capacitor (*Cvolume*) representing the size of the chamber into which the sound is radiated. *Rnozzle* and *Lnozzle* represent the resistance and inertance of the cylindrical receiver port. The receiver may be included or excluded from the model, and the input to the model may be adjusted to include or exclude external ear effects (spherical head diffraction, pinna flange, and concha effects are discussed later) or an amplifier with a variable amount of gain. The output from the receiver feeds into a system of tubes, each modeled as a right circular cylinder using Gardner and Hawley's (1972) techniques, modified by adding a resistance to simulate frictional losses in the tube (Olson, 1957). Using two sections per cm of tubing extends the accuracy of the simulation well beyond the highest frequency calculated (6100 Hz). The length and diameter of each tube can be specified, and most tubes can be terminated with an optional damper. The receiver tube, earhook, and parallel vent are each modeled as a single tube. The earmold tubing can have as many as four separate segments, the ear canal can have three. The model can be terminated in either a simulated real ear, a 2-cc coupler, or a simple resistance. The coupler is a 0.7 cm long, 1.9 cm diameter cylinder, with a hard termination (10,000 ohms).

Because each element of the model can be included or excluded, a variety of simulations can be created. For example, the ear canal-to-eardrum transform can be simulated by excluding the receiver from the model, using a constant voltage

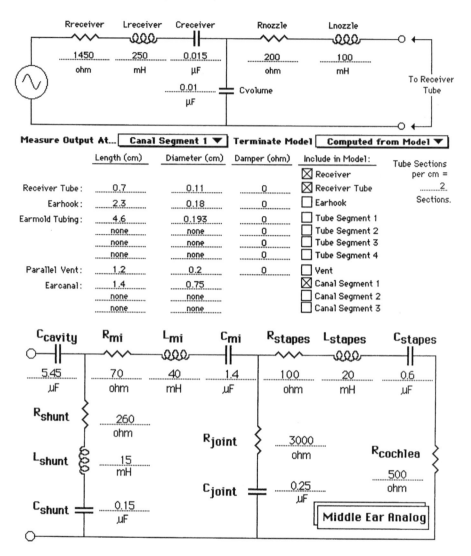

**Figure 2–1.** The electrical analog model of the hearing aid receiver, coupling tubing, vent, and ear canal is given in the top of the figure. The canal was terminated with a slightly modified version of Zwislocki's normal middle ear (Zwislocki, 1962) as shown in the bottom of the figure.

input, and terminating the model with a normal ear. Including the receiver, receiver tube with a parallel vent, and adding a canal segment emulates an ITE aid. Adding an earhook and tubing segment simulates a BTE aid. The output can be measured at the eardrum, or at a variety of other locations to simulate the effects of changing the location of a probe microphone.

The model also contains a slightly modified version of Zwislocki's (1962) electrical analog of the middle ear. The circuits representing the middle ear cavities and portions of the eardrum have been simplified. A similar model is discussed by Zwislocki (1976) briefly, but *Rcochlea* is the resistance of the cochlea. *Rstapes*, *Lstapes*, and *Cstapes* represent the equivalent resistance, inductance, and compliance associated with the structure of the stapes and annular ligament. *Rjoint* and *Cjoint* is a parallel branch representing the coupling of the incudostapedial joint. *Rmi*, *Lmi*, and *Cmi* indicate frictional, mass, and compliance effects associated with the malleoincudal complex and that portion of the eardrum tightly coupled to the malleus. *Rshunt*, *Lshunt*, and *Cshunt* represents shunting effects of those portions of the eardrum whose movements are not effective in driving the malleus. And, finally, *Ccavity* is a capacitor representing the combined volume of the tympanum, epitympanum, and mastoid antrum. Together, these structures combine to give a total resistance (R) and reactance (X) of a typical normal ear (Møller, 1974; Shaw, 1974b), as illustrated in Figure 2–2. The model's results (shown as the thick curves) compare well to the median values for a majority of studies (thin curves in shaded areas) of normal middle ear resistance and reactance as summarized by Shaw (1974b).

Figure 2–3 illustrates how a tube can be modeled as an electrical transmission line. The canal, as other tubes in the model, is treated as an electrical analog transmission line after Gardner and Hawley (1972). In the top panel, a 0.5-cm section of tube is shown with the formulas for acoustic resistance (Ra), inductance (La), and capacitance (Ca). Also shown is the coefficient of viscosity μ = 0.000186 g/(cm sec), density ρ = 0.00121 g/cm³, and the speed of sound c = 34400 cm/sec. The length of the canal is 2.57 cm, diameter 0.75 cm. Curve A (thin line) shows results for the canal terminated with a 300 ohm resistance, curve B (thick line) is

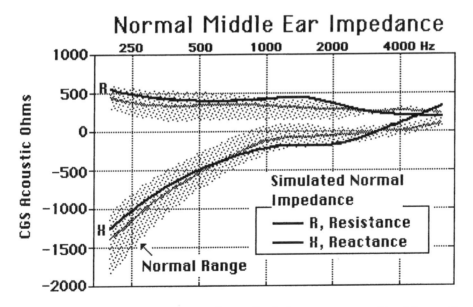

**Figure 2–2.** Normal middle ear impedance. Shaded area covers results of the median values for a majority of studies of normal middle ear resistance (R) and reactance (X) according to Shaw (1974b). The solid lines give computed R and X values according to the electrical analog model of the middle ear.

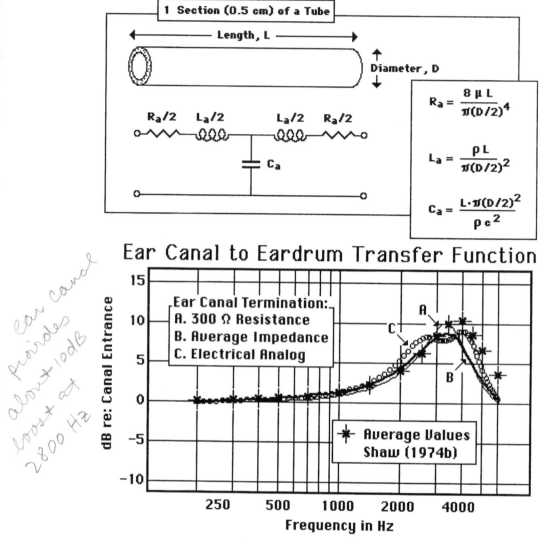

*ear canal provides about +10dB boost at 2800 Hz*

**Figure 2–3.** Modeling tubes as electrical analog transmission lines and the simulated ear canal-to-eardrum transfer function.

for the canal terminated with average impedance values for the middle ear (see Figure 2–2), and curve C (circles) is for terminating impedance values calculated from the electrical analog in Figure 2–1. Data points (crosses) are taken from average values for subjects given in Figure 13 by Shaw (1974b). There is good agreement between the model's predictions and average ear canal entrance-to-eardrum transfer functions obtained from subjects of several studies (Shaw, 1974b). Individual subject variation is usually at least as large as the difference between the model's predictions and average values. By manipulating or fine tuning parameters of the model it is possible to improve or reduce agreement.

## Measuring Hearing Aid Performance in a Coupler

Traditionally, the frequency response and saturation sound pressure level (SSPL) of a hearing aid are described in terms specified by the current ANSI standard (ANSI S3.22-1987, 1987). The ANSI standard calls for measurements to be performed under conditions that are quite different from those in which the hearing aid will actually be worn. The hearing aid is placed in a test box that simulates a free field condition that is devoid of the diffraction effects that are normally present when the hearing aid is worn on the head. The output of the hearing aid is measured on either an HA-1 or HA-2 version of the 2-cc coupler. For a BTE aid using the HA-2 configuration, the earhook of the instrument is coupled to 25 mm of #13 tubing (1.93 mm internal diameter, ID). The tubing ends in a simulation of an earmold with a bore 18 mm long with an ID of 3 mm. The earmold is not vented. The output of the earmold simulator ends in a cylindrical cavity approximately 19 mm in diameter by 7 mm long. The HA-1 coupler, used for ITE aids, is similar to the HA-2 coupler but lacks the earmold simulator.

The actual earmold, or ITE shell, worn may be quite different from the 2-cc coupler. In the case of BTE instruments, it is more common to run the #13 tubing to the tip of the mold, thus eliminating the 3-mm horn effect of the earmold. Venting effects on the actual mold, either intentional or the inevitable slit leaks, will change load impedance and, therefore, the output SPL in the coupler will not be the same as that developed in the real ear. Differences in load impedance between the ear canal/middle ear system of the individual will be different from that of the 2-cc cavity. For this reason, too, the coupler output will differ from that in a real ear. Consequently, it may be expected that the coupler specifications supplied by the manufacturer may have little to do with the real ear performance of the hearing aid. Figure 2–4 shows the difference between the simulated response of a hearing aid in an average real ear and in an HA-1, 2-cc coupler. The length from the shell tip to the eardrum was 1.4 cm, the canal diameter was 0.75 cm. The real-ear coupler difference (real ear minus coupler SPL) is also illustrated. Positive values indicate a greater SPL in the real ear than in the coupler. The model's predictions are similar to the data on real ears reported by Sachs and Burkhard (1972), but are somewhat different from those reported by Hawkins, Cooper, and Thompson (1990). Possible causes for these differences will be discussed later.

## KEMAR, the "Average Person"

The Knowles Electronics Manikin for Acoustic Research (KEMAR) effectively deals with differences between 2-cc coupler and real-ear measures for a typical, median individual. Dirks and Gilman (1979) demonstrated that KEMAR shows head shadow and diffraction effects that are in good agreement with Shaw's (1974a) data representing average human subjects, especially if a pink noise is used to smooth sharp antiresonances, which occur in the higher frequencies. KEMAR has the average dimensions of an adult human, based upon a survey of over 4000 male flying personnel, and 852 WAF trainees. The height and breadth of KEMAR's head, neck diameter, shoulder breadth, and chest width are all within 4% of normal. The size and shape of the pinna is both acoustically and

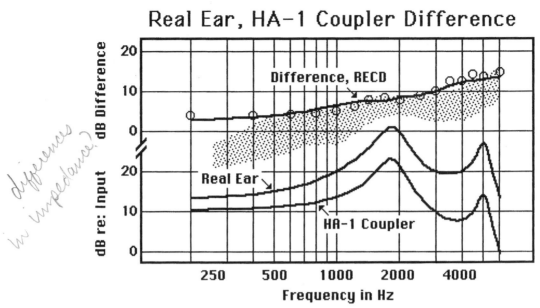

**Figure 2–4.** Simulated difference between the real ear and 2-cc coupler (HA-1), the real-ear coupler difference (RECD). Circles are data points for 11 ears from Sachs and Burkhard (1972). The shaded area represents ±1 standard deviation from the mean RECD (Hawkins et al., 1990).

dimensionally average. The concha connects to a 7.5 mm diameter canal with a length that gives an ear canal resonance that matches the average ear. A Zwislocki ear simulator terminates the canal. The Zwislocki coupler offers an acoustic impedance typical of the average ear. The KEMAR manikin looks human, can wear hearing aids, clothing, wigs, and does a remarkable job of simulating the acoustic behavior of a median individual (Burkhard and Sachs, 1975).

KEMAR greatly simplifies the process of determining how a hearing aid will perform on a typical individual. Rather than undergoing the tedious, time consuming process of averaging measures made upon a number of individuals, the output of the hearing aid can be measured directly upon a KEMAR. It is possible to determine a correction curve that will translate the 2-cc coupler response to a median real-ear response, at least for a closed earmold condition (Burnett and Beck, 1987; Bentler and Pavlovic, 1989, 1992). Although this correction curve will vary with the type of hearing aid (i.e., BTE versus ITE), it should be possible to apply the same curve to all BTE aids and all ITE aids, providing the physical construction of the aids are similar. The microphones should be in comparable positions; the residual volume of the canal from earmold (or shell) tip to eardrum should be similar. To determine how a particular hearing aid will perform on a median adult, it is, therefore, not necessary to actually measure the aid on a KEMAR. The real-ear response can be calculated from the 2-cc coupler response. This greatly facilitates the process of estimating the real-ear performance of a hearing aid from a manufacturer's 2-cc coupler data.

The inference that emerges from much of the previous discussion is that the same hearing aid, if placed on a different individual, will perform differently.

The frequency response of the hearing aid (and saturation level) is inextricably tied to the ear to which it is coupled. Each person will differ by some degree from normal (i.e., KEMAR). The size and shape of the head, torso, pinna, as well as clothing effects could produce differences. Differences from the normal length and diameter of the ear canal and middle ear impedance could create additional variation from normal. Although KEMAR data do predict the median response, they do not adequately address the issue of normal variability. KEMAR data may not be used to confidently predict how a hearing aid would respond upon children whose physical dimensions are much different from adults or to ears that have been surgically altered. Ears that exhibit pathology are likely to demonstrate load impedance differences even greater than would be expected to occur from normal variability. This produces a dilemma for the audiologist dispensing a hearing aid according to a prescription. Unless it is possible to accurately measure diffraction and load impedance effects prior to fitting the instrument, it is not possible to know beforehand how a hearing aid will perform on the one individual who will be wearing that hearing aid.

### Real-Ear Probe Microphone Measures

Real-ear measures using a calibrated sound source, reference microphone, and probe tube microphone are a potential solution to the problem of measuring how the individual differs from the group. Commercially available systems can rapidly and efficiently measure the SPL present at a reference microphone location on the head (usually over the ear, or under the cheek), and compare this SPL to that developed in the ear canal, close to the eardrum. Depending upon the test protocol utilized, it is possible to measure the combined effects of virtually any variable unique to the individual being tested: head, neck, torso, pinna, concha, ear canal, or middle ear impedance. Whether or not the desired prescription is being met can be verified, and if not, steps can be taken to adjust the hearing aid until it is.

Whenever a probe microphone system is used, the measurement obtained is, in part, due to the unique individual characteristics of the person being tested. In part, the measure is going to be contaminated by error, as any measurement will be. There are many possible sources of error (Tecca, 1991). The examiner may be less than meticulous and fail to control important test variables such as keeping placement depth of the probe tube constant or location of the reference microphone. The subject may move during the test, changing either the elevation or the azimuth of the sound source so that one measure (i.e., the real-ear unaided response, REUR) is not comparable to another (the real-ear aided response, REAR) giving an erroneous derived REIR (real-ear insertion response). Placing the loudspeaker too far from the subject can create measurements that are contaminated by reverberation. In some instances, fairly large frequency specific differences in probe tube output can occur between a test booth environment and a reverberant room (Hawkins and Mueller, 1986). The probe microphone measures can be susceptible to errors from subject vocalizations, or measures can be contaminated from ambient noise. Amplified sound radiated from the ear canal of an open mold fitting can be sensed by the reference microphone and alter gain measures. For example, Moskal and Goldstein (1992) obtained REAR and REIR curves for 12 adult ears using a substitution, modified comparison, and ipsilateral comparison method. Each subject was seated 1.25 m from a loudspeaker located at 0° azimuth in a sound-treated room. A linear BTE aid was used in both a closed- and open-mold condition. The REAR differed for each of the three methods, regardless of whether the mold was open or closed. This would be expected, because the modified comparison method excludes the head baffle, and the ipsilateral comparison method excludes the REUR. The REIR was not significantly different across the three methods for the closed-mold condition, but the modified comparison method showed less REIR for the open-mold condition. The authors indicated that sound radiating from the open mold could have increased the input SPL at the reference microphone, causing the loudspeaker output to drop, reducing the REIR.

Inherent system noise, calibration error, or equipment tolerances can limit the ultimate accuracy of the measurements. Hawkins and Mueller (1986) demonstrated that the one-probe microphone system was able to give fairly accurate measurements when compared to the Zwislocki coupler output as measured in a KEMAR. However, the probe system levels were consistently about 2 to 6 dB higher than the coupler levels. In a similar study, probe microphone levels were virtually identical to the SPLs developed in KEMAR's Zwislocki coupler (Dirks and Kinkaid, 1987). Several studies (see Tecca, 1991) have shown that the standard deviations (SD) for test-retest reliability are approximately 2 to 3 dB. Variability is usually less for the lower frequencies, greater for the higher frequencies, and likely to be greater if the test is repeated on a different day. This provides a 95% confidence interval of roughly 4 to 6 dB. Whenever a probe microphone measurement is obtained, it may be viewed as merely one instance of a population of possible responses. This makes the interpretation of individual differences problematic for the audiologist. When differences between the individual measurement and the expected KEMAR response are obtained, are those differences real or merely measurement error? If the difference between target and actual gain were the manifestation of a real individual difference, then it would seem logical to correct the hearing aid's response. If the difference were only measurement error, then the adjustment would probably be detrimental.

It has been suggested that a more accurate, individualized fit could be obtained if certain sources of individual variability could be controlled, such as the REUR, RECD, and load impedance (Mueller, 1989; Larson et al., 1991; Fikret-Pasa and Revit, 1992). This represents a more proactive approach to dealing with individual differences. Instead of ordering a hearing aid, then finding an inappropriate fit, and making changes after the fact (or returning the aid), a hearing aid with a more appropriate response could be ordered initially. A system that could measure the load impedance of the ear canal/middle ear system for the individual could accurately predict the SPL developed at the eardrum. Both the REUR and the real-ear coupler difference show variation between individuals, and methods have been proposed to measure and compensate for these differences when ordering a hearing aid from 2-cc coupler specifications (Byrne and Upfold, 1991). Moodie, Seewald, and Sinclair (1994) successfully used a measure of RECD, head diffraction, and microphone location to correct the 2-cc coupler response to predict the REAR and the real-ear saturation response (RESR). For one individual, the mean prediction error was 0.95 dB, and the largest error was 3.2 dB for REAR. For RESR the mean prediction error was 0.51 dB, and the largest error was 2.8 dB. Seewald, Sinclair, and Moodie (1994) found correlation coefficients between measured and predicted REARs typically exceeded 0.95 for 15 subjects ranging in age from 5 to 39 years. Good test-retest reliability for RECDs has been reported for both very young children (e.g., 0 to 10 months) and adults; however, these results indicated lower correlation coefficients for children who were more difficult to test, those with a high degree of activity (Sinclair et al., 1994). Ideally, measurement error should be very low in these circumstances. Otherwise, the hearing aid would be ordered with potentially unusual characteristics that are based on assumptions that are neither valid, reliable, nor reproducible.

As Killion and Revit (1987) pointed out, ". . . Modifying the response of the hearing aid based on a particular insertion gain measurement is risky business, however, if the measurement itself may be at fault rather than the hearing aid." Sources of individual differences, problems with measurement error, and modification of the target 2-cc coupler response were further discussed by Killion and Revit (1993), and a 1/2-correction suggestion was made. Instead of correcting the average CORFIG (coupler response for flat insertion gain) by the full amount of individual difference, a 1/2-correction compromise would help to adjust for measurement error. When repeated measurements are made, an individual result that is initially quite different from the mean, on subsequent measurements tends to regress toward the mean.

## Probe Microphone Measurement Error

The standard deviation of the absolute differences in SPLs obtained during repeated measurement of the same experimental condition is a commonly used index of measurement variability. The standard deviation is often multiplied by 1.96 to give the 95% confidence interval, the range over which 95% of the differences in repeated measurements would expect to fall. When the measurement is repeated for the same subject, it is presumed that all significant variables unique to that subject (i.e., baffle effects, ear canal dimensions, middle ear impedance) are held constant. This intrasubject (or within subject) standard deviation is a direct measure of the error inherent in the measurement procedure and its reliability. Presumably, only when an actual measurement falls outside the 95% confidence interval can one be fairly certain that a true individual difference exists. When measures are repeated for different subjects (intersubject, between subject) the variability measure includes both subject differences and measurement error.

### Test-Retest Reliability

Using laboratory equipment, rather than a commercially available system, Ringdahl and Leijon (1984) indicated a 95% interval for intrasubject variability to range from ±2 dB to ±8 dB in the frequency range from 250 to 4000 Hz. The greater variability was typically associated with the higher frequencies. Dillon and Murray (1987) compared the accuracy of a variety of methods for estimating the real-ear gain of hearing aids. It was measured subjectively using functional gain measures, objectively using one of four commercially available probe microphone systems, or using coupler-based measures. Eight subjects were tested repeatedly on five separate occasions over a two-month period. Results indicated that each technique gave somewhat different estimates of real-ear gain. Consequently, deciding what is the "true" gain becomes somewhat difficult. However, five of the methods (two functional gain, three probe microphone systems) gave consistent results, and the average gain of these five methods was used to estimate true gain. Standard error of estimates (the standard deviation of the differences between measured and true gain) were between 1 and 2 dB; higher values were associated with higher frequencies. This suggests that there is an ultimate limit to the accuracy of insertion gain measures. Concerning within subject test-retest reliability of the measures, the probe tube systems gave standard deviations averaging about 2.5 to 3.4 dB across frequency. Typically, variability was lowest for the lower frequencies; standard deviations were about 2 dB, increasing to 4 to 7 dB at 5000 and 6000 Hz. These data indicate that 95% confidence intervals of roughly 4 to 10 dB are not unusual. These conclusions are comparable to subsequent findings obtained by Humes, Hipskind, and Block (1988). Insertion gain was obtained for three probe tube systems for 12 female subjects, each of whom was tested twice. Differences between systems were not statistically significant. The intrasubject 95% confidence intervals ranged from 2.8 to 8 dB, depending upon the system used.

Nelson Barlow, Auslander, Rines, and Stelmachowicz (1988) examined 15 hearing-impaired children (ages 3 to 15 years) and 15 hearing-impaired adults using probe tube microphone measures. The same examiner repeated the measures three times within the same session. Mean intrasubject standard deviations were roughly 1 dB at the lower frequencies, increasing to no more than 2.5 dB at the higher frequencies. The authors stated that mean standard deviations across frequency never exceed 2.8 dB for the children and 2.2 dB for the adults, at least up to 4000 Hz. This suggests 95% confidence intervals no more than about 4.5 to 5.5 dB and indicate that the reliability of these procedures is similar for both children and adults. Feigin, Kopun, Stelmachowicz, and Gorga (1989) examined test-retest reliability in 22 children and 21 adults. Mean standard deviations ranged from a low of about 0.5 dB to a high of 2 dB. Variability was greater for the higher frequencies. Interestingly, and in contrast to the other studies, the lowest frequencies showed almost the same amount of variability as the high frequencies. Because custom earmolds were not used, the authors felt that differences in the acoustic seal on repeated measures could account for the variability.

Valente, Meister, Smith, and Goebel (1990) compared insertion gain measures for two examiners in a study using 28 subjects. This study gave similar, although slightly lower intrasubject 95% confidence intervals, averaging 3.3 dB across frequency. The largest interval was 4.1 dB at 3000 Hz. Average differences in gain were not statistically significant for the two people performing the measurements. These findings are in contrast to those of Hawkins (1987) who compared the reliability of six audiologists who were routinely making probe tube measurements for at least six months prior to the study. The investigator obtained repeated measures on KEMAR and found mean intertrial differences of 0 dB at 500 Hz, 1 to 2 dB at 1000 to 4000 Hz, and 2.4 dB at 6000 Hz. Each of the 6 audiologists tested the same subject (Hawkins) on 5 separate occasions using the same hearing aid with the volume control taped to a fixed position. The audiologists gave mean intertrial differences ranging from 2.2 dB at 1000 Hz to 4.7 dB at 4000 Hz. At 6000 Hz the difference was 7 dB. At 1000 Hz 80% of the measures were within ±3 dB. At 6000 Hz 25% of the measures differed by more than 10 dB. Hawkins concluded that some of the audiologists were more careful than others. Probe insertion depth varied widely. Some audiologists were careful to maintain the probe in the same location for the aided and unaided measurements, while others were not. For the probe microphone measurement to be within 6 dB of the SPL at the eardrum (for frequencies up to 6000 Hz), Chan and Geisler (1990) found that the probe must be no further than 6 mm from the top of the eardrum. Previously, it had been demonstrated that error in the insertion response could be as great as ±8 dB at 5000 Hz if the probe location changed between the aided and unaided conditions (Hawkins and Mueller, 1986). Some of the audiologists failed to properly seat the tight fitting mold, creating unintentional vent effects, contributing to low-frequency variability. Hawkins indicated that probe tube microphone measures should not be viewed as invariant measures simply because the behavioral response of the listener has been removed. Care should be taken to minimize sources of variability to enhance the value of these measures.

## Probe Microphone Placement

Proper placement of the probe tube in the ear canal is an important consideration for probe microphone measurements. At the tip of the earmold, or ITE shell, there is a circular opening. For the ITE, this opening is the end of the receiver tube. Sound emerging from this tube, into the ear canal, encounters a transition zone. The sound wave changes from a spherical wave to a planar wave. Within this zone, the SPL varies with radial distance from the center of the opening to the canal wall. The examiner should avoid placing the probe tip within this zone to avoid erroneous measurements. The transition zone varies with frequency and size of the opening, but at 10,000 Hz it is essentially complete at a distance of about 4 mm from the earmold tip (Burkhard and Sachs, 1977). To avoid measurement error, extending the tip of the probe tube a distance of 5 mm, or more, beyond the most medial point of the shell should be adequate.

Whether the ear canal is open or closed by an earmold, the SPL measured in the canal changes with distance from the eardrum (Gilman and Dirks, 1986; Dirks and Kincaid, 1987). The ear canal can be viewed as a tube closed at the medial end by the tympanic membrane. The acoustic impedance of the canal is relatively small (92 cgs, centimeter-gram-sec, ohms), compared to the impedance of the middle ear system; therefore, the system will resonate to a frequency with a wavelength four times the length of the "tube." This resonance is a prominant component of the free field-to-eardrum transform, and changes with the effective length of the canal. For any frequency, a pressure maximum will exist at the eardrum, and a pressure minimum will be present at a location approximately 1/4 wavelength from the eardrum. This difference has been termed the standing wave ratio (SWR). Magnitudes of SWRs for frequencies between 5000 and 8000 Hz ranging from about 10 to 25 dB have been reported (Stinson et al., 1982; Stinson, 1985). An 8000 Hz tone will have a pressure minimum located about 11 to 12 mm from the eardrum, and the SPL at the 12 mm distance will be about 12 dB less than at the eardrum. A 6000 Hz tone will have a minimum located at 16 mm from the eardrum with a SPL about 11 dB less than the eardrum SPL. For example, relative to the eardrum SPL a probe measurement taken at a location 10 mm distant will differ by 10 dB at 8000 Hz, 7 dB at 7000 Hz, 5 dB at 6000 Hz, and 1 dB at 3000 Hz. The exact location of the pressure minimum and its absolute magnitude depends upon the terminating impedance. Because middle ear impedance varies, the location and magnitude of the pressure minimum is subject to individual variation. Gilman and Dirks (1986) found that a high impedance termination would shift the minimum closer to the eardrum, a low impedance termination would move it further away. For a 6000 Hz tone, the magnitude of the effect was only about 2.5 mm. They found that the maximum changes in SWR produced by varying eardrum impedance varied with frequency. The change was 1 dB or less below 1000 Hz. The greatest increases were 6 dB for frequencies close to 3000 Hz. Beyond 5000 Hz the differences diminished to about 3 dB. For absolute measures, REUR, REAR, and RESR, maintaining a location close to the eardrum, would minimize variability. A probe location 5 mm from the eardrum would be expected to have less than a 1 dB effect upon frequencies up to 8000 Hz. For a relative measure like the REIR, the absolute position of the probe is less important than maintaining a constant insertion depth for both the REUR and REAR.

Changes in REUR produced by varying the distance from the probe tip to the eardrum are illustrated for a single subject (the author) in Figure 2–5. The probe tube was marked in approximately 5 mm increments, beginning at 5 mm from the tip of the probe and ending at 35 mm. The distance from the eardrum to the most lateral point of the tragus was about 35 mm. Location A is at the eardrum (thin line), B is 10 mm from the eardrum (circles), C is 15 mm (thick line), and D is 20 mm lateral to the eardrum (thin line). All locations are approximate. The bottom portion of the figure shows the difference between the REUR at the eardrum and the different distances from the eardrum. Negative values indicate an SPL less than that measured at the eardrum. Curves were obtained using the Fonix 6500 under typical clinical conditions. The loudspeaker was located at a distance of 30 cm from the head and an azimuth of approximately 45°. Gain is plotted relative to the sound field leveled at a reference microphone location above the pinna. Probe locations within about 5 to 8 mm of the eardrum accurately reflect eardrum SPL for frequencies up to 6000 Hz. Greater distances have a tendency to underestimate the REUR for frequencies above 2000 Hz.

A similar experiment was performed on the same subject to illustrate the effect of probe depth on the RECD using a slightly modified version of the procedure described by Fikret-Pasa and Revit (1992). Rather than threading the probe tube through the 12 mm long foam earplug attached to the ER-3A earphone, the probe was placed between the canal wall and the foam plug. The real-ear SPL developed at different probe depths was determined and compared to the earphone output in an HA-1 coupler to determine the RECD. Results are displayed in Figure 2–6 and are qualitatively similar to the results for the REUR. The high-frequency components of the RECD beyond 2000 Hz can be underestimated by a

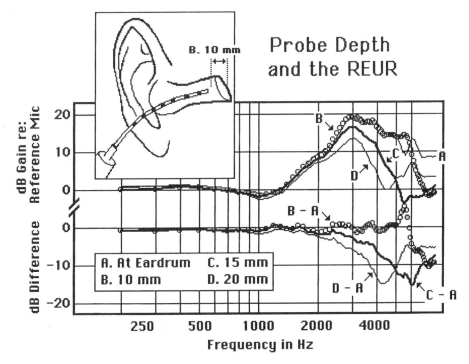

**Figure 2–5.**   Real-ear unaided responses for a single subject at different probe locations.

probe located too far removed from the eardrum. The last curve (F) indicates an attenuated response produced by a probe location estimated to be 25 mm from the eardrum. This placed the probe tip between the foam plug and the canal wall. It would be important not to mistake this placement error for an actual individual difference in RECD.

To evaluate the effects of middle ear impedance on probe depth, a simulation of an otosclerotic ear and an ear with an ossicular discontinuity was created. The low-impedance discontinuity and the high-impedance otosclerotic ear represent extremes in variability in middle ear impedance. Impedance values for the simulations along with subject data are shown in Figure 2–7. Heavy solid curves represent a simulation of resistance and reactance for the otosclerotic ear. Thin solid curves represent a simulation of resistance and reactance for the ossicular discontinuity. The shaded area covers results of the median values for the majority of studies of normal middle ear resistance and reactance (Shaw, 1974b). Figure 2–8 shows that these extremes produce predictable, yet small, effects on the REUR measured at the eardrum versus that measured at a location 20 mm distant. When compared to a more typical 6- to 8-mm probe depth, larger differences would be expected at the 20-mm location. Consequently, normal variation in middle ear impedance should not be a major source of variability with regard to probe insertion depth.

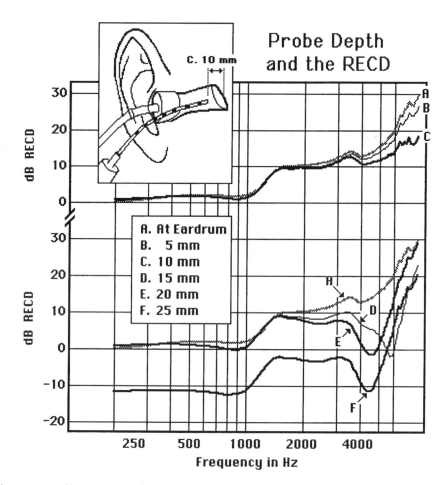

**Figure 2–6.**  Changes in RECD produced by different probe locations for the same subject as in Figure 2–5. The last position F is actually between the foam earplug and the canal wall.

## Loudspeaker Location and Head Movements

Killion and Revit (1987) investigated the effects of loudspeaker location on the reliability of insertion gain measurements. In particular, they were concerned with differences in SPL produced by small head movements that would likely occur during a typical clinical procedure. Insertion response measures were obtained five times from each of 10 subjects. Loudspeaker locations were 0°/0°, 0°/45°, 45°/45°, 90°/0°, where the first number of each pair represents the elevation, the second number the azimuth. Subjects were asked to control head position by a visual fixation procedure. Their results indicated that the mean insertion gain obtained across subjects did vary with loudspeaker location, particularly for high frequency gain for the 45° and 90° elevations. Across-subject standard deviations varied with frequency from a low of approximately 2 dB at frequencies up to 1000 Hz, and up to 5 dB for the higher frequencies, and about 7 dB for 6000 Hz. Within-subject variation was smaller but depended upon loudspeaker location.

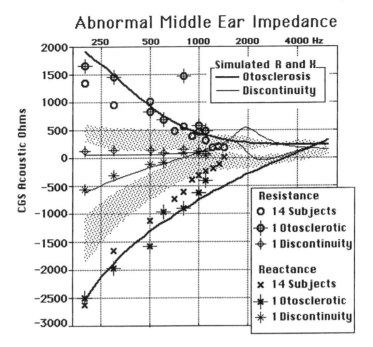

**Figure 2–7.** Mean values are shown for resistance and reactance for 14 subjects with otosclerosis taken from Zwislocki, 1957, 1 typical subject with otosclerosis, and an ossicular discontinuity (Zwislocki, 1963).

Variability was smallest, about 0.5 to 1 dB less, for the 0°/45°, 45°/45° locations, and greatest for the traditional 0°/0° position. Again, standard deviations were smallest for the lower frequencies, slightly less than 1 dB, and greater with increasing frequency, up to 3 dB at 6000 Hz. This would indicate 95% confidence intervals ranging from about 1.5 to 6 dB. When the experiment was repeated using KEMAR, 5 test-retest replications gave across-frequency standard deviations of only 0.33 to 0.43 dB. It was concluded that head movements appeared to be a primary source of variability. This also suggests that when extreme care is taken in the measurement, it is possible to have 95% confidence intervals of less than 1 dB. The authors also compared their variability estimates to those obtained by other researchers for the ear canal SPL developed by an insert earphone. They concluded that approximately half the total variation is from external ear effects, while the other half is from closed ear impedance effects.

Tecca (1991) reviewed several studies dealing with the reliability of probe tube microphone measures. When the measurement was repeated within the same test session, standard deviations of within-subject variability, averaged across frequency, ranged from 1.1 to 3.4 dB, with a mean value of almost 2 dB (95% confidence interval of 3.8 dB). When the testing was performed on different days, the average standard deviations were greater, 3.01 to 3.71 dB (95% confidence interval of 7.3 dB for the larger value). Tecca concluded that variability increased when testing was performed on different days or when the testing environment became less laboratory-like and became more clinical. Also, variability is usually

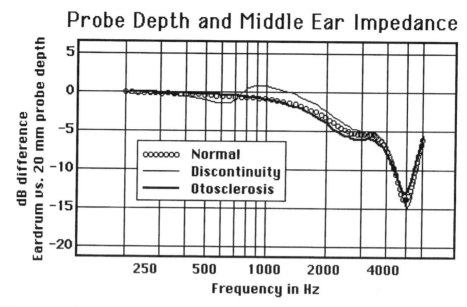

**Figure 2–8.** Simulated changes in REUR produced by a probe location 20 mm from the eardrum for a normal ear (circles), an otosclerotic ear (heavy line), and an ear with an ossicular discontinuity (thin line). Negative values indicate an SPL less than that obtained at the eardrum.

much less for the lower frequencies and greater for frequencies above 1000 Hz. To minimize variability, he suggested inserting the probe to within 6 to 8 mm of the eardrum, orienting the loudspeaker to a 45° azimuth, using a modified comparison method with an active control microphone to minimize head movement effects, test in a sound treated room, avoid slit leaks in a closed mold by drilling a special channel for the probe tube, and using a broad-band test signal. Many unusual, large diffraction effects (antiresonances) occur in the higher frequencies in narrow frequency regions. Using a spectrally dense broad-band stimulus (many closely spaced frequencies), in conjunction with a wider bandwidth measurement filter, tends to smooth responses and minimize this effect.

When a probe tube microphone measurement is made, the measurement is expected to conform to what one would expect for a typical person, modified by the unique characteristics of the individual being evaluated. However, the measurement is confounded by measurement error, and it could be possible to mistake these errors for individual difference. The mistake would be compounded by applying an unwarranted correction. It appears that much error can be avoided by meticulous attention to detail, but a certain irreducible minimum remains of about 4 to 7 dB. It is important to judge the magnitude of individual differences in terms of how large they are relative to measurement error.

*The Free/Diffuse Field-To-Eardrum Transformation*

The free and diffuse field-to-eardrum transformation, as a function of frequency $T_d(f)$, describes the sum total of all acoustic diffraction effects presented by the environment the listener is in, the head, neck, torso, pinna flange, concha, ear canal, and input impedance to the middle ear. The transform has been thoroughly investigated and excellent summaries of these results have been presented (see Shaw, 1974a, 1974b, 1980; Kuhn, 1979, 1980). Numerical values for the free field transform as a function of azimuth have been supplied by Shaw and Vaillancourt (1985). Modified transforms obtained in slightly different fashions are clinically referred to as the REUR. This unaided response is often used as the reference to which subsequent aided measures are compared, so it is useful to investigate how it might be impacted by individual differences. The following section briefly describes the average transform with particular attention to the magnitude of the above effects, likely sources of individual variability, and the magnitude of the individual effects.

In an ideal situation, the free-field measurements would be made in an anechoic chamber, i.e., a free-field environment with no echoes, so only the SPL at a particular frequency developed by the incident wave need be considered. A loudspeaker would serve as a sound-source generating frequencies covering an appropriate range (say, 100 Hz to at least 8000 Hz, or higher), and a microphone would sample the sound field. The field would be leveled to as great an extent as practical, all frequencies developing close to but slightly different SPLs, $L(f)$ at a microphone location that would later correspond to a point at the center of the subject's head. With the subject's head at this reference point, a probe microphone would sample the SPL developed in close proximity to the eardrum, $L_d(f)$. The dB level at each frequency for the transform would be:

$$T_d(f) = L_{Md}(f) - L(f)$$

The transform is sensitive to the azimuth, $\theta$, of the sound source in the horizontal plane and the elevation in the vertical plane. Azimuth is usually described in such a way that $0°$ is directly in front of the listener, $90°$ would be directly toward the ear being measured with the probe microphone, and $180°$ would be directly behind the listener, etc. Elevation is given as a vertical displacement from the horizontal. Occasionally transforms are obtained for points of interest other than the eardrum, such as locations corresponding to hearing aid microphones or the ear canal entrance.

The concept for the transform would be similar for a diffuse field, except that measurements would be obtained in a reverberation chamber. In this case, the SPL of the incident wave and that of the reflections are nearly equal so the sound source loses directionality and the azimuth becomes random. Kuhn (1979) measured the diffuse field transform for KEMAR and two subjects using a fairly spectrally dense 1/3-octave band noise source centered at frequencies from 200 Hz to 10,000 Hz. Killion and Monser (1980) used amplitude modulated tones warbled over a range of ±50 Hz.

Figure 2–9 depicts a typical transform and its components (Shaw, 1974a). Curve A is the pinna flange; B is the contribution of the torso and neck; C is the effect of the head modeled as a rigid sphere. The concha is represented by curve D; E is the ear canal contribution calculated from the model (3.2 cm long, 0.75 cm diameter), terminated with the normal analog middle ear; F is the total free field-to-eardrum transform (45° azimuth) obtained by summing curves A–E; and G is

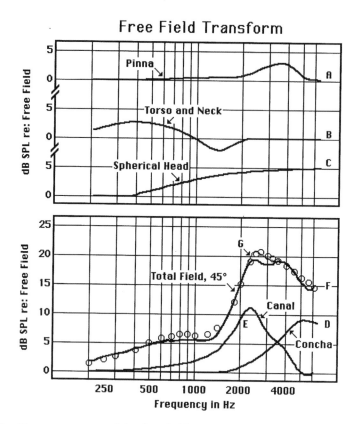

**Figure 2–9.** The components of the free field-to-eardrum transform at 45° azimuth. The ear canal contribution is calculated from the model terminated with the normal analog middle ear. Curve F is the total free field-to-eardrum transform obtained by summing curves A–E; and G is the same as F, except the thin line represents the calculated response for a slightly wider canal. The circles are data points plotted from the numerical values given by Shaw and Vaillancourt (1985).

the same as F, except the thin line represents the calculated response for a slightly wider canal 3.2 cm long, 0.82 cm diameter. Curve E is the contribution to this transform made by a cylindrical ear canal with an effective length of 3.2 cm and a diameter of 0.75 cm. The canal is terminated with an impedance calculated from the electrical analog model of the middle ear given in Figure 2–1. The agreement between the model's predictions and actual values (shown by the circles in Figure 2–9) given by Shaw and Vaillancourt (1985) is good. The agreement can be made better by slightly changing canal diameter to 0.82 cm, as shown in curve G.

The transforms displayed usually represent average data that has been smoothed. When results were plotted for individuals (10 individuals, Shaw, 1966; 12 males and 12 females, Burkhard and Sachs, 1975) in the free field, it can be seen that many subjects deviate from the average, primarily in the frequency region above 2000 Hz. At the higher frequencies, resonances and antiresonances associated primarily with the complex and unique shape of each pinna occur, often at very narrow and specific locations in the spectrum. The transforms can change dramatically with azimuth. At any one frequency, say 4000 Hz, the range of differences for the individuals could easily be 15 to 20 dB. By adjusting the frequency position of the individual curves (i.e., sliding the curves slightly left or right), peaks could be aligned, reducing this variability. Using 1/3-octave band noise, or a warble tone, in a diffuse field similarly tends to smooth these differences. Apparently, details of the measurement procedure can affect the examiner's perception of the amount of individual variability present. A separate issue would be whether it is practical, or even feasible, for the manufacturer to incorporate such individual differences into the fabrication of a custom hearing aid.

Killion and Monser (1980) describe a fairly large, over 15 dB, notch at 8000 Hz in the KEMAR free field, 0° azimuth CORFIG response. This notch, attributed to a sharp concha antiresonance, was not present in the diffuse field response. When the concha is filled with an earmold, or ITE shell, the effect is lost. They describe the dilemma faced by the designer of a broadband hearing aid, as to whether this effect should be compensated or not. Under typical conditions, the listener's environment is reverberant, and the notch will be "filled in" by reflected background sound, so that it might be ignored. However, the notch may serve as a vital perceptual cue in vertical localization so should be included in free field listening. For many hearing-impaired with poor sensitivity above 3000 to 4000 Hz, the argument is probably moot because, even when aided, the cue would be imperceptible. Shaw (1980) states that the diffuse field response may be more appropriate for a listener's appreciation of sound quality in enclosed rooms, whereas a free-field response could be more appropriate for face-to-face speech communication within the critical distance, where the SPL of the incident sound is more intense than reflections.

### Sources of Individual Variability

Figure 2–9 illustrates the separate components of the average 45° azimuth free-field response. Discussing each component represents a convenient means for addressing individual variability. Several of these issues were investigated by Kuhn (1979). Using KEMAR as a reference, the transformation from the diffuse field to the surface of the head (torso absent) is very similar to theoretical predictions for a rigid sphere. The SPL developed at the top, front, and rear pinna notch were judged to be equal, and the average value is generally no more than about 1 to 1.5 dB higher from the ideal sphere. Scattering of sound produced by adding a bare torso increases the level slightly, by perhaps an additional 1 dB. Adding clothing (a T-shirt, shirt, necktie, and sport coat) reduces the level back to the case without the torso, and even reduces the high-frequency (beyond 5000 Hz) response to a level up to 4 dB less than the theoretical predictions for the sphere. The pressure transformation from the diffuse field to the tragus was also investigated with 6 different sized pinna adapted to KEMAR intended to simulate small and large male and female ears, and 2 human male subjects with pinna length and breadth within the range encompassed by the artificial pinna. The transform showed differences between pinna less than 2 dB, and the results of the 2 human subjects were similar. Because results for KEMAR and the two subjects were so similar to theoretical predictions (a simple sphere), it was concluded that pressure buildup on the surface of the head is quite insensitive to individual fine facial features below 10,000 Hz and surface impedance (i.e., skin texture, hair) below 7000 Hz. This conclusion is also supported by data presented by Shotland and Hecox (1990) that showed no significant differences in the SPL developed slightly off of and in front of the head for 9 subjects.

Changing pinna had a slightly greater effect on the diffuse field-to-eardrum transform in KEMAR, although below 1000 Hz effects were negligible. From 1000 Hz to 2000 Hz the range of differences from the smallest to largest pinna were about 1.5 to 3.5 dB, 3 dB from 2000 Hz to 6000 Hz, increasing to about 5 dB at 8000 Hz (Kuhn, 1979). Because all other factors, head size, facial features, ear canal length and diameter, and eardrum impedance were held constant, it can be assumed that variation in pinna contours, such as concha volume, were solely responsible for these differences. Up to 6000 Hz the effects were usually no more than a few dB.

Teranishi and Shaw (1968) found that a fairly simple model consisting of a rectangular pinna containing a cylindrical concha cavity (22 mm diameter, 10 mm depth), elevated 30° from a large rigid plane accurately simulated the average response from a group of six subjects. Adding a 22.5 mm long, 7 mm diameter cylindrical cavity perpendicular to the plane, terminated with a 400 cgs ohm resistance and 0.193 cm$^3$ cavity, completed the model by adding an ear canal and middle ear impedance. The response of the model gave a good simulation of the data for Teranishi and Shaw's six subjects, and the average response of Wiener and Ross' (1946) six to 12 male subjects, up to at least 6000 Hz. Being able to model the ear canal as a simple cylinder is fortunate because the ear canal, like the pinna, has an unusual shape that is difficult to easily specify.

Wiener and Ross (1946) showed a free field-to-eardrum transform very similar to the subsequent results given by Shaw (1974a). The transform was shown to be sensitive to azimuth, and variations in azimuth were generally larger than individual variability, which had standard deviations that increased gradually with frequency from a value of about 1 dB to about 6 dB at 6000 Hz. The transform from the ear canal entrance to the eardrum was independent of azimuth, as would be expected, because head diffraction is believed to be responsible for these effects. Standard deviations of the canal entrance-to-eardrum transform were only slightly less than standard deviations given for the free field-to-eardrum transform, suggesting that perhaps effects related to individual differences in ear canal geometry and middle ear impedance have the greatest effect upon the entire transform. For this experiment, all subjects had the position of their head maintained by a rigid apparatus, thus minimizing head movements. A subsequent report (Wiener, 1947) showed similar standard deviations but also gave the ranges for the left ears of six male subjects. Variability was greatest above 2000 Hz, and at a frequency approximating the peak in the free field-to-eardrum transform (slightly less than 3000 Hz); the range was 15 dB, which is considerable given only six ears. Bryant (1972), citing an unpublished study by Zwislocki, showed ranges of 10 dB for seven subjects in the transform for the ear canal entrance to the eardrum.

## Variability in Real-Ear Unaided Responses

REURs obtained clinically for the purpose of hearing aid fitting are similar to the field-to-eardrum transform, with some notable exceptions. The environment is typically neither free field, nor diffuse field, but somewhere in between. Maintaining a close distance between the loudspeaker and listener (30 to 40 cm) tends to minimize reflections and create more of a free-field condition. Averaging and smoothing options, like that present on the Fonix 6500, simulate a warble tone and tend to minimize effects produced by sharp antiresonances. REURs are not usually obtained using a substitution method, as proper use of this procedure requires a controlled acoustic environment. Instead, a reference microphone, placed either over the ear on the head or slightly under the pinna on a hanger, is used to both level the sound field and to serve as a comparison to the probe microphone. During REUR measurement the SPL developed at the reference microphone is subtracted from that developed at the probe microphone. Therefore, head diffraction effects are minimized in the measurement, and differences can occur due to exact reference microphone placement. Major effects related to pinna, concha, ear canal resonances, and middle ear impedance are included.

Fikret-Pasa and Revit (1992) compared REURs on KEMAR using a Fonix 6500 system with the loudspeaker placed at either a 0° or 45° azimuth using both an under- and over-the-ear (UTE, OTE) location for the reference microphone. These REURs were compared to results obtained for a substitution method, as would be used to describe a field-to-eardrum transform. Results indicated that at 0° azimuth both the UTE and OTE locations gave results comparable to the substitution method within about ±3 dB. REUR values were consistently less, by about 3 to 10 dB, than what would have been obtained with the substitution method for both the UTE and OTE location when the azimuth was 45°. The OTE gave slightly less error than the UTE location, but both gave slightly different results, depending upon the location of KEMAR in the test room, because the environment was not free field. Feigin, Nelson Barlow, and Stelmachowicz (1990) compared differences between the SPL developed at the microphone of a BTE hearing aid and the SPL developed at an OTE or a UTE reference microphone position for 20 subjects. Differences were greater with the UTE position. Standard deviations of the differences between the hearing aid microphone and UTE reference microphone ranged from 1.2 dB at 500 Hz to a maximum of 3.6 dB at 3000 Hz. For the OTE reference, the standard deviations were 0.5 dB at 500 Hz to 1.9 dB at 3000 Hz. All subjects showed at least a 3 dB difference between the hearing aid microphone and the reference microphone for at least one frequency, and 35% of the subjects had differences greater than 7 dB. A 95% confidence interval of about ±3.7 dB would describe the relationship between an OTE reference microphone SPL and the SPL present at the hearing aid microphone of a BTE aid. The authors pointed out that these differences would affect the REIR of a compression aid, where gain varies as a function of input level, more so than that of a linear aid.

Gartrell and Church (1990) compared the difference in SPL developed at the microphone of a BTE aid versus an ITE aid for 20 subjects. The SPL was higher for the ITE location and was greatest at 3000 Hz where the average difference was 6.3 dB, standard deviation of 4.2 dB. There was considerable variability in the data; often the standard deviations were equal to or greater than the mean differences. Fikret-Pasa and Revit (1992) also found that variability was present in the SPL developed between the typical location for a BTE versus ITE hearing aid. Across subject standard deviations of the differences between these locations varied with frequency from a low of 1 to 2 dB for frequencies less than 4000 Hz, to roughly 6 to 7 dB from 5000 to 8000 Hz. They suggested that this variability in the higher frequencies could have been exaggerated by the placement of the reference microphone over the hair of the subjects. It was found that the practice of placing the reference microphone over (rather than under) the hair of KEMAR wearing a wig increased the differences between microphone location at the high frequencies.

Variation in free-field pressure along contours located above and behind the pinna of KEMAR has been investigated by Kuhn and Burnett (1977). With the sound source located at 0° azimuth, there was a smooth decrease in pressure from the front to back at frequencies below 2000 Hz. Below 4000 Hz, variation in SPL was less than 6.5 dB. At higher frequencies the pinna casts an appreciable shadow, often 12 to 25 dB deep. These differences were minimized by using 6% to 29% bandwidth (of the center frequency) pink noise rather than pure tones. They gave results that did suggest that variation in placement of an OTE reference microphone could affect the REUR, although differences would likely be small, less than 2 dB, for frequencies up to 4000 Hz. Movement to a new position less than 3 cm forward of a position above the pinna and directly over the canal opening changed the SPL by as much as 5.5 to 8 dB for frequencies between 5 and 8000 Hz. Shotland and Hecox (1990) used digitally synthesized white noise from a loudspeaker located at 0° azimuth to assess the effects of reference microphone location for a group of 9 subjects. The least intersubject variability occurred for a reference microphone positioned slightly forward of the pinna but 2 to 4 cm away (lateral) from the head surface.

Typical REURs have been reported for individuals with normal middle ear function. Upfold and Byrne (1988) measured REURs for 20 male and 20 female subjects. They identified the frequency of the peak as 2968 Hz with a standard deviation of 361 Hz, peak height as 18 dB with a standard deviation of 3.3 dB. The bandwidth (defined as the difference between those frequencies 6 dB less than the peak) surrounding the peak was 1.225 octaves with a standard deviation of 0.438 octaves. Rodrigues and Gerhardt (1991) found a peak of 2810 Hz (range of 2000 to 3500 Hz), with an amplitude of 20.6 dB (range of 14 to 25 dB) for 31 subjects with a mean age of 21 years. Valente, Valente, and Goebel (1991) evaluated 49 ears of 25 subjects with a mean age of 64.4 years. Estimates of test-retest reliability were also available, because the same examiner repeated the measurement 1.5 to 2 weeks later. The repeated measures were on average quite similar to each other, peak frequency of 2585 Hz, peak amplitude of 18.5 dB, with a standard deviation across subjects of 3.3 dB. Standard deviations at higher frequencies were only slightly greater, 3.9 dB. Therefore, the 95% range in across subject variability would be expected to be 15.3 dB at 3000 and 4000 Hz. The repeat measure of the peak frequency was within 300 Hz of the initial measure in 93% of the measures, indicating good agreement. The average within-subject standard deviation of the absolute differences between repeated measures was 2.02 dB (3.95 dB for the 95% confidence interval). At 3000 and 4000 Hz, the intrasubject standard deviations were 2.33 and 3.41 dB, giving 95% confidence intervals of approximately 4.6 to 6.7 dB (average value of 5.65 dB). The variability in repeated measures was about 37% of that across subjects. So, measurement error can account for an appreciable part of the differences observed across subjects in the magnitude of the REUR.

### REURs in Children

The preceding discussion focused upon REURs obtained for adults. It would be anticipated that anatomical differences could produce substantial differences in children. Kruger (1987) summarized results for 34 ears of 26 children from ages birth to 3 years. She reported that the REUR decreased from approximately 6000 Hz in the newborn to a normal adult value of 2700 Hz by age 20 months, or earlier. This result was explained as an increase in the effective ear canal length from roughly 12 mm at birth to a normal adult value of 32 mm by 20 months. The actual physical length of 25 mm in the adult (Shaw, 1974a) is increased somewhat by the presence of the concha. Bentler (1989) found that the REURs of children from ages 3 to 13 years did not differ appreciably from those in adults. Peak frequency was 2848.8 Hz (standard deviation of 490.8 Hz, range 1774 to 4039 Hz), peak amplitude was 18.9 dB (standard deviation of 3.5 dB, range 11.3 to 27 dB). The average canal opening was 37.5 mm$^2$, with a standard deviation of 9.5 mm$^2$. Although there were slight negative correlations between peak resonant frequency and age, height, and weight, there was no significant correlation with head circumference or size of the canal opening. It was interesting that she could find no other physical measure that correlated significantly with the amplitude of the resonant peak. Dempster and Mackenzie (1990) found that the peak resonant frequency decreased systematically until it reached the typical adult value of 2700 Hz by 7 years. The effect they reported was a decrease of about 300 Hz (3002 Hz for their 15 subjects under the age of 4 years, to 2707 for 16 subjects, 9 years old). They noted considerable variability in the data; standard deviations ranged from 178 to 428 Hz for different age groups, so even the youngest children overlapped with the adults.

### Abnormal Ears and the Effects of Load Impedance

Goode, Friedrichs, and Falk (1977) evaluated the effects of modification of external ear anatomy produced by tympanomastoid surgery for 30 ears, four fresh cored temporal bones, and also simulated these effects using a KEMAR manikin. Varying the ear canal length had predictable effects on the frequency of the ear canal resonance; shorter canals had higher frequency resonances. They found that the presence of small experimentally induced perforations (0.75, 1 mm diameter) had little effect upon the REUR, whereas larger perforations (2 mm diameter) tended to reduced the magnitude of the REUR in the range from 300 to 3000 Hz by 3 to 4 dB, and produced sharp high-frequency antiresonances.

Figure 2–10 shows REURs for four young (20s to 30s) female patients, with perforations, who were seen in our clinic. Each REUR was obtained with the Fonix 6500 with the loudspeaker located about 30 cm from the ear at an azimuth of 45°.

# REURs in Perforated Eardrums

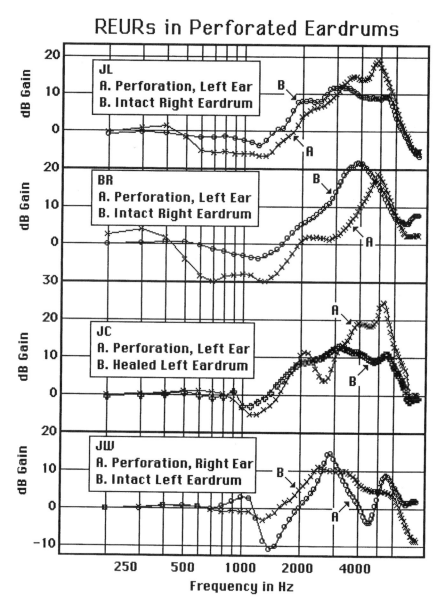

**Figure 2–10.** The real-ear unaided responses for four individuals with perforated eardrums.

The probe tip was placed into the ear canal at a position close to the eardrum, about 30 mm from the most lateral point of the tragus. Patient JC had the left ear perforate following inflammatory disease of the middle ear. Approximately two weeks later, the perforation healed, and the tympanogram and hearing had returned to normal. The effect of the perforation was to reduce the REUR for the midfrequencies and shift the response peak to a fairly high frequency, about 5000 Hz. A similar pattern was seen for both JL and BR, both of whom also have normal hearing. JL's perforation was about two months' duration; however, she has a long history of middle ear problems. A tympanic membrane reconstruction was performed at age 9 years in the left ear. At age 16, a right fascia graft tympanoplasty was initiated for a panperforation. BR has had a perforated left ear for years. In all cases, the perforations were small. JC's equivalent "ear canal" volume (i.e., ear canal plus middle ear) was only 1.5 ml, BR's was 3.4 ml, and JL's was large and exceeded the ability of the equipment to measure it. JW had a longstanding, small perforation associated with 35 dB HL hearing loss. Her REUR is qualitatively different from the other three, although, except for the hearing loss, there are no obvious differences in the physical characteristics of her ear that would explain the difference.

These REURs, especially the reduced response in the ear with the perforation, are consistent with the observations of Goode, Friedrichs, and Falk (1977). They also noted an appreciable effect produced by surgical changes in the volume terminating the ear canal. When the medial end of the canal was increased in size, or communicated with the mastoid, the peak frequency of the response was reduced. Figure 2–11 shows the REURs, also obtained from our clinic, for two young adults with modified radical mastoidectomy of the right ear. SO's right ear had a flat tympanogram with a physical volume of 2.7 ml. The left ear was normal, physical volume of 1.0 ml, except for a slightly negative tympanometric peak pressure (TPP) of –126 daPa. Hearing for both ears was within the normal range. For KD the right ear physical volume was 4.0 ml and the left ear was normal at 1.1 ml. Hearing in the unoperated ear was normal, but the right ear had a 50 dB HL conductive hearing loss. The most striking feature of both REURs is the reduction in frequency of the peak to about 1,500 Hz.

Figures 2–12 to 2–17 illustrate the effects of load impedance on either the REUR or the free-field transform. The difference between the REUR obtained with a normal middle ear pressure (ambient) and a severely reduced middle ear pressure is shown in Figure 2–12. By reversing a normal Valsalva procedure, it is possible to evacuate the middle ear cavities. For one subject (the author), tympanometry performed immediately after the REUR was obtained verified that the TPP was more negative than –500 daPa. The change in REUR (6–7 dB) was most pronounced between 2000 and 3000 Hz, but for most of the frequency range changes were less than 3 dB. The stiffening effect produced by changing middle ear pressure is qualitatively similar to that produced by a simulated otosclerotic ear. The thick and thin lines of Figure 2–13 represent simulations of an otosclerotic ear and an ossicular discontinuity with impedance values shown in Figure 2–7. Whereas the stiffening pathology tends to slightly increase the eardrum response, the ossicular discontinuity tends to produce the opposite effect, reducing the response between 800 and a little over 2000 Hz. These pathologic effects are relatively small and suggest that normal variation in middle ear impedance probably does not effect significant variation in the REUR.

Little is known about the effects of middle ear effusion on the REUR. As illustrated in Figure 2–14, the model predicts an enhanced REUR between 2000 and 3000 Hz for simulations of the effects of middle ear fluid. The curves in the bottom panel of the figure were created by increasing $Rmi$ to 100 ohms, increasing Lmi to 700 mH, and reducing $Cmi$ to 0.01 µF. These changes were intended to

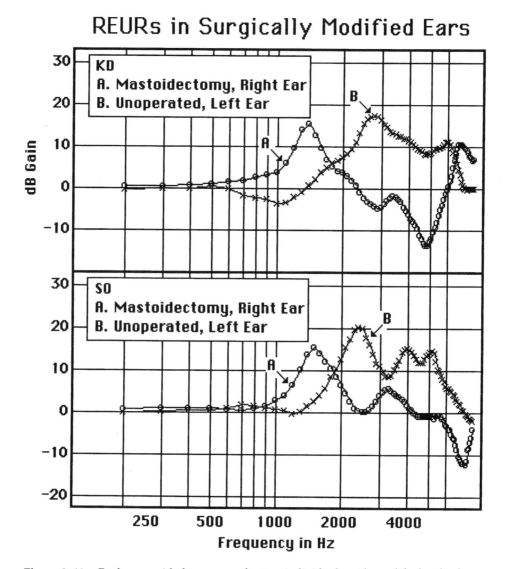

**Figure 2–11.**   Real ear unaided responses for two individuals with modified radical mastoidectomies.

mimic the effects upon the middle ear of the presence of fluid and the tension induced by negative middle ear pressure. *Ccavity* was varied over a range of 5.45 μF (7.8 ml) to 0.15 μF (.21 ml) to simulate the reduction in volume of the middle ear spaces created by the presence of fluid. As this volume is reduced, the REUR peak increases in a predictable fashion.

The top panel of Figure 2–14 shows the results for DS, a 6-year-old girl with a history of middle ear disease. Results for the left ear were consistent with effusion: a 20 dB HL conductive hearing loss, a flat tympanogram with a peak admittance of 0.1 mmho, and absent acoustic reflexes. The right ear had better, but not

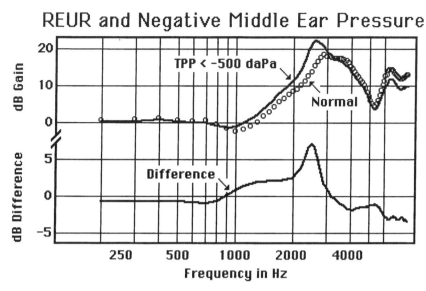

**Figure 2–12.**  Difference in REUR for a single subject with normal tympanometric peak pressure (TPP), and an induced TPP less than –500 daPa. The negative middle ear pressure was generated by performing a "reverse" Valsalva procedure. Probe was located at the eardrum.

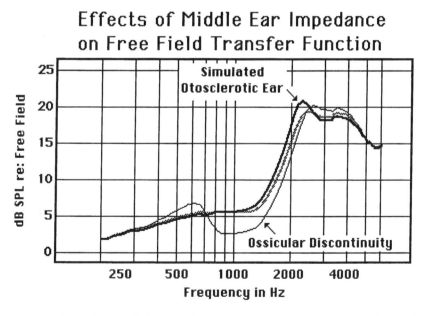

**Figure 2–13.**  The effects of changes in middle ear impedance on the free-field-to-eardrum transform. The dotted line is a normal transform for an ear canal 3.2 cm long, 0.75 cm diameter, terminated with a simulated normal middle ear.

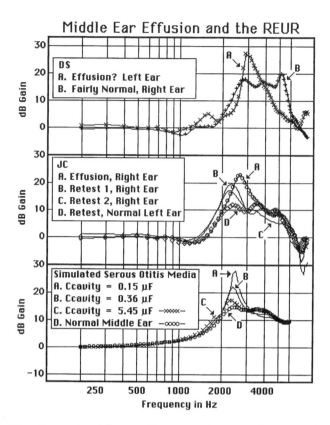

**Figure 2–14.** The effects of middle ear effusion on the REUR for two individuals and for predictions from the computer simulation.

entirely normal, hearing (5 to 10 dB HL) and middle ear function. The tympanogram was shallow, with a negative tympanometric peak pressure (–200 daPa) and a peak admittance of 0.2 mmho. The REUR for the right ear is not unusual, but the left ear shows a rather high amplitude peak (27.4 dB) at 2900 Hz. Although it is not certain that this effect is related to effusion, the results are suggestive.

The middle panel of Figure 2–14 shows three REURs for JC's right ear and a repeat REUR for the left ear (see Fig. 2-10). The right ear had an acute otitis. The presence of effusion was apparent otoscopically and was documented by her physician. At the time curve A was obtained, the audiogram showed a 30 dB HL conductive hearing loss, and the tympanogram was flat, with a peak admittance less than 0.1 mmho. Curve C was obtained when hearing had improved to about 20 dB HL; the tympanogram was still flat, with a peak admittance of 0.1 mmho. Curve B was associated with only a 10 dB HL loss, and the tympanogram had improved to a peak admittance of 0.5 mmho with a TPP of –246 daPa and a tympanometric width of 108 daPa. Although the difference between curve A and B is small, because B was associated with better middle ear functioning, it was anticipated that it would have a slightly lower amplitude peak than C. Instead, the reverse was found. Although this phenomenon needs to be investigated in more patients, it appears that inflammatory disease of the middle ear can have an appreciable influence on the REUR peak.

Figures 2–15 and 2–16 illustrate the simulated effect on the free-field transfer function of changing ear canal length and diameter by ±1 and ±2 standard deviations (Kates, 1988b). In the bottom of Figure 2–15, the thin line is the transform for a normal canal (3.2 cm long, 0.75 cm diameter). Thick lines represent long (3.6 cm) and short (2.8 cm) canals with normal diameter. The long canal is +2 SDs longer, and the short canal is –2 SDs shorter than normal. The maximum difference is about 5.8 dB at 4000 Hz. The upper part of the figure shows the difference between ear canals that are ±2 or ±1 SDs longer or shorter than normal, but each canal had a normal diameter. The +1 SD length was 3.4 cm, –1 SD was 3.0 cm. In Figure 2–16, the thin line represents the normal canal (3.2 cm long, 0.75 cm diameter). Thick lines represent wide (1.03 cm) and narrow (0.47 cm) canals with normal length. The maximum difference between the responses is about 13.8 dB at 2580 Hz. The difference between a canal diameter +1 SD wider (3.2 cm long, 0.89 cm diameter) and –1 SD narrower (3.2 cm long, 0.61 cm diameter) is also shown in the upper part of the graph. Variation within ±1 standard deviation predicts changes less than about 5 dB, which are confined to frequencies greater than 1000 Hz. More extreme changes, such as varying diameter by two standard deviations, can create differences in excess of 10 dB.

### Ear Canal Taper

Gardner and Hawley (1972) modeled the ear canal as both a cylinder and one with taper, and suggested that variation in ear canal geometry might account for some cases of individual variation in the ear canal entrance to eardrum transform. Using the model, they determined the difference between a canal that was larger at the entrance, smaller at the eardrum, as compared to a reversed taper (i.e., an abnormal canal, larger at the eardrum and smaller at the ear canal entrance). The reversed taper showed a lower frequency for the resonance peak, and less high frequency output, both for theoretical calculations and for physical measurements taken from a manikin fitted with models of tapered canals. Johansen (1975) obtained ear impressions taken all the way to the eardrum from 10 cadavers (six males, four females). Changes in cumulative volume were recorded as distance increased from the eardrum to the canal opening. Johansen's volume data was used here to derive changes in a cross-sectional area and equivalent diameter for a circular section. These values are shown in the upper portion of Figure 2–17, and the variation was modeled as four sections of tubing with different lengths and diameters. The lower part of Figure 2–17 illustrates the effects of canal taper on the ear canal entrance to eardrum transfer function. Tapering the canal (larger at entrance, narrower at the eardrum) causes the transform peak to be shifted upward in frequency. Reversing the taper (larger diameter at the eardrum) lowers the frequency of the peak and creates a slight reduction in peak height. Hudde's (1983a) work suggests that the ear canal is tapered in both directions, narrowing toward the middle, whereas Johansen's (1975) data indicate a uniformly tapered canal, narrower at the eardrum. Perhaps the complex contour

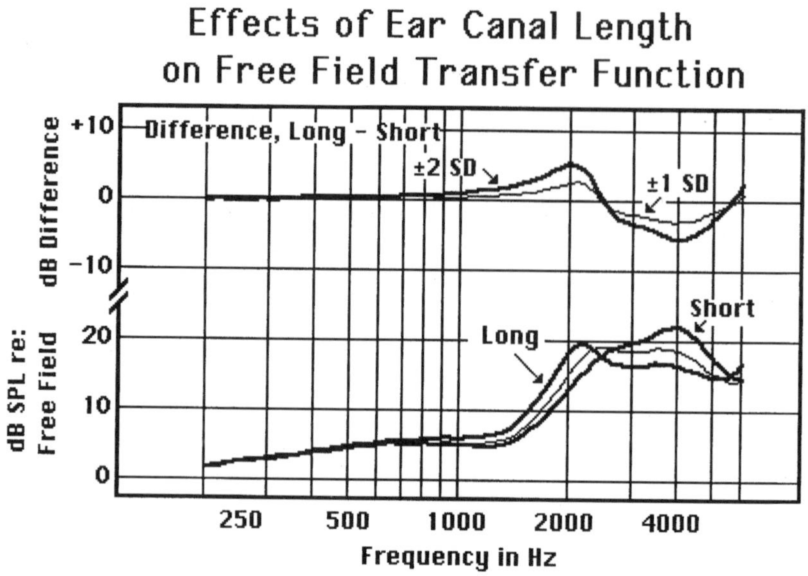

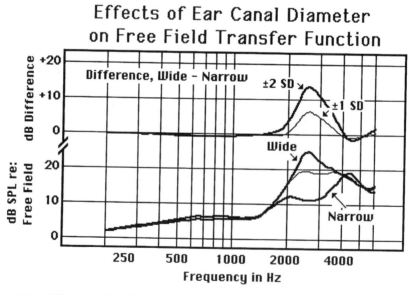

**Figure 2–15.**   Effects on the free-field-to-eardrum transform of changing ear canal length ±2 and ±1 standard deviations (SD).

of the canal and the large angle at which the eardrum ends the canal makes the exact shape of the canal in the vicinity of the eardrum difficult to determine. Regardless, it seems that changes in taper can effect changes in the ear canal transform, and perhaps account for some of the changes seen in the surgically modified ears of Figure 2–11.

**Figure 2–16.**   Effects on free-field-to-eardrum transform of changing ear canal diameter ±2 and ±1 standard deviations.

The REUR can be a considerable source of individual variability. Although part of this variability might be attributed to measurement error, most of the differences seen across subjects are large enough to reflect true differences in acoustic response produced primarily by resonances associated with the pinna, concha, ear canal, and middle ear impedance.

### Effects of Load Impedance on the Occluded Ear Response

From an acoustic impedance point of view, the geometry of the ear canal can be specified by its area function; that is, how the cross-sectional area of the canal varies with distance from the eardrum to the canal opening in the concha. When a hearing aid is worn, it is the area function from the tip of the ITE shell (or BTE mold) to the eardrum that is relevant. Hudde (1983a) used an acoustic method to estimate the area function for six individuals. Although it was not possible using this method to give absolute measures, relative measurements showed a slight decrease in area from the entrance to midcanal, then a slightly greater increase in area at the eardrum. Johansen's (1975) average canal length was 2.57 cm, with a standard deviation of 0.19 cm. The diameter varied fairly uniformly from 0.43 cm at the eardrum to about 0.8 cm at the entrance (as shown in Figure 2–17). At midcanal (about 1.2 cm) the diameter was calculated as 0.67 cm. Stinson (1985)

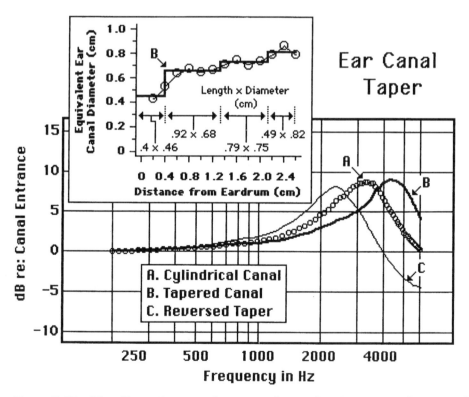

**Figure 2–17.** The effects of ear canal taper on the canal entrance-to-eardrum transfer function.

reported an area function obtained from an ear replica made from a cadaver impression. Although the volumetric method was slightly different from Johansen's, the qualitative shape of the function, tapering toward the eardrum, was similar. Based upon ear impressions, or fitting spheres of graduated radii, for 39 subjects Gerhardt, Rodriquez, Hepler, and Moul (1987) measured a diameter at the canal entrance to be 0.86 cm with a standard deviation of 0.105 cm, and a range of 0.66 to 1.04 cm. Kates (1988b), reporting unpublished work by Horbach, indicated an average canal radius of 0.33 cm at the second bend. Standard deviations of 0.2 cm for canal length and 0.07 cm in equivalent radius at the second bend agree quite well with the data derived from Johansen. Keefe, Bulen, Arehart, and Burns (1993) reported ear canal dimensions for both children and adults. They found slightly shorter adult ear canal length (2.3 cm) and wider canal diameter (1.04 cm) at the midcanal location. Ear canal diameter ranged from 0.44 cm to 0.77 cm for 1-month and 24-month-old children, respectively. Canal length changed from 1.4 cm to 2.1 cm for the same age groups. Zemplenyi, Gilman, and Dirks (1985) used an optical method (an operating microscope with a narrow depth of field) to estimate mean ear canal length at 2.5 cm for five males and 2.4 for five females. The smallest canal was 2.2 cm long; the longest was 3.0 cm. The authors believed these results to be in good agreement with typical estimates of 2.3 to 2.7 cm. Chan and Geisler (1990) replicated these results for seven males and seven females. Measuring from the canal entrance to the umbo, the mean canal length was 2.55 cm. However, male ears were about 0.4 cm longer than the female ears (2.76 cm versus 2.34 cm). The ear canal in KEMAR is a cylinder (Zwislocki coupler) 2.15 cm long and 0.75 cm in diameter (Burkhard and Sachs, 1975). The length is less than average to account for the greater sound velocity at normal body temperature and the compliance of the coupler microphone. Oliveira, Hammer, Stillman, Holm, Jons, and Margolis (1992) reported that the cartilaginous outer 1/3 of the canal can change shape during jaw movements. They demonstrated a change from 5.1 to 6.3 mm in the anterior–posterior direction at a location between the first and second bend as the jaw changed from a closed to 35 mm open position. If a typical earmold is 14 mm from the eardrum, most of these changes should not produce too great an effect on this residual volume.

**Residual Ear Canal Size**

Figures 2–18 and 2–19 show the effect produced on the occluded real-ear response (essentially an REAR with the SPL at the microphone held constant) of changing the length and diameter of that portion of the ear canal between the tip of the simulated ITE shell and the eardrum. In Figure 2–18, curve D is the normal length (thick line), and the difference between curves C and E (crosses) represents ±2 standard deviations. The difference between curves B and F (circles) represent extremes. In Figure 2–19, the thick curve, C is the normal canal width of 0.75 cm. Curves B and D are diameters ±1 standard deviation below and above average. Curves A and E are ±2 standard deviations below and above the average width. The curves representing the difference between B and D (circles) and A and E (crosses) are given in the upper part of the figure. In extreme cases, espe-

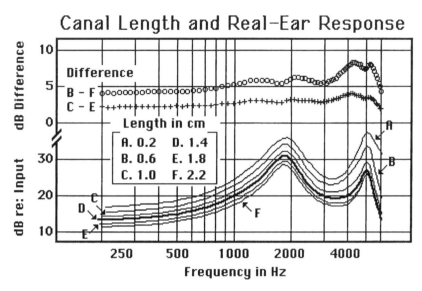

**Figure 2–18.** The effects of residual ear canal length (ITE shell tip to eardrum) on the simulated real-ear response.

cially for the higher frequencies, these differences can become large, approaching 15 dB.

The SPL developed in an ear canal is proportional to its size. Shorter, narrower ear canals have a greater output SPL at the eardrum and longer, wider canals have a lower SPL. However, the effect is more prominent for the higher frequencies. The larger canals lose high-frequency output to a greater extent than low frequency output. Having a small canal in effect creates a mild high-frequency

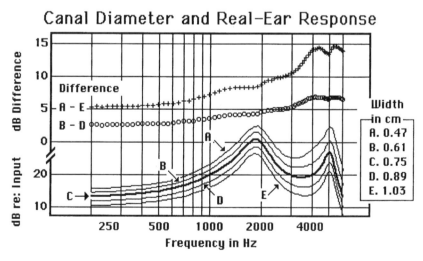

**Figure 2–19.** The effects of residual ear canal diameter on the simulated real-ear response.

emphasis condition (Egolf et al., 1980; de Jonge, 1983). A similar result was reported by Kates (1988a, 1988b). For a closed-mold simulation where canal dimensions varied over a normal range, the corresponding change in hearing aid response was 5.5 dB at 500 Hz, but amounted to about 10 dB between 3000 and 4000 Hz. Because these changes vary with frequency, they cannot be completely compensated by volume control wheel adjustment. Changing the diameter of the ear canal has a greater effect than changing ear canal length.

Because changes in ear canal size affect both the REUR and the REAR, it is interesting to determine whether these changes will be canceled or magnified in the REIR. Figure 2–20 shows changes in the REIR for "big" and "small" canals with lengths and diameters ±1 and ±2 standard deviations from normal. Each curve represents the difference between itself and the normal REIR. The normal REUR is based on a canal 3.2 cm long, 0.75 cm diameter, and the REAR is computed from a distance from the shell tip to eardrum of 1.4 cm, and a canal diameter of 0.75 cm. Curves B1 and S1 were computed from canal lengths and diameters ±1 standard deviations larger and smaller than normal. Curves B2 and S2 are ±2 SDs larger and smaller. This simulation suggests that the effect of canal size is preserved and the REIR of small ears tends to be greater than normal, whereas the REIR of larger ears is less, in extreme cases by more than 10 dB at the higher frequencies. Also, the effect is not entirely uniform with respect to frequency.

### Middle Ear Impedance

Average impedance values have been determined for the middle ear, and the results can be summarized as resistance and reactance curves that are a function of frequency, such as those given previously in Figure 2–2 (Møller, 1974; Shaw, 1974b). Zwislocki (1957) obtained acoustic impedance data for frequencies up to 2000 Hz for nine normal ears, 14 ears with otosclerosis, and one ear with an ossicular discontinuity (see Fig. 2–7). Normal resistance was about 500 ohms and varied

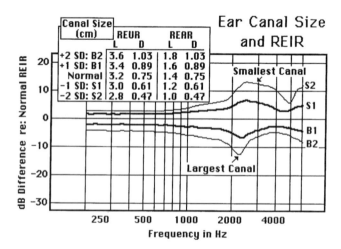

**Figure 2–20.** Effects of changes in canal length and diameter on the real-ear insertion response.

little across frequency. Normal reactance varied from about −2700 ohms at 100 Hz to almost 0 at 1000 Hz, suggesting a stiffness dominated system for the lower frequencies, beginning to resonate at approximately 1000 Hz. The otosclerotic ears had higher resistance values and smaller (i.e., large negative) reactance values, particularly for the lower frequencies. The ear with the ossicular discontinuity showed the opposite effect; resistance values were much lower, and the reactance was greater. The results of this and subsequent work (Zwislocki, 1962) were used to develop a theoretical model, an electrical analog of the middle ear. Onchi (1961) measured acoustic impedance of 24 cadaver middle ears, 17 to 64 years of age, for frequencies up to 10,000 Hz. Although there were marked individual differences, resistance values were fairly uniform across frequency, usually between 200 to 1700 ohms. Reactance values were large and negative, particularly for the lower frequencies, becoming progressively smaller as frequency increased. When the malleus handle was removed from the tympanic membrane in one specimen to simulate a discontinuity, resistance and reactance curves maintained their typical shape but became very small, and reactance values were much less negative, indicating a low impedance ear. Similar results have been found by Zwislocki (1963) and Feldman (1963). In an experiment designed to develop a network model of the middle ear, Møller (1961) obtained results from six living subjects that were qualitatively similar to those obtained by Zwislocki (1957) and Onchi (1961), although the living ears exhibited much less stiffness for the lowest frequencies. It has been suggested that measurements carried out on cadaver ears are not comparable to those of living ears dues to postmortem changes primarily increasing low-frequency impedance (Hudde, 1983b). Mehrgardt and Mellert (1977) used a technique that allowed middle ear impedance to be calculated for the frequency range from 2000 to 15,000 Hz. Generally, these results were comparable to those of previous studies for the lower frequencies and suggested that at the higher frequencies reactance becomes positive, and the impedance, although low, becomes dominated by resistance. Rabinowitz (1981) demonstrated that eardrum impedance data could be used to accurately calculate ear canal entrance to eardrum transfer functions.

Modeling studies have investigated the effects of changing middle ear impedance to simulate pathological ears (Lutman and Martin, 1979). de Jonge (1983) found that abnormally high (i.e., an "otosclerotic") or low (a simulated "ossicular discontinuity") load impedance had predictable effects upon the SPL developed at the eardrum for frequencies less than 2000 Hz. These effects were similar, producing SPL changes in the same direction as Gilman, Dirks, and Stern (1981) found using low- and high-impedance ear couplers. Increasing middle ear impedance increased the frequency response relative to normal, whereas reducing impedance produced less output in the lower frequencies. Egolf, Feth, Cooper, and Franks (1985), using a different modeling technique, found similar results for the effects of high- and low-impedance ears for the lower frequencies. Because these effects are frequency dependent, a simple adjustment in the volume control cannot completely compensate.

Figures 2–21 and 2–22 illustrate the effects upon the real-ear response and the REIR produced by changing the terminating impedance from normal to simulate either an otosclerotic ear or an ear with an ossicular discontinuity. Changes are

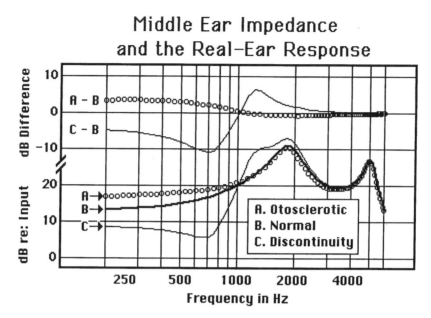

**Figure 2–21.** The effects of simulated changes in middle ear impedance on the real-ear response.

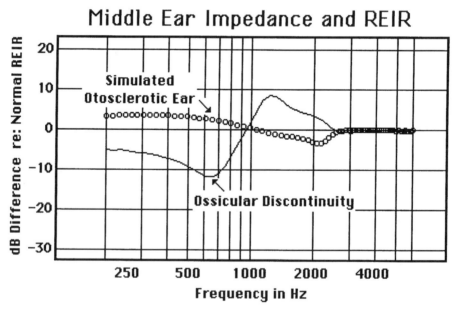

**Figure 2–22.** The effects of middle ear impedance on the REIR. The curves are plotted relative to the normal REIR. Positive values indicate gain greater than normal, negative values gain less than normal.

more prominent for the lower frequencies and, in the case of the high-impedance ear, did not exceed 5 dB. The low-impedance ear produced changes which, at the extremes, could change the REIR by as much as ±10 dB.

## Vent Effects

Earmolds, or ITE shells, often contain a cylindrical channel, running parallel to the main sound bore, that connects the residual ear canal volume to the outside environment. This vent modifies the hearing aid frequency response (Lybarger, 1985). The general effect of the vent is to create a low-impedance path for sound to flow away from the ear canal. Because the impedance of a tube decreases with frequency, the low-frequency portion of the response (below roughly 1000 Hz) is more affected by the vent than the higher frequencies. Figure 2–23 shows the simulated effect of venting a normal sized ear canal (1.4 cm from shell tip to eardrum, 0.75 cm canal diameter) with a parallel vent 1.2 cm long with a 0.2 cm internal diameter. Below 600 Hz the vented response is less than the unvented, and above 2000 Hz the two responses are essentially the same. Between these two points, the vented response is greater than the unvented. The peak of this resonance (about 850 Hz for the normal ear canal) is affected by several variables: the length and diameter of the vent, the size of the ear canal, and the impedance of the middle ear.

Figure 2–23 also shows the effect upon the vent response produced by changing the size of the residual ear canal volume (the volume between the shell tip and the eardrum). For the ear canal B2, which is 2 standard deviations larger than normal (see Fig. 2–20 for the canal dimensions of B2 and S2), the resonant peak is shifted downward from 850 Hz to 600 Hz, and only frequencies less than 400 Hz are attenuated. The reverse effect is seen for the small canal S2; only frequencies less than 1000 Hz are attenuated, and the resonant peak is shifted upward in frequency. The addition of a vent is usually thought of as a way of reducing the low-frequency response of the hearing aid, thereby providing a high frequency emphasis. Actually, the presence of the vent can enhance the hearing aid output between 500 and 1000 Hz. This effect is exaggerated for larger ear canals.

Figure 2–24 shows the simulated vent responses for the model terminated with abnormal middle ears. In each case, the residual ear canal size is normal. Qualitatively, the effect of reducing the impedance of the middle ear is similar to increasing the size of the ear canal. The model suggests that increasing the impedance of the middle ear will increase the magnitude of the resonance peak, particularly for middle ear effusion. Perhaps this sharp peak could increase the tendency of the hearing aid to feedback.

## Variability in the RECD

As part of a project for the fabrication and evaluation of the Zwislocki coupler, SPLs were measured on 11 human ears, converted to eardrum SPL and compared to SPLs developed in a 2-cc coupler (Sachs and Burkhard, 1972). The Zwislocki coupler response agreed with the mean real-ear data within ±2 dB up to 7000 Hz. Variability across subjects was lowest below 1000 Hz (standard

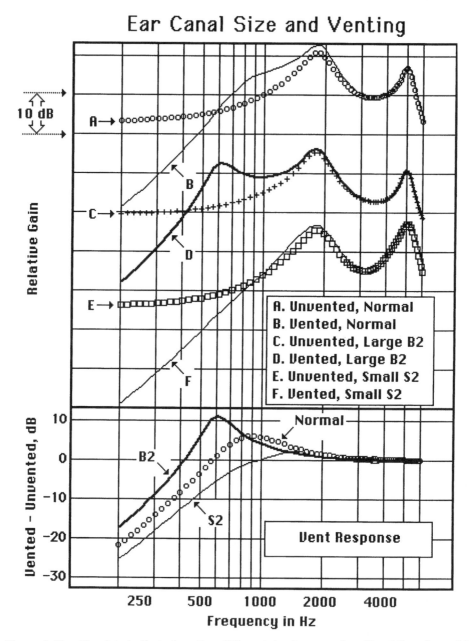

**Figure 2–23.**   Simulated effect of venting different sized ear canals with a 1.2 cm long, 0.2 cm diameter parallel vent.

deviation of about 1.5 dB), and increased to standard deviations of 3.5 to 5 dB for the higher frequencies. The mean response (see Fig. 2–4) indicated real-ear SPLs about 3.5 dB greater than coupler SPLs up to 800 Hz, then gradually increasing to about 8 dB at 2000 Hz, 14 dB at 6000 Hz. Subsequent research has generally been in agreement with these findings, except for the lower frequencies where slit

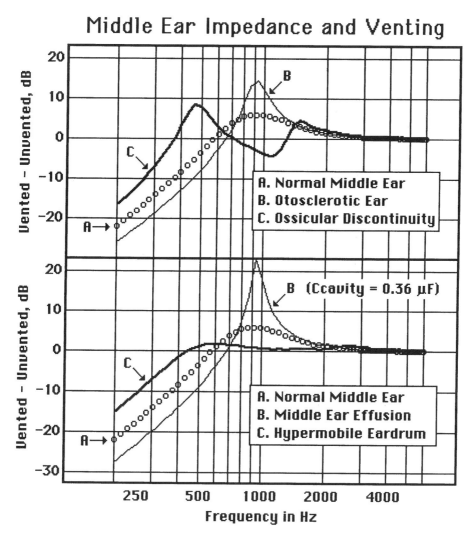

**Figure 2–24.** Simulated effect of venting different middle ears with a 1.2 cm long, 0.2 cm diameter parallel vent. Ear canal size was normal.

leaks have been implicated as a cause for reduced real-ear SPL (Larson et al., 1977). Hawkins, Cooper, and Thompson (1990) obtained RECDs for 30 normal adults, 25 females and 5 males, aged 23 to 56 years. The results ranged from about –6 dB at 250 Hz, 0 dB at 500 Hz to 12 dB at 6000 Hz, indicating greater SPL in the real ear than in the coupler, except for the lowest frequencies. They suggested that leakage around the foam earmolds may have reduced the real-ear output and, because earmolds are seldom airtight, this might be a more realistic estimate of typical performance. Standard deviations across subjects ranged from 2 to 5 dB. In contrast, Fikret-Pasa and Revit (1992), also using a foam earmold, reported a mean RECD virtually identical to that obtained by Sachs and Burkhard (1972).

Figure 2–25 illustrates the models predictions regarding small leaks, which were simulated as narrow diameter parallel vents. The ear canal, terminated by a normal middle ear, is slightly wider than normal (0.82 cm). The ER-3A foam earplug is assumed to be 1.2 cm long, so the distance from the earplug to the eardrum is 2.0 cm. The leaks were simulated by equivalent vents 1.2 cm long, and 0.075 (V1) and 0.15 cm (V2) diameter. In the top panel, the real-ear response, both sealed and leaking, is compared to a closed HA-1 coupler. In the bottom panel, the coupler response, closed and leaking, is compared to a sealed real ear.

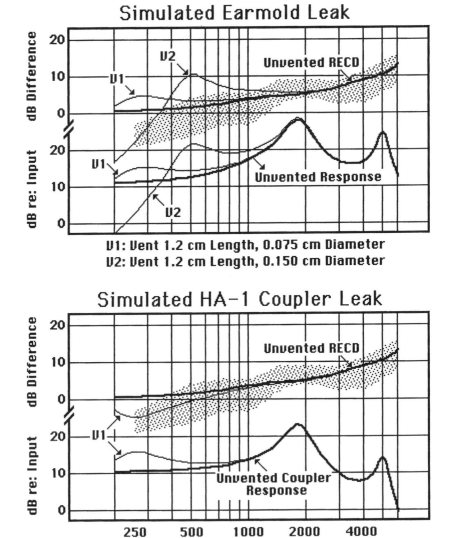

**Figure 2–25.** Simulated effect of earmold and coupler leaks on the real-ear coupler difference.

The shaded area represents ±1 standard deviation from the mean for the real-ear HA-1 coupler difference (Hawkins et al., 1990). Venting the real-ear response increased the low-frequency portion of the RECD curve or produced unusual resonances that were not like the data reported by Hawkins, Cooper, and Thompson (1990). However, slightly increasing the diameter of the ear canal to 0.82 cm, and adding a slight leak to the coupler produced a simulated RECD that was quite similar to their data.

The top portion of Figure 2–21, in addition to showing the effects on real-ear response, also illustrates the difference from normal that would be expected in the RECD. The otosclerotic ear would have a slightly larger low-frequency RECD, whereas the ear with the more mobile system would have a RECD curve less than normal for the low frequencies, and slightly greater than normal between 1000 and 2000 Hz. Figure 2–26 shows the changes produced in the RECD for one subject (the author) when a large negative middle ear pressure was induced by a reverse Valsalva procedure (TPP < –500 daPa). The difference between the two curves (before and after the creation of the negative middle ear pressure) is given in the bottom of the figure. Positive dB values indicated greater ear canal SPLs with the reduced middle ear pressure. The stiffening effect is similar to that obtained for the otosclerotic ear simulation. The method for measuring the RECD was the same as that described by Fikret-Pasa and Revit (1992), except that the probe tube was not threaded through the foam ER-3A plug, but was placed between it and the canal wall. The probe tip was located at the eardrum.

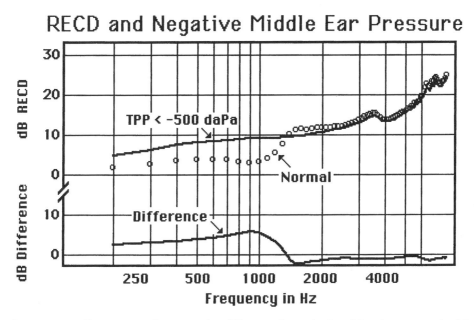

**Figure 2–26.** Change in real-ear coupler difference for a single subject for a normal middle ear pressure (circles) versus a negative middle ear pressure (thick line).

Fikret-Pasa and Revit (1992) obtained RECD measurements on 18 ears of 15 (9 male, 6 female) subjects aged 43 to 86 years seen consecutively for hearing aid selection at a university clinic. Although most diagnoses indicated presbycusis, there were middle ear anomalies such as a neomembrane of the eardrum, otosclerosis, perforated eardrum, large canal volumes, and both increased and decreased middle ear admittance. As might be expected, larger intersubject standard deviations (than found by other authors) were obtained, roughly 5 to 8 dB across frequency. One subject, with a perforation, had an RECD more than 20 dB less than normal for the lower frequencies, another subject had an RECD about 7 dB higher than normal for all frequencies. Many subjects, however, had RECDs comparable to the norm, or what would be expected from changes in probe depth (e.g., curves D and E of Fig. 2–6).

Figure 2–27 shows the RECDs obtained for three individuals with unilateral perforations. These subjects' REURs were given in Figure 2–10, and their tympanometric and audiometric results were described in the text associated with this figure. Perhaps the most prominent feature of the RECDs for the perforations is the approximate 15 dB reduction in low-frequency response. The greatest reduction occurred at 500 Hz for BR and JL, who both had similar RECDs. For JW the maximum reduction was at 1300 Hz, and her RECD was qualitatively different from the others, as was the REUR. JW's tympanometric results were not obviously different from the others, but she did have a hearing loss (35 dB HL) in the perforated ear. It is not clear why the conductive hearing loss would precipitate this difference. Figure 2–28 shows the RECD for KD's ear with the modified radical mastoidectomy (see Fig. 2–11 for this subject's REUR). Compared to the unoperated left ear, the RECD for the right ear is about 20 dB less. It is interesting that a prominent notch in the RECD for the right ear occurs at 4500 Hz. Normally, a notch like this would be expected if the probe were placed about 20 mm from the eardrum. KD's REUR shows a peak at 1400 Hz which, from the computer model, would suggest an effective canal length of approximately 5.7 cm. Because the probe was placed 30 mm from the tragus, it is possible that this notch could be explained as the result of probe placement depth.

Using functional gain measures, it has been determined that some individuals have RECDs that are statistically significantly different (Shum, 1986). Zelisko, Seewald and Gagné (1992) calculated within-subject, across-session standard deviations in real-ear SPL used to determine the RECD. They found an average standard deviation of about 1.5 dB across frequency; the largest mean standard deviation was about 2 dB at a frequency just less than 6000 Hz.

Children tend to have RECDs that are greater than adults (Feigin et al., 1989). Presumably, this is due to the smaller size of the ear canal. They compared 31 children under the age of 5 years to 21 adults, and found the mean RECD for children to be 5 dB greater than the adult over the range from 1000 to 3000 Hz. There was slightly more variability across subjects for the children (standard deviation of 2.6 dB), than the adults (1.9 dB). Variability was less in the midfrequencies, and greatest for the lower and higher frequencies (standard deviations of about 4.5 to 6 dB). They predicted that the children's data would fall within 1 standard deviation of the adults by 7.7 years of age. A tympanometrically measured ear canal volume could account for only 49% of the total variance in the

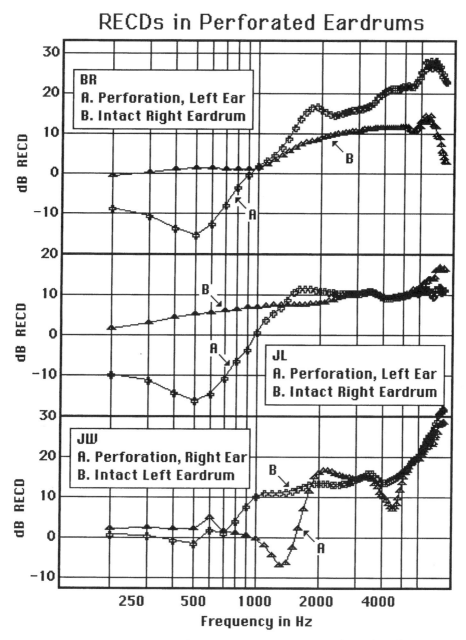

**Figure 2–27.**   Real-ear coupler differences for subjects with perforated eardrums as compared to their intact eardrums.

data, and they suggested that ear canal length and middle ear impedance may interact with volume to influence the RECD. Figure 2–29 shows that the model predicts changes in RECD as the ear canal size changes and that these changes are generally consistent with the differences Feigin, Kopun, Stelmachowicz, and Gorga (1989) found between adult and children's ears. Standard deviations of 2.9

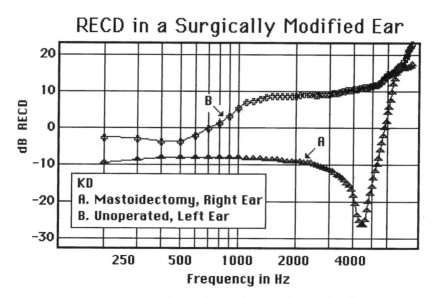

**Figure 2–28.** Real-ear coupler difference for a subject with a modified radical mastoidectomy in the right ear as compared to the unoperated left ear.

to 5.8 dB have been reported for the intersubject variation in the real-ear SPL developed by ER-3A earphones (Valente et al., 1994). These values are similar to those shown in Figure 2–29, suggesting that variation in canal size could have accounted for at least part of the measured differences. All curves in the figure are plotted relative to the normal RECD associated with a residual canal size of 1.4 cm in length and 0.75 cm diameter. Curves B1 and S1 were computed from

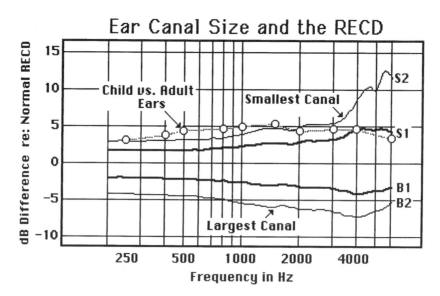

**Figure 2–29.** Changes in RECD produced by varying the size of the ear canal.

canal lengths and diameters ±1 standard deviations larger and smaller than normal. Curves B2 and S2 are ±2 SDs larger and smaller (see Fig. 2–20 for canal dimensions). Data points (circles) are the mean differences between child and adult RECD (Feigin et al., 1989). Positive values indicate a greater SPL in the ear canal than normal.

Nelson Barlow, Auslander, Rines, and Stelmachowicz (1988) also found that a tympanometric ear canal volume (Vec) estimate obtained at –400 daPa was a poor predictor of the RECD. Possible reasons for this might include Vec not being sensitive to variation in ear canal diameter versus ear canal length, because the model predicts that canal diameter affects the hearing aid response differently from length. It is possible that the residual ear canal volume at the immittance probe tip would be different from the volume created with the earmold. Although a –400 daPa pressure significantly stiffens the eardrum, middle ear impedance is not driven to infinity. Consequently, Vec is an overestimate of true ear canal volume; Vec is contaminated by the residual compliance of the middle ear. This is unfortunate because it would be desirable to have a simple measure that could account for the effects of ear canal size.

RECDs for nine adolescents were reported by Zelisko, Seewald, and Gagné (1992). Across subjects, differences ranged to almost 12 dB, in contrast to intra-subject standard deviations of 1.5 dB (95% confidence interval of about 2.9 dB) obtained by testing each subject on three separate occasions. It appears that when measures are carefully performed, measurement error can be much less than intersubject variability.

## Summary

Compensating for individual variation identified by probe microphone measurements holds the promise of a more accurate fit and increased patient benefit from the hearing aid. Prior to ordering the hearing aid, probe microphone measurements, such as the REUR and RECD, can be performed to verify that the individual ear is typical or deviates significantly enough to justify modifying the hearing aid response. From 2-cc coupler data it is possible to predict the performance of this hearing aid on the average individual and to use probe microphone measures to verify or disprove this assumption. Depending upon the flexibility of the hearing aid being fit, it may be possible to compensate for any differences. However, it is important to realize that any corrections made are only valid if the measurements are reasonably accurate. Measurement error can be quite small if reasonable precautions are taken, or quite large with careless inattention to detail. Use of a quiet environment, careful positioning of the probe microphone (within approximately 8 mm of the eardrum), maintaining the loudspeaker location at a 45° azimuth and 30-cm distance from the subject's head, use of a reference microphone to help control for head movements, and reflections from movements of obstacles in the sound field can all help to minimize measurement error.

Fine facial details, the size of the head, presence of hair, and clothing are likely to produce minimal amounts of individual variation, up to at least 6000 Hz. Figure 2–30 compares the average human free-field transform (Shaw and

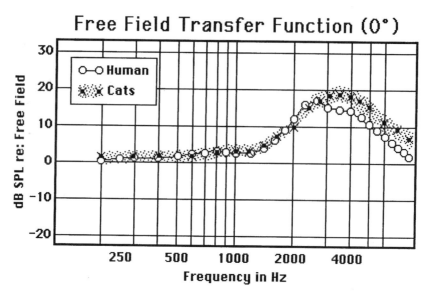

**Figure 2–30.** The 0° azimuth free-field-to-eardrum transform for humans (circles, connected by thin lines), and data for five cats (crosses, approximate range given by shaded area). Human data is from Shaw and Vaillancourt (1985), feline data is from Wiener, Pfeiffer, and Backus (1966).

Vaillancourt, 1985) with that obtained from five cats (Wiener et al., 1966). Despite obvious differences in head and body size, facial features, etc., the cat data is remarkably similar to the human data. This was also noted by other researchers who performed similar measures on domestic cats (Musicant et al., 1990). Major differences are in the higher frequencies and are presumed to relate to differences in ear canal size and larger cat middle ear impedance (Møller, 1974). The size and shape of the human pinna and concha are difficult to quantify and, therefore, it is difficult to specify their effect. Sharp antiresonances produced by these structures are usually beyond 6000 Hz. Whereas these antiresonances may be important cues for localization, present hearing aid technology would make it difficult to preserve these cues and perhaps unnecessary, considering the poor high-frequency sensitivity of most hearing aid wearers. The length, diameter, and taper of the ear canal can have a pronounced effect on both unaided and aided measures. Differences in ear canal size can effect changes in real-ear SPL and could account for some of the variability in subjective measures used to fit hearing aids, such as the loudness discomfort level. Variation in ear canal diameter seems to be one variable with the potential for eliciting the most dramatic effects. Stiffening pathology of the middle ear (i.e., otosclerosis and reduced middle ear pressure) seems to have minimal effects upon either the RECD or REAR. However, under certain circumstances, especially with middle ear effusion, fairly large changes can be observed in the REUR. Middle ear effusion is a common occurrence, especially in children, yet it seems that little is known about its effects. The model predicts that the REAR is probably not severely affected when effusion is simulated by reducing middle ear volume. However, as can be seen in

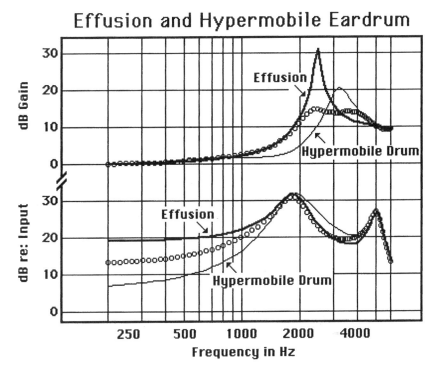

**Figure 2–31.** Model predictions for the normal ear (circles), middle ear effusion (thick line), and a hypermobile eardrum (thin line).

Figure 2–31 (and discussed previously in Fig. 2–14), potentially large increases in the REUR are predicted in the vicinity of 2000 to 3000 Hz by reducing *Ccavity* to 0.12 µF. This would correspond to a volume of only 0.17 ml for the entire middle ear space, and the total input admittance to the middle ear at 250 Hz was only 0.11 mmho. It would be interesting to experimentally verify this effect, especially because many children with effusion have unusual audiograms, that is, "inverted notches" with peaks of good hearing close to 2000 Hz. A common sequel of middle ear disease is an atrophic or hypermobile tympanic membrane that is characterized by a tympanogram with a high peak admittance. For the example in Figure 2–31, admittance at 250 Hz was 2.51 mmho for the hypermobile eardrum as compared to 0.89 mmho for the normal ear (curve shown by the circles). Simulation suggests that this effect on the impedance of the ear changes the REUR and REAR in a manner similar to that produced by a (more rare) ossicular discontinuity. This, too, deserves experimental verification so that common conditions affecting hearing aid performance might be better understood.

## References

American National Standards Institute. (1987). American National Standard Specifications of Hearing Aid Characteristics. (ANSI S3.22-1987). New York: ANSI.

Bade P, Engebretson AM, Heidbreder AF, Niemoller AF. (1984). Use of a personal computer to model the electroacoustics of hearing aids. *J Acoust Soc Am* 75:617–620.

Bentler RA. (1989). External ear resonance characteristics in children. *J Speech Hear Dis* 54:264–268.

Bentler RA, Pavlovic CV. (1989). Transfer functions and correction factors used in hearing aid evaluation and research. *Ear Hear* 10:58–63.

Bentler RA, Pavlovic CV. (1992). Addendum to "Transfer functions and correction factors used in hearing aid evaluation and research." *Ear Hear* 13:284–286.

Bryant HW. (1972). Comparable coupler and real-ear measurements on supraaural and insert-type earphones. *J Acoust Soc Am* 52:1599–1606.

Burkhard MD, Sachs RM. (1975). Anthropomorphic manikin for acoustic research. *J Acoust Soc Am* 58:214–222.

Burkhard MD, Sachs RM. (1977). Sound pressure in insert earphone couplers and real ears. *J Speech Hear Res* 20:799–807.

Burnett ED, Beck LB. (1987). A correction for converting 2 $cm^3$ coupler responses to insertion responses for custom in-the-ear nondirectional hearing aids. *Ear Hear (Suppl)* 8:89S–94S.

Byrne DB, Upfold MA. (1991). Implications of ear canal resonance for hearing aid fitting. *Semin Hear* 12:34–41.

Chan JCK, Geisler CD. (1990). Estimation of eardrum acoustic pressure and ear canal length from remote points in the canal. *J Acoust Soc Am* 87:1237–1247.

de Jonge RR. (1982). *Computer Simulation of Differences Between Coupler and Real-Ear Gain.* Presented at the meeting of the American Speech-Language-Hearing Association, Toronto, November, 1982.

de Jonge RR. (1983). Computer simulation of hearing aid frequency responses. *Hear J* 35(4):27–31.

Dempster JH, Mackenzie K. (1990). The resonance frequency of the external auditory canal in children. *Hear Instrum* 11:296–298.

Dillon H, Murray M. (1987). Accuracy of twelve methods for estimating the real ear gain of hearing aids. *Ear Hear* 8:2–11.

Dirks DD, Gilman S. (1979). Exploring azimuth effects with an anthropometric manikin. *J Acoust Soc Am* 66:696–701.

Dirks DD, Kincaid GE. (1987). Basic acoustic considerations of ear canal probe measurements. *Ear Hear (Suppl)* 8:60S–67S.

Egolf DP. (1977). Mathematical modeling of a probe-tube microphone. *J Acoust Soc Am* 61:200–205.

Egolf DP. (1980). Techniques for modeling the hearing aid receiver and associated tubing. In: Studebaker GA, Hochberg I, eds. *Acoustical Factors Affecting Hearing Aid Performance.* Baltimore: University Park Press, pp. 297–319.

Egolf DP, Feth LL, Cooper WA, Franks JR. (1985). Effects of normal and pathologic eardrum impedance on sound pressure in the aided ear canal: A computer simulation. *J Acoust Soc Am* 78:1281–1285.

Egolf DP, Haley BT, Larson VD. (1986). The constant-volume-velocity nature of hearing aids: Conclusions based on computer simulations. *J Acoust Soc Am* 79:1592–1602.

Egolf DP, Haley BT, Bauer DM, Howell HC, Larson VD. (1988a). Experimental determination of cascade parameters of a hearing-aid microphone via the two-load method. *J Acoust Soc Am* 83:2349–2446.

Egolf DP, Haley BT, Howell HC, Larson VD. (1988b). A technique for simulating the amplifier-to-eardrum transfer function of an in situ hearing aid. *J Acoust Soc Am* 84:1–10.

Egolf DP, Haley BT, Howell HC, Legowski S, Larson VD. (1989). Simulating the open-loop transfer function as a means for understanding acoustic feedback in hearing aids. *J Acoust Soc Am* 85:454–467.

Feigin JA, Kopun JG, Stelmachowicz PG, Gorga MP. (1989). Probe-tube microphone measures of ear-canal sound pressure levels in infants and children. *Ear Hear* 10:254–258.

Feigin JA, Nelson Barlow NL, Stelmachowicz PG. (1990). The effect of reference microphone placement on sound pressure levels at an ear level hearing aid microphone. *Ear Hear* 11:321–326.

Feldman AS. (1963). Impedance measurements at the eardrum as an aid to diagnosis. *J Speech Hear Res* 6:315–327.

Fikret-Pasa S, Revit LJ. (1992). Individualized correction factors in the preselection of hearing aids. *J Speech Hear Res* 35:384–400.

Gardner MB, Hawley MS. (1972). Network representation of the external ear. *J Acoust Soc Am* 52:1620–1628.

Gartrell EL, Church GT. (1990). Effect of microphone location in ITE versus BTE hearing aids. *J Am Acad Audiol* 1:151–153.

Gerhardt KJ, Rodriguez GP, Hepler EL, Moul ML. (1987). Ear canal volume and variability in the patterns of temporary threshold shifts. *Ear Hear* 8:316–321.

Gilman S, Dirks DD, Stern R. (1981). The effect of occluded ear impedances on the eardrum SPL produced by hearing aids. *J Acoust Soc Am* 70:370–386.

Gilman S, Dirks DD. (1986). Acoustics of ear canal measurement of eardrum SPL in simulators. *J Acoust Soc Am* 80:783–793.

Goode RL, Friedrichs R, Falk S. (1977). Effect on hearing thresholds of surgical modification of the external ear. *Ann Otol* 86:441–450.

Hawkins DB. (1987). Variability in clinical ear canal microphone measurements. *Hear Instrum* 38(1):30–32.

Hawkins DB, Mueller HG. (1986). Some variables affecting the accuracy of probe tube microphone measurements. *Hear Instrum* 37(1):8–12, 49–50.

Hawkins DB, Cooper WA, Thompson DJ. (1990). Comparisons among SPL in real ears, 2 cm³ and 6 cm³ couplers. *J Am Acad Audiol* 1:154–161.

Hudde H. (1983a). Estimation of the area function of human ear canals by sound pressure measurements. *J Acoust Soc Am* 73:24–31.

Hudde H. (1983b). Measurement of the eardrum impedance of human ears. *J Acoust Soc Am* 73:242–247.

Humes LE, Hipskind NM, Block MG. (1988). Insertion gain measured with three probe tube systems. *Ear Hear* 9:108–112.

Johansen PA. (1975). Measurement of the human ear canal. *Acustica* 33:349–351.

Kates JM. (1988a). Acoustic effects in in-the-ear hearing aid response: Results from a computer simulation. *Ear Hear* 9:119–132.

Kates JM. (1988b). A computer simulation of hearing aid response and the effects of ear canal size. *J Acoust Soc Am* 83:1952–1963.

Keefe DH, Bulen JC, Arehart KH, Burns EM. (1993). Ear-canal impedance and reflection coefficient in human infants and adults. *J Acoust Soc Am* 94:2617–2638.

Killion MC, Monser EL. (1980). CORFIG: Coupler response for flat insertion gain. In: Studebaker GA, Hochberg I, eds. *Acoustical Factors Affecting Hearing Aid Performance.* Baltimore: University Park Press, pp. 149–168.

Killion MC, Revit LJ. (1987). Insertion gain repeatability versus loudspeaker location: You want me to put my loudspeaker WHERE? *Ear Hear (Suppl)* 8:68S–73S.

Killion MC, Revit LJ. (1993). CORFIG and GIFROC: Real ear to coupler and back again. In: Studebaker GA, Hochberg I, eds. *Acoustical Factors Affecting Hearing Aid Performance,* 2nd ed. Boston: Allyn and Bacon, pp. 65–85.

Kruger B. (1987). An update on the external ear resonance in infants and young children. *Ear Hear* 8:333–336.

Kuhn GF, Burnett ED. (1977). Acoustic pressure field alongside a manikin's head with a view towards in situ hearing-aid tests. *J Acoust Soc Am* 62:416–423.

Kuhn GF. (1979). The pressure transformation from a diffuse sound field to the external ear and to the body and head surface. *J Acoust Soc Am* 65:991–1000.

Kuhn GF. (1980). Some effects of microphone location, signal bandwidth, and incident wave field on the hearing aid input signal. In: Studebaker GA, Hochberg I, eds. *Acoustical Factors Affecting Hearing Aid Performance.* Baltimore: University Park Press, pp. 55–80.

Larson VD, Studebaker GA, Cox RM. (1977). Sound levels in a 2-cc cavity, a Zwislocki coupler, and occluded ear canals. *J Am Audiol Soc* 3:63–70.

Larson VD, Egolf DP, Cooper WA. (1991). Application of acoustic impedance measures to hearing aid fitting strategies. In: Studebaker GA, Bess FH, Beck LB, eds. *The Vanderbilt Hearing Aid Report II.* Parkton, MD: York Press, pp. 165-174.

Lutman ME, Martin AM. (1979). Development of an electroacoustic analogue model of the middle ear and acoustic reflex. *J Sound Vibr* 64:133–157.

Lybarger SF. (1985). Earmolds. In: Katz J, ed. *Handbook of Clinical Audiology,* 3rd ed. Baltimore: Williams and Wilkins, pp. 885–910.

Mehrgardt S, Mellert V. (1977). Transformation characteristics of the external human ear. *J Acoust Soc Am* 61:1567–1576.

Møller AR. (1961). Network model of the middle ear. *J Acoust Soc Am* 33:168–176.

Møller AG. (1974). Function of the middle ear. In: Keidel WD, Neff WD, eds. *Handbook of Sensory Physiology.* Vol. 1. Berlin: Springer Verlag, pp. 491–517.

Moodie KS, Seewald RC, Sinclair ST. (1994). Procedure for predicting real-ear hearing aid performance in young children. *Am J Audiol* 3:23–31.

Moskal NL, Goldstein DP. (1992). Probe tube systems: Effects of equalization on real ear insertion and aided gain. *Ear Hear* 13:46–54.

Mueller HG. (1989). Individualizing the ordering of custom hearing instruments. *Hear Instrum* 40(2):18–22.

Musicant AD, Chan JCK, Hind JE. (1990). Direction-dependent spectral properties of cat external ear: New data and cross-species comparisons. *J Acoust Soc Am* 87:757–781.

Nelson Barlow NL, Auslander MC, Rines D, Stelmachowicz PG. (1988). Probe-tube microphone measures in hearing-impaired children and adults. *Ear Hear* 9:243–247.

Oliveira RJ, Hammer B, Stillman A, Holm J, Jons C, Margolis RH. (1992). A look at ear canal changes with jaw motion. *Ear Hear* 13:464–466.

Olson HF. (1957). *Acoustical Engineering.* Princeton, NJ: D. Van Nostrand, pp. 17–24, 89, 116–117.

Onchi Y. (1961). Mechanism of the middle ear. *J Acoust Soc Am* 33:794–805.

Rabinowitz WM. (1981). Measurement of the acoustic input immittance of the human ear. *J Acoust Soc Am* 70:1025–1036.

Ringdahl A, Leijon A. (1984). The reliability of insertion gain measurements using probe microphones in the ear canal. *Scand Audiol* 13:173–178.

Rodriguez GP, Gerhardt KJ. (1991). Influence of outer ear resonant frequency on patterns of temporary threshold shift. *Ear Hear* 12:110–114.

Sachs RM, Burkhard MD. (1972). *Zwislocki coupler evaluation with insert earphones. Report No. 20022-1.* Franklin Park, IL: Knowles Electronics.

Schum DJ. (1986). Inter-subject variability effects on coupler to real ear correction curves. *Hear Instrum* 37(3):25–26.

Seewald RC, Sinclair ST, Moodie KS. (1994). *Predictive accuracy of a procedure for electroacoustic fitting in young children.* Presented at the meeting of the American Academy of Audiology, Richmond, VA, April, 1994.

Shaw EAG. (1966). Earcanal pressure generated by a free sound field. *J Acoust Soc Am* 39:465–470.

Shaw EAG. (1974a). Transformation of sound pressure level from the free field to the eardrum in the horizontal plane. *J Acoust Soc Am* 56:1848–1861.

Shaw EAG. (1974b). The external ear. In: Keidel WD, Neff WD, eds. *Handbook of Sensory Physiology.* Vol. 1. Berlin: Springer Verlag, pp. 455–490.

Shaw EAG. (1980). The acoustics of the external ear. In: Studebaker GA, Hochberg I, eds. *Acoustical Factors Affecting Hearing Aid Performance.* Baltimore: University Park Press, pp. 109–125.

Shaw EAG, Vaillancourt MM. (1985). Transformation of sound-pressure level from the free field to the eardrum presented in numerical form. *J Acoust Soc Am* 78:1120–1123.

Shotland LI, Hecox KE. (1990). The effect of probe tube reference placement on sound pressure level variability. *Ear Hear* 11:306–309.

Sinclair ST, Beauchaine LK, Moodie KS, Feigin JA, Seewald RC, Stelmachowicz PG. (1994). *Repeatability of real-ear to coupler difference measurement as a function of age.* Presented at the American Academy of Audiology Meeting, Richmond, VA, April, 1994.

Stinson MR, Shaw EAG, Lawton BW. (1982). Estimation of acoustical energy reflectance at the eardrum from measurements of pressure distribution in the human ear canal. *J Acoust Soc Am* 72:766–773.

Stinson MR. (1985). The spatial distribution of sound pressure within scaled replicas of the human ear canal. *J Acoust Soc Am* 78:1596–1602.

Studebaker GA, Cox RM. (1977). Side branch and parallel vent effects in real ears and in acoustical and electrical models. *J Am Audiol Soc* 3:108–117.

Tecca JE. (1991). Reliability of insertion gain measures. *Semin Hear* 12:15–25.

Teranishi R, Shaw EAG. (1968). External-ear acoustic models with simple Geometry. *J Acoust Soc Am* 44:257–263.

Upfold G, Byrne D. (1988). Variability of earcanal resonance and its implications for the design of hearing aids and earplugs. *Aust J Audiol* 10:97–102.

Valente M, Meister M, Smith P, Goebel J. (1990). Intratester test-retest reliability of insertion gain measures. *Ear Hear* 11:181–184.

Valente M, Potts G, Valente M, Vass W, Goebel J. (1994). Intersubject variability of real-ear sound pressure level: Conventional and insert earphones. *Am J Audiol* 5:390–398.

Valente M, Valente M, Goebel J. (1991). Reliability and intersubject variability of the real ear unaided response. *Ear Hear* 12:216–220.

White REC, Studebaker GA, Levitt H, Mook D. (1980). The application of modeling techniques to the study of hearing aid acoustic systems. In: Studebaker GA, Hochberg I, eds. *Acoustical Factors Affecting Hearing Aid Performance.* Baltimore: University Park Press, pp. 267–296.

Wiener FM, Ross DA. (1946). The pressure distribution in the auditory canal in a progressive sound field. *J Acoust Soc Am* 18:401–408.

Wiener FM. (1947). On the diffraction of a progressive sound wave by the human head. *J Acoust Soc Am* 19:143–146.

Wiener FM, Pfeiffer RR, Backus ASN. (1966). On the sound pressure transformation by the head and auditory meatus of the cat. *Acta Otolaryngol (Stockh)* 61:255–269.

Zelisko DLC, Seewald RC, Gagné JP. (1992). Signal delivery/real ear measurement system for hearing aid selection and fitting. *Ear Hear* 13:460–463.

Zemplenyi J, Gilman S, Dirks D. (1985). Optical method for measurement of ear canal length. *J Acoust Soc Am* 78:2146–2148.

Zwislocki J. (1957). Some impedance measures on normal and pathologic ears. *J Acoust Soc Am* 29:1312–1317.

Zwislocki J. (1962). Analysis of middle-ear function. Part I: Input impedance. *J Acoust Soc Am* 34:1514–1523.

Zwislocki J. (1963). An acoustic method for clinical examination of the ear. *J Speech Hear Res* 6:303–314.

Zwislocki J. (1976). The acoustic middle ear function. In: Feldman AS, Wilber LA, eds. *Acoustic Impedance and Admittance—The Measurement of Middle Ear Function*. Baltimore: Williams and Wilkins, pp. 66–77.

# 3

## Microphone, Receiver, and Telecoil Options: Past, Present, and Future

### PETER L. MADAFFARI
### W. KENT STANLEY

### Introduction

In this chapter, the authors will describe the role transducers play in the performance of a hearing aid. The transducer is defined, and an overview is given of the history of transducer development. This is followed by a description of how transducers work and the various technologies that are applicable to the fitting of hearing aids. In a later section, the performance of transducers is described as well as the difference between active, that is, internally amplified, versus passive devices.

Of practical interest to an audiologist, the limitations in performance as well as the causes of malfunction and failure are explained. Some discussion is provided of the future development of transducers. Finally, a synopsis of options is presented as a possible guide to the audiologist so that the information may be used to provide more successful hearing aid fittings.

### Transducer: Definition and Function

Just what is a transducer? A transducer is, by definition, a device that transforms energy in one energy system to energy in another. In this sense, an electrical motor is a transducer, transforming energy in the electrical system to energy in the mechanical system.

The transducers used in a hearing aid provide the internal electronic circuits a means of communicating with the outside world—their ears and voices. In the specific case of hearing aids, the transducers presently used for ears are microphones and telecoils; the ones used for voices are receivers.

A microphone is a device that converts the acoustical energy of a sound field to electrical energy. A telecoil, or telephone pickup coil, is a device that converts the energy in an electromagnetic wave into electrical energy. A receiver is a device that converts electrical energy into acoustic energy of a sound field.

The jargon of various industries uses these terms in somewhat different ways. For example, in the hearing aid industry, the word "microphone" is almost universally used for the device converting acoustic energy to electrical energy. However, the telephone industry often uses the word "transmitter" for this conversion device.

The word "telecoil," which seems to be unique to the hearing aid industry, is a shortening of the term "telephone pickup coil." This term derives from the usage of the device to "pick up" the magnetic field produced by every telephone handset and to transform that signal into a corresponding electrical signal.

The word "receiver" is also used in many ways (e.g., TV receiver) but, in the hearing aid industry, it is used, as in the telephone industry, to designate the device used to transform the electrical output of the amplifier to acoustic pressure at the ear.

When used in hearing aids, these transducers function as interfaces between the hearing aid electrical circuits and the outside world. A close analogy is a sound-reinforcing or public address system. In this situation, microphones pick up the various sources of sound and send corresponding electrical signals to the amplifiers. The amplifiers alter the input signals to produce an electrical output that will drive the loudspeaker to produce the desired acoustic sound levels.

The hearing aid microphones in current use are electret devices that have rather good linear behavior over a frequency range of 50 Hz to 6000 Hz, and the technology is available to extend this to a range of 20 Hz to 20,000 Hz and beyond. This range can be modified somewhat by the acoustic connections used to couple the microphone to the incoming sound wave or by modifications internal to the microphone. Figure 3–1 shows the frequency response characteristics for six commercially available microphones.

The other input device is the telecoil. Telephone handsets are required to produce some minimum level of external electromagnetic field in order to provide a nonacoustic link to the hearing aid. This is the dominant United States application while, in Europe, telecoils are generally used with loop transmission signals in conjunction with public address systems. The telecoil is designed to detect the electromagnetic fields radiating from telephones and originated by loop transmission fields. The telecoil transforms these signals into an electrical signal that can drive the amplifier of a hearing aid. For a constant field strength, the output signal has a frequency response that rises at 6 dB/octave. Telecoils are also made with integral amplifiers to both raise the level of the output signal and to alter the frequency response (e.g., The Tibbetts Industries PowerCoil™). Some representative response curves are shown in Figure 3–2.

Most hearing aid designers prefer that the input transducer (i.e., the microphone or telecoil) has a frequency response that is either flat (horizontal) or rising to, at most one peak. In that situation, the amplifier does not have to be designed to compensate for a multitude of frequency-dependent irregularities from the input transducer. The designer of the amplifier has enough problems providing compensation for the wide variability of the intersubject frequency sensitivity of hearing-impaired ears and the inescapable peaks and troughs in the frequency

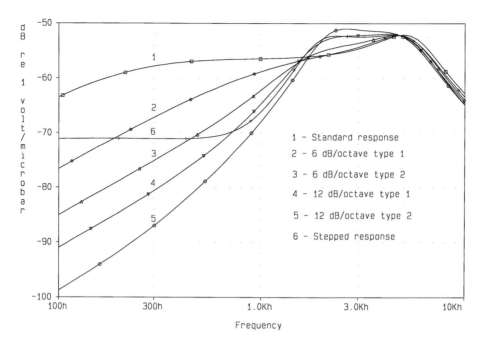

**Figure 3–1.** Microphone frequency response.

response of the combination of the receiver, as well as the acoustic coupling to the ear canal.

The receiver is usually a balanced armature magnetic transducer. These transducers contain a plethora of electrical, mechanical, and acoustical reactive elements with coupled resonances. This results in a transducer that is highly "colored." That is, when driven with a constant-current electrical signal and coupled directly to an acoustic cavity, such as the ear canal or an artificial one of similar size, these transducers show one major peak in acoustic output caused by the receivers natural resonance followed by a smaller peak caused by the acoustic path required to couple the receiver to the acoustic load. Often the receiver is some distance from the ear canal, as in behind-the-ear (BTE) applications. The extra tubing connecting the receiver to the canal will cause additional resonant peaks. Figure 3–3 shows the acoustic pressure obtained when a typical receiver is coupled to a 2-cc earphone coupler (ANSI S3.7, 1973) with various tubing lengths. The locations of the peaks and valleys are dependent upon the internal construction of the receiver. Diffraction about the human head (Madaffari, 1974) and, in addition, resonances of the ear canal (Shaw, 1974) will also affect the frequency response. In addition, location of the aid as, for example, BTE versus in-the-ear (ITE), will modify these conditions to different extents, and it is partially a responsibility of the aid to compensate for these effects.

All the transducers (Figs. 3–1, 3–2, and 3–3), and particularly the receivers (Fig. 3–3), have considerable influence on the design requirements for the hearing aid electrical circuits and for the acoustic connection to the ear.

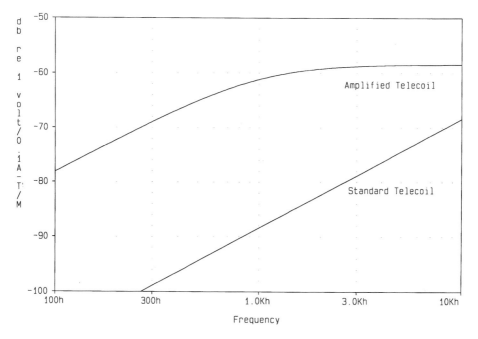

**Figure 3–2.**  Standard and amplified telecoil.

## Transducer History

The design of transducers for hearing aids has always been driven by the technological changes in the means of amplification available, and the aim in hearing aid development has been to reduce size, increase reliability, and provide better hearing for the user. These aims are very often incompatible. What can be accomplished with a rack full of electronic equipment, several microphones, and high fidelity earphones cannot yet be duplicated with a device small enough to be buried in the ear.

Rehabilitation for hearing has a long history and has always been limited by technological development. The earliest documented help was that provided by various acoustic devices, primarily in the form of some sort of horn that had a large collecting area and tubulation causing acoustic resonances that amplified specific frequencies. Speaking tubes were also used, but it is obvious that the person with a hearing handicap was really handicapped.

It would require the long fumbling growth in the understanding of electrical effects to bring relief. That growth had, by the mid-1800s, set the stage for realization of the goal of speech transmission by electrical current. In 1846, Alexander Graham Bell achieved this with two moving armature magnetic transducers, one for a microphone and one for a receiver, wire connections, and a battery.

The development of the carbon microphone during the next few years led to the design of electrical amplifiers using the carbon microphone coupled to the moving armature receiver. All the elements for sound reinforcement were now in

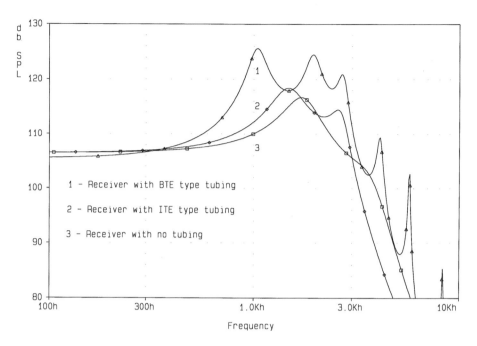

**Figure 3–3.** Tubing effects on receiver frequency response.

place: microphone, amplifier, and receiver. What came after were improvements in these three elements.

The tremendous flurry of inventive activity in the late 1800s unveiled all the transduction principles in use today for electro-acoustic transducers. Microphones using the electrostatic principle, often referred to as condenser microphones, were described by both Edison and A. E. Dolbear. Dolbear completed an electrostatic demonstration telephone at the Paris Electrical Exhibition of 1881 (Hunt, 1982, p. 41). The piezoelectric effect was discovered by Jacques and Pierre Currie in 1880, but remained a scientific curiosity until 1912 with Langevin's work with quartz ultrasonic transducers for the detection of submarines in WWI. The concept of a moving coil or dynamic transducer first appeared in Ernst Werne Siemens' 1874 patent filing. This was 2 years before Bell's telephone, and the Siemens' patent seemed to have telegraph relays in mind—not acoustic transducers. The year after the Bell filing, Charles Cuttriss and Jerome Redding filed an 1877 application for what seems to be the first electro-acoustic moving coil transducer. Two weeks later, Siemens' applications were filed in Germany and England for electro-acoustics, using many of the fundamentals of today's typical dynamic transducers.

Siemens' 1877 specification also disclosed the other transducer of interest to us, the balanced armature magnetic transducer—although not in the form in use today. T. A. Watson, in 1882, and Frank L. Capp, in 1890, obtained patents on balanced armature devices with operative methods more nearly like those in use today. Both patents expired before any commercial use was made of them.

In the early 1900s, an electrically powered hearing aid was introduced. This aid was simply a telephone system enclosed in a box. It consisted of a battery, a carbon granule microphone, sometimes a carbon amplifier, and a telephone-type magnetic receiver, with all the inherent distortion problems of these transducers.

The introduction of the thermionic triode in 1907 opened a new avenue of approach for electrical amplification of sound. It had the potential of amplifying an electrical signal without the gross distortion of the carbon amplifier. It also opened up possibilities of utilizing transduction methods developed during those fruitful years in the late 19th century.

Despite the widespread use of the vacuum tube amplifier in other fields, it was not until 1921 that a hearing aid using a vacuum tube amplifier was commercially available. In that year, Western Electric produced one for Globe Earphone Company (Hodgson and Skinner, 1977). This aid was portable but far from wearable—it resembled one of the early radios produced by Western Electric. During the 1920s, vacuum tubes became smaller and more reliable, and, as a consequence, wearable hearing aids appeared. They were usually contained in two boxes, one for the amplifier and one for the batteries.

The high gain of the vacuum tube amplifier allowed the use of much less sensitive microphones. The technology of choice for this was the piezoelectric crystal with its ability to produce electrical signals when mechanically stressed. The lower sensitivity of devices using the technique was accompanied by the potential of greater linearity and a better impedance match to the vacuum tube circuit.

Of the available materials, Rochelle salt had the highest sensitivity. With an upper curie point of 120°F, the fragility and unfortunate propensity to become liquid above 80% relative humidity (RH), and turn to powder below 40% RH, Rochelle salt presented a real challenge to transducer developers. During the 1920s, all too little was known about the crystal axes that might be exploited and uniformly pure and homogeneous crystals were difficult to obtain in useful size and quantity. The Brush Development Company was the major developer, working with Rochelle Salt devices before WWI. It developed or acquired a mass of patents during the 1930s and the post-WWII period. At Brush, engineers developed methods for growing crystals witih useful sizes and predictable axis orientations and methods for cutting crystals, thus providing the materials for their development of the two-element cantilevered "bender" and torsional "twister" devices, terms later copyrighted by Brush.

The development of the miniature vacuum tube in England in 1934–1935 made possible the construction of truly wearable aids. These smaller devices obviously were in need of smaller sensitive microphones. At Brush, means had been developed to produce very thin crystals and transducers developed to drive these crystals with direct pressure, thereby eliminating the need for auxiliary mechanical drive mechanisms allowing the drastic reductions in transducer size needed for these smaller hearing aids.

Developments during WWII in the miniaturization of electrical circuits and, particularly, reduction in transducer and battery size set the stage for the really usable hearing aids.

By about 1943 the first single unit wearable aids were being introduced, using the more compact batteries and the smaller lower current consumption tube made first by Hytron and, later, Raytheon. The WWII development and use of the mercury battery invented by Samuel Rubin gave further impetus to size reduction.

The fragile crystal microphone and its physical limitations was still the only choice for a microphone. The bandwidth limitations imposed by the mass of the driving mechanism, the problem of protecting the microphone from the environment, and reducing the susceptibility to shock damage received considerable attention from the producers of crystal devices.

A concept differing from the conventional method of driving the crystal in a bending mode appeared in the patent application of Dr. Raymond W. Tibbetts, filed in 1942 (Tibbetts, 1945). The scheme placed a thin flat crystal plate in tension across one diagonal and in compression across the other diagonal.

The new device alleviated the fragility problem but not the environment sealing one. It was not a completely practical solution, and was never used in practical devices. George Tibbetts, home on Thanksgiving vacation in his second semester at Harvard University, discussed this shortcoming with Dr. Tibbetts and developed a concept to eliminate it. The idea was to use a uniquely formed set of surfaces attached to the frame around the crystal to apply stress to the diagonals. A rapid reduction to practice was achieved, and an application for a patent filed in 1944 (Tibbetts, 1946). The term diabow was applied to the structure, and the first of these Tibbetts diabow devices were sold to Beltone in June of 1946. Various modifications with shrinking sizes were marketed in quantity for as long as the vacuum tube circuit was used in hearing aids.

During this period, the most common principles for receiver operation were the bipolar metal diaphragm devices of telephone ancestry and the balanced armature devices following the work done for the military in WWII. A fine wire cable connected the body-worn amplifier to the receiver, which was snapped into a connector at the earmold. Crystal receivers were also used. Both Tibbetts and Brush developed and produced them.

The next technical breakthrough in sound amplification came with the invention of the point contact transistor in 1947 and the junction transistor in 1952.

This development posed a new set of problems for the transducer designer. The transistor had both a low input impedance and a low output impedance. This required that the microphone and receiver also have low impedances.

Initially, the receiver presented no great problem; the coils could be wound with fewer turns of heavier wire. Microphone manufacturers had more of a problem, and the solution was to incorporate a small transformer in the microphone housing—which was gargantuan by today's standards.

This solution was short-lived. Within a few years, the hearing aid had been reduced in size to the point where a head-worn aid was feasible. With this decrease in size, the microphone designer no longer had the luxury of space. With smaller size came smaller batteries, and the demand for greater transduction efficiencies for both microphone and receiver.

The only device that had this potential seemed to be the balanced armature transducer. Historically, commercial use of the principle did not occur until Nathaniel Baldwin's patent (Baldwin, 1915) resulted in the "Baldwin" headphones so dear to amateur radio operators for years. Over the years, improvements were made on devices using this principle, and microphones were designed for use by the Navy and Air Force during WWII. The usual construction consisted of a pair of "U"-shaped pole pieces and a permanent magnet. A cantilever armature with one end fixed between a set of poles and the other end free to move in the air gap of the other set of poles was inserted through a wire coil. This is often referred to as a parallel configuration.

The structure had some very serious problems. One was metallurgical. The same metal path carried both the high density permanent magnet flux and the low density signal flux. A metal optimized for high flux densities is a poor candidate for carrying low flux densities. In addition, the high-flux level itself shifts the material characteristics to the detriment of its small signal handling ability. A second problem was, with the advent of the head-worn aid, two transducers with similar resonant frequencies were in close proximity. Extraneous magnetic fields produced by the receiver could easily be picked up by the microphone, adding to the already annoying problem of mechanical and acoustic feedback.

The first problem was one that begged for a solution, regardless of the end use of the transducer. The approach used by designers was to find ways to separate the polarizing flux path from the signal flux path.

Benjamin B. Bauer, of Shure Brothers, Inc., devised a structure (Bauer, 1948) that brought the coil and an "E"-shaped armature structure outside the magnet and pole structure. This removed much of the high flux biased pole assembly from the signal flux path. In an article in *The Journal of the Acoustical Society of America* he describes a small commercial microphone made for transistorized amplifiers and developed with the participation of Elmer V. Carlson and R. Carr (Bauer, 1953).

Further developments addressed this problem by optimizing the magnetic materials for signal flux handling and making the polarizing flux path that would be compromised by this as short as possible.

The designers were also much concerned about the second problem, the generation of or influence from external magnetic fields. At Industrial Research Products, with the patents of Hugh S. Knowles and William A. Plice (Knowles and Plice, 1959) and that of Knowles and Joseph E. Mullen (Knowles and Mullen, 1959) and, at Tibbetts Industries, with the patent of Raymond W. Tibbetts and George C. Tibbetts (Tibbetts and Tibbetts, 1961), a new class of structure evolved.

These, like the Bauer device, were parallel constructions; that is, they were not designed for the signal flux to pass through the magnets. The shielding effect was achieved by using a long magnet or magnets running the length of the armature and large area pole structures reduced to small area poles at the armature tip. The Knowles and Plice concept used one magnet and could use separate return paths for the signal flux. As a microphone, it provided partial shielding from the AC power fields in the environment and, as a receiver, some shielding of the internal generated leakage fields. The introduction of the Knowles Model AH and AJ microphones in 1955 and 1954 were based on this concept.

The Knowles AO and AR microphone and receiver were introduced in 1955, and all subsequent transducers until 1960 were based on the concepts described in the 1959 Knowles and Mullen patent. This structure used two long permanent magnets, one on each side of a symmetrical device with the pole structure spanning the space between the magnets, with space cut out for the coil in their centers. The use of shunt bars for the signal flux provided shielding of the coil. Armature magnetic centering was achieved by bending the armature. These devices are reported to have reduced external "hum" pickup by 6–8 dB (Egolf, Carlson, and Mostardo, 1989).

Introduced in 1956, the Tibbetts Industries Model 80 and Model 82 microphones and the Model R2 receivers were based on a similar structure and resulted in the 1961 Tibbetts and Tibbetts patent. These devices did not use a separate signal flux path shunt. Instead, the pole assembly covered the top and bottom, enclosing the entire structure for improved magnetic shielding. Magnetic centering was fine tuned by means of tabs at the fixed end of the armature, which could be bent toward either of the fixed end poles to shunt flux and establish a neutral point commensurate with the mechanical centering.

Devices with this construction were reduced in size to meet the demand of smaller hearing aids, and culminated in the M4 and R4 series. The R4 series was the first of them to use an external flap and tube arrangement to attach the receiver to the acoustic tube leading to the ear mold.

Despite the gains in the magnetic shielding in all these devices, the closer proximity of the two transducers in the smaller aids required better shielding to prevent feedback.

At Industrial Research Products, Elmer Carlson (Carlson, 1963) developed a better-shielded structure. This transducer used the Bauer "E"-shaped armature, but brought the external magnets into a position over the pole faces, providing a compact structure. The magnets were attached to a case structure of magnetic material, which provided an equi-potential exterior surface at the polarizing flux potential. Egolf (Egolf et al., 1989) reports that this achieved an order of magnitude reduction in magnetic "leakage." The Knowles Model BA and BB transducers using this configuration were introduced in 1960.

Further reduction in size along with reduced magnetic interference came with Tibbetts Industries introduction in 1950 of the M6 and R6 microphone and receiver. Developed by George C. Tibbetts, these employed a concept differing from that used in the previously described transducers. Instead of a "parallel" magnetic path, this transducer used a "series" path. The signal flux now went through the magnet. The general construction, shown in Figure 14, is described in detail in the patent (Tibbetts, 1970).

This type of magnetic path had been used earlier by Dyna Magnetics Devices. Howard Fener describes such a device in a patent filed in 1959 and issued in 1963 (Fener, 1963).

The Tibbetts transducer design, developed independently, was radically different in construction. A similar device developed by Carlson, Cross, and Killion at Knowles Electronics is described in a 1971 patent (Carlson et al., 1970). This was marketed as the Knowles BJ/BK series.

All subsequent receiver modifications at Knowles used the "series" magnetic path (Egolf et al., 1989). Tibbetts Industries continued using the "series" circuit but changed the armature configuration after the M6/R6 series. These structures are described in patents (Tibbetts and Sawyer, 1972; Tibbetts, 1983; Stanley and Tibbetts, 1985).

A completely new concept for using the balanced armature principle for acoustic transduction was developed at Tibbetts Industries in the early 1990s. The impetus for the development was the need for receivers that would not so easily be plugged with wax, a problem that has plagued hearing aid users since receivers were placed in the ear. The new structure developed to accomplish this was called a balanced armature transducer with a transverse gap. The structure is described in patents (Tibbetts and Madaffari, 1993; Tibbetts, 1994).

The development in the late 1960s of the junction field effect transistor (JFET) and the availability of reasonably sensitive piezoelectric ceramics provided the opportunity for transducer developers to eliminate the use of magnetic microphones and their sensitivity to stray magnetic fields and inherent narrow bandwidth. These ceramics made it possible to utilize the piezoelectric phenomena with its linearity and potentially greater bandwidth without all the disadvantages of Rochelle salt. The JFET provided a tiny impedance-matching device between the transducer and the amplifier input.

At Knowles Electronics, Elmer Carlson and Mead Killion developed a microphone using the piezoelectric ceramics in flexure and an enclosed JFET (Carlson and Killion, 1972). This was marketed as the Knowles Model BL microphone and was introduced commercially in 1968 (Egolf et al., 1989).

At Tibbetts Industries, a ceramic/JFET microphone, the Model 133, was developed using the "Diabow" structure of the earlier Rochelle salt era driving two ceramic struts across the diagonals. The microphone is described in Whitney (1973) and Flint and Tibbetts (1972).

Use of the ceramic microphone was short-lived. The availability of relatively stable electret materials in the early 1970s sparked renewed interest in condenser microphones using these materials to provide the polarizing field, and the JFET to provide the impedance match. Earlier efforts were hampered by inadequate electret materials. One of the earliest electret microphones, built in 1928, used the same scheme used today, an electret backplate with a nonelectret diaphragm (Sessler and West, 1973). These authors also report that microphones with wax backplates were offered commercially in the United States in the late 1930s under the name "NuVoltage Velatron." This type of microphone was used in large quantities by the Japanese military for field communication in WWII.

By the early 1970s, miniature microphones had been produced using these new electret materials. Fraim and Murphy had developed a microphone using a Teflon electret diaphragm (Fraim and Murphy, 1974). The disadvantage of the competing electret and mechanical properties of a Teflon electret diaphragm led Knowles Electronics to develop a microphone using an electret-coated backplate (Schmitt, 1973), and an unstressed Mylar diaphragm supported on protrusions on the backplate (Carlson and Killion, 1973). This microphone was introduced as the Knowles Model BT in 1972. Somewhat smaller microphones were designed over the next decade and a half. Size reduction, unfortunately, was usually accompanied by a reduction in signal level or signal-to-noise ratio. However, a breakthrough in electret microphone design (Carlson and Madaffari, 1988) improved signal level by 6 dB and improved the signal-to-noise ratio by 2 dB or better, allowing the smaller devices to compete with their older and larger predecessors.

Hearing aids have become progressively smaller and been pushed further into the inhospitable environment of the ear. Knowles Electronics has produced successively smaller receivers and microphones, culminating at present in the Model EM microphone and the Model EH receiver.

Tibbetts Industries introduced in 1993 an extremely miniature electret microphone using a stretched diaphragm rather than an unstressed supported one. Developed by Peter L. Madaffari, this microphone, the Model 2515, has the smallest volume yet achieved without reducing the sensitivity compared to larger microphones. This is the latest but, in all likelihood not the last, reduction in microphone size.

The telecoil, which works on the principle of magnetic induction, also has a relatively long history. The earliest use in a hearing aid seems to be the use by Sam Lybarger of an air core coil in a body aid at Radioear in 1947 (Marshall, 1992). Subsequent use of metal cores, usually nickel-iron, permitted reductions in size such that it was feasible to use them in head-worn hearing aids. Several manufacturers including Stanton Magnetics, Vicon, Microelectric, Dyna Magnetics, and numerous hearing aid manufacturers produced these coils at one time or another through the 1970s. Tibbetts Industries, in the early 1970s, began manufacturing coils to customer specifications, and in 1974 introduced telecoils of its own design. Subsequently, the sensitivity for a given volume of coil has been increased by a factor of two. Because the sensitivity is a function of the square of the volume, this has allowed the design of much smaller telecoils. The expanded and more sophisticated use of telecoils led to the development of amplified telecoils where the output level and frequency response could be tailored to the needs of the hearing aid designers. The Tibbetts' PA-1 was introduced in 1991 and was followed by the current Model PA-3. One of the authors (Stanley, 1977), in an article on transducers, commented that size reduction in transducers was reaching the limit of practical need. The intervening years have proved only that prophecy was not one of his strong points. He is only willing to say that vanity will push for less obtrusive devices and that the transducers will change in unpredictable ways.

## Transducer Technologies and Processes

Almost all transducer technologies depend upon acoustical to electrical or electrical to acoustical conversion of energy. The one exception is the telecoil. The members of the main group are, therefore, defined by the method used for mechanical to electrical or electrical to mechanical conversion. This is because they all have in common a means to convert acoustical to mechanical or mechanical to acoustical energy. This conversion is accomplished by the use of a diaphragm. The diaphragm is normally a membrane sealing a volume within the transducer. The membrane is moved by the sound wave (acoustical to mechanical) or the moving membrane produces a sound wave (mechanical to acoustical).

There are many different technologies that could be and have been used for hearing aid transducers. However, only two, magnetic and electret, are currently being used and a third, piezoelectric, was used until recently. For the time being, other technologies are of academic interest only, but this could change quickly if the appropriate technology provided the appropriate benefits.

## Piezoelectric Transducers

Piezoelectric transducers make use of the principle that a crystal of piezoelectric material will produce an electrical potential across two sides of the crystal when stressed. Conversely, when a potential is placed across the appropriate faces of the crystal, flexure will occur. Unfortunately, crystals are fairly massive, even when sliced into thin sections. As such, they are sensitive to mechanical vibration, so much so that this transducer is often used today as an accelerometer. Also, the piezoelectric materials were such relatively poor transducers that magnetic receivers superseded them as output devices and electret microphones replaced them as input devices.

## Electret Transducers

In an electret transducer or, more properly, an electret condenser transducer, the diaphragm (either microphone or receiver) is also one plate of an electrical element, a condenser. Condenser is the original term used for what is today called a capacitor. Normally capacitors are used with both plates fixed, unless they are used as tuning elements. In an electret microphone, a fixed charge is placed on this capacitor so that as the plates move relative to each other the capacitance and, consequently, the voltage, are varied. Conversely, if a time-varying voltage is placed on the plates, the plates will also move toward and then away from each other in the same fashion and the device is useful as a receiver. When the DC potential is supplied externally by a power supply, the device is a simple condenser transducer, and this external potential may run about 150 to 200 volts. If the charge is supplied by an electret material, the device is termed an electret condenser transducer, and no external potential need be supplied. As noted, electrets have the ability to accept and maintain a charge or a charge separation within its material which, in turn, produces a potential.

For a hearing aid-sized electret microphone, the devices are so tiny and the capacitance is so small that a very high input impedance amplifier must be used to prevent signal degradation. A special transistor, the Junction Field Effect Transistor (JFET) is often used.

Electret technology can also be used for receivers but, in general, this requires signal levels far in excess of what can be provided by the single-cell power supply normally found in a hearing aid.

## Magnetic Transducers

In discussing magnetic transducers, it would be necessary to enumerate the various forms of magnetic technology. Keep in mind that magnetic transducers, just as condenser transducers, are inherently bidirectional; that is, they will transform acoustic energy to electrical, as in a microphone, and electrical energy to acoustical, as in a receiver.

The basic form of a magnetic transducer requires a coil of wire and a magnetic field. The coil carries the electrical current. The magnetic field is most often provided by a permanent magnet, although at one time a second coil carrying a constant current was used instead of the magnet. Obviously, a permanent magnet is preferable because it requires no power for its operation.

The transduction principle is based on the fact that a current is induced in a coil of wire, if the coil is moved so that the magnetic field strength through the coil changes. Conversely, current flowing through a coil of wire immersed in a magnetic field will cause displacement of the coil if properly oriented with respect to the magnetic field. Therefore, if you connect a diaphragm to such a coil, the diaphragm will move with the coil and perform the mechanical/acoustical conversion while the coil and magnetic field will perform the mechanical/electrical conversion. Such a transducer is called an *electrodynamic magnetic transducer* and may be either microphone or receiver.

Placing a shaped element of magnetic material called an armature within the moving coil improves the efficiency of the transducer. Using such an arrangement, the coil could remain stationary because the armature or a portion of it could then become the important moving element. Such a transducer is termed a moving armature magnetic transducer, and the diaphragm is now connected to the armature. Again, both receivers and microphones are possible with this technology.

It was found that the use of a second magnet provided symmetry and improved the linearity of the transducer. Furthermore, the arrangement of the magnets could be such that there was no net force on the moving piece, the armature, unless the armature was displaced as in a microphone or current was passed through the coil as in a receiver.

In general, magnetic transducers have low electrical impedance and are normally connected to amplifiers using common bipolar transistors.

**Telecoil Transducers**

The telecoil is a transducer in its own right. It is differentiated from other hearing aid transducers in that it converts electromagnetic energy to electrical energy. It is, therefore, primarily an input device. The telecoil works in a manner similar to an antenna. It is usually composed of a bar of metal, normally a nickel-iron alloy, wound with many turns of fine wire. An electromagnetic wave will induce a time-varying magnetic field in the bar, which will, in turn, produce a time-varying voltage at the two terminals of the telecoil. The induced voltage has very similar signal properties to the electromagnetic wave and can, in turn, be processed by the hearing aid amplifier and receiver to reproduce a sound.

*Transducer Response Shapes*

Transducers have an intrinsic frequency response shape that is modified in two ways. First, there are the requirements for operation. For example, microphones and receivers require a housing as well as an inlet or outlet for the acoustic energy, and terminals for the electrical energy. These constraints cause limitations in the performance of the transducer.

Second, there are elements that are added to the basic transducer to purposely modify the performance, either to compensate for an intrinsic limitation or to provide an improvement in performance or some combination of the two.

It has been known for many years that the acoustical, mechanical, and electrical systems have analogous basic elements. These elements are often referred to as *resistance, inductance,* and *capacitance* because electrical circuit theory is so common today. In the mechanical system, the terms would be *resistance, mass,* and *compliance.* In the acoustical system, they would be *resistance, inertance,* and *compliance.*

A transducer changes energy from one system to another. Microphones and receivers use all three systems. However, in their simplest form they have a frequency response that starts out flat, then rises to a peak, then declines. The height of the peak is controlled by resistance, while the frequency of the peak is controlled by both the inductive and capacitive elements in whatever system or systems they lie.

Figures 3–1, 3–2, and 3–3 show the basic frequency responses of the most popular transducers: the electret microphone, the telecoil and the balanced armature magnetic receiver, respectively.

As noted above, aspects of the casing and the outlet/inlet of the transducer affect the frequency response. By purposely augmenting or, at least, modifying these structures it is possible to purposely modify the frequency response.

## Receiver Frequency Response

Magnetic receivers almost always have an intrinsic peak in the center of the audible frequency spectrum and at least one secondary peak somewhat higher in frequency due to the housing and sound outlets. Electret transducers have their intrinsic peak near the upper limit or above the range of hearing, but the casing and inlet cause a resonance within this audio spectrum, although at the higher frequencies. The telecoil, as it does not use the acoustic system, has no secondary peak and the primary peak is far beyond the range of hearing. However, the telecoil is a far more basic transducer and, for most applications, is best represented as an inductor only. As such, its intrinsic response shape is best represented as a straight line rising at 6 dB per octave.

BTE hearing aids require additional tubing to conduct the sound from the receiver inside the case of the hearing aid to the earhook, tubing of the earmold and, finally, the ear canal. Such tubing has natural resonances that result in additional peaks in the receiver frequency response curve and extend the high-frequency performance. Unfortunately, additional peaks also result in troughs between the peaks, and the amplified sound may not appear natural. The addition of some resistance to the tubing, also referred to as a damper, reduces the amplitude of the peaks and partially increases the amplitude of the troughs to result in a smoother frequency response. This is covered in great detail in Chapter 6.

As acousticians became more experienced, it was realized that by the using tubes of differing diameters and lengths, and using suitable damping elements, the peaks could be suppressed and the high frequency performance could be extended. This topic is also covered in great detail in Chapter 6.

For in-the-ear (ITE) and in-the-canal (ITC) hearing aids, the connecting tubing or plumbing, as it is sometimes called, is not sufficiently long enough to provide significant peaks. It is, therefore, important that the two peaks in the frequency response be properly located so as to maximize the performance of the receiver. With the ear canal filled or at least blocked by the shell of the hearing aid, the natural resonance of the canal is eliminated. Therefore, it is useful to have the lower peak of the receiver occur at about 2800 Hz, the approximate frequency of the natural canal resonance (Shaw, 1974). The second peak extends the frequency response to between 4000 and 6000 Hz.

For completely-in-canal (CIC) hearing aids, it is possible that the natural functioning of the outer ear structure and, possibly, the ear canal itself will be unimpeded. Such applications essentially reduce the receiver to its bare essentials because of the restrictions of space. For such applications, new designs have been generated, such as the Knowles OV receiver, which uses the shell of the hearing aid rather than its own casing for extending the output level. Also, the Tibbetts 321 receiver, which has no diaphragm cover or tubing, is a viable option for CIC hearing aids (Tibbetts and Madaffari, 1993).

**Telecoil Frequency Response**

The telecoil, as has been described above, has an intrinsic frequency response with only electronic filtering as the means for modifying its frequency response. Fortunately, the 6 dB/octave rise of the telecoil response shape is appropriate for hearing aid users with predominantly high-frequency hearing loss. Also, this telecoil response is similar to the 6 dB/octave frequency response of so-called *ski-sloped* microphones as well as *first-order gradient directional microphones*, both of which will be discussed shortly. The most common microphone frequency response is basically flat at the higher frequencies with some small rolloff at frequencies below 1000 Hz. A reasonably similar frequency response may be easily achieved by using an operational amplifier to modify the basic telecoil frequency response.

**Microphone Frequency Response**

Receivers generally show little variation in frequency response shape within a model line. Microphones, on the other hand, show great variation, with the differences intentional. This gives the hearing aid manufacturer and, ultimately, the hearing aid dispenser greater control of the frequency response by the choice of microphone model. The intrinsic microphone frequency response is essentially flat from low (300 Hz) through midband acoustical frequencies to the higher frequencies (4000 to 7000 Hz) where a peak occurs due to the casing and inlet. The low to midfrequencies may be modified by the choice in size of the *internal microphone vent*. A sealed diaphragm will experience unequalized pressure against its faces unless some form of venting is used. In its simplest form, the vent is a small hole, normally less than 0.1 mm in diameter. This vent can allow sound to equalize across the diaphragm, particularly at low frequencies. The vent diameter can be made small enough that no appreciable modification of low frequencies occurs. However, some low-frequency modification may be desirable and, in such instances, larger vent diameters are used.

In general, low-frequency sounds, up to about 100 Hz, tend to have a mechanical origin and are not useful for communication. Therefore, a minimal diameter vent can be used to prevent the amplification frequencies below 100 Hz. However, hearing loss in most individuals tends to occur at the higher frequencies and, therefore, a uniform level of gain will cause the low frequencies to dominate. By using a microphone where the diameter of the vent is greater than necessary for barometric pressure relief, it is possible to attenuate the low frequencies to a lesser or greater degree, depending on the diameter of the vent. Whole families of frequency–response curves may be generated, depending on the venting used, as previously shown in Figure 3–1. The particular curves shown are for the Tibbetts Industries' model series 251-20 microphones. A set showing essentially the same frequency response could have been generated for the Tibbetts' 251-01 series, the Knowles' EM and EK series, as well as for microphones made by PI-AC of the Netherlands and Lectret of Switzerland. It should be noted that the EK is a larger device than the EM, yet the frequency responses are very similar. In an effort to provide a complete model line, most manufacturers of transducers will closely match a competitor's transducer size, shape, and performance.

Note on Figure 3–1 that, at the very low frequencies, the slope of the response is 6 dB/octave for all microphones, even the so-called flat microphone (#1 in Fig. 3–1). It is possible to make the vent appear inductive rather than resistive at higher frequencies by using an elongated tube rather than a hole in the diaphragm. The result is a change in the frequency response from a 6 dB to a 12 dB/octave slope at the higher frequencies. Because of the inductance, a peaking of the frequency response may occur. In the neighborhood of the peak, the slope may rise at more than 12 dB/octave. Indeed, an 18 dB/octave designation has been used, but this is a misnomer, as it applies only to a narrow frequency range for this microphone.

In general, a *pressure microphone*, that is, a single sound inlet microphone with a 6 dB or greater rising low-frequency response, is often referred to as a "ski-slope" microphone. This is actually a slang term not in formal use by transducer manufacturers, but very descriptive of the frequency–response shape and easily remembered.

The 6 dB and 12 dB response shapes also occur for another type of microphone, the *directional microphone,* which will be discussed shortly. However, these microphones have more than one inlet in addition to their directional properties. Before moving on, the *stepped response microphone* (trademark of Knowles Electronics) will be discussed.

The stepped response microphone, developed by Mead Killion, is especially tailored to produce a relative constant level at low frequencies and another, higher level, at high frequencies with a rapid transition point in between. This transition is generally in the neighborhood of 1000 Hz. The purpose of this microphone is to prevent complete loss of the lower frequencies as would be caused with a large vent, yet achieve a rapid transition in level as the higher frequencies are approached. The structure is fairly complex compared to a pressure microphone, as it requires an auxiliary diaphragm and special internal signal routing.

As just noted, another means of attenuating low frequencies is accomplished by a vent in the hearing aid shell from the ear canal to the outside world. Because of the high impedance of the ear canal and ear drum, such a vent attenuates the receiver output. This is the most common method of attenuating the low frequencies, but it can result in feedback. Various methods have been devised to minimize this tendency to feedback, some of them quite ingenious, involving active signal suppression.

## Directional Microphones

Directional microphones will be given a greater emphasis in this text than would be warranted by their usage in the hearing aid industry. This will be done because their benefits are often overlooked by hearing aid professionals. A directional microphone is a microphone with an electrical output level that varies with both the amplitude and the direction of the sound source relative to the microphone. The logical application is the differentiation between wanted and unwanted sounds by proper orientation of the microphone with respect to the sound sources.

For example, a listener is at a cocktail party and wishes to hear the person he is facing. Sounds from behind the listener are unwanted, but sounds from the side are moderately important, as they may become part of the conversation with an interjection. In this application, a *cardioid directional microphone* might be suitable. For this particular situation the pickup of the directional microphone is maximum at 0° incidence, reduced by 6 dB at ±90° (sides) and by 20 dB or more, from 180° (rear).

It should be noted that this is a true "noise reduction" capability as long as wanted or unwanted noises are defined by spatial orientation. In a perfect directional microphone, the directional properties are frequency invariant. However, the signal spectrum is altered so that, for a flat input, the electrical signal is generated at the output at 6 dB/octave. For a practical device, the directional properties of the microphone may be compromised at the low frequencies due to head diffraction effects. In addition, at the high frequencies, the directivity of the microphone is reduced due to a failure of the acoustical network within the microphone that develops the directional properties. However, head diffraction at high frequencies causes a shadowing effect that, in itself, is a useful directional property.

In an *anechoic room*, with only the directional microphone or only the directional aid, the benefits of a directional microphone can be very dramatic. In a *reverberant room*, sound comes with equal intensity from all directions, and the directional microphone is unable to differentiate. Most listening environments are somewhere in between. That is, sounds from *low-priority directions* are somewhat attenuated, but are rarely reduced to zero. [This practical limitation is in a sense valuable because a "blind spot" in our sensory input may prevent perception of a rare, but necessary, signal.] In fact, some wearers of directional hearing aids show concern for this.

All microphones can be referred to as *gradient microphones.* The order of the microphone depends on the number of sound inlets and the manner in which the sound from these inlets is added or subtracted. A microphone with a single sound inlet is termed a *zero order gradient* or *pressure microphone.* There may be some directional characteristics due to the housing but, in general, for microphones with small housings, as would be used in a hearing aid, the directional effects are very small.

A microphone with *two sound inlets* is a *first-order gradient microphone.* It may be constructed from two pressure microphones by subtracting one signal from another electrically. A first-order gradient microphone may also be made from a single casing with sound entrance on both sides of the diaphragm. In the latter case, the one acoustic signal is subtracted from the other acoustically and the resultant is transformed from acoustical to electrical energy.

Whether done electrically or acoustically, this effect is essentially the same as the method used to determine the slope or gradient of a line, either straight or curved. For low frequencies, the slope of the sine way is more gradual than it is at high frequencies, and because the gradient is lower at the low frequencies, so is the output signal. The frequency response for sound arriving from the front of the microphone is 6 dB/octave, that is, directly proportionate to frequency up to the frequency where the directional properties fail. This can be as low as several hundred hertz or as high as 6000 Hz, depending on the design of the microphone.

Some classical first-order directional patterns are the *cosine, cardioid, super cardioid,* and *hypercardioid microphone.* For the cosine microphone, the two signals are simply subtracted. For the cardioid microphone, a time delay is introduced for one signal that is equal to the time delay of the sound wave moving from one inlet to the other. For the super cardioid and hypercardioid microphone, the internal time delays are less than for the external maximum delay.

Higher order directional microphones require additional sound inlets. At least three sound inlets are required for a second-order directional microphone, but most often, four sound inlets are used. As before, pressure microphones may be used for each sampling point, or a single casing with multiple sound inlets or a combination of these two approaches. The second-order microphone essentially measures the slope of the slope of the sound field, so that low frequencies are more attentuated than for a first-order microphone. The frequency response rises at 12 dB/octave. Directional microphones emphasize the high frequencies, a characteristic often used by audiologists to compensate for high-frequency hearing loss.

The real merit of the higher order microphones is their increased focusing power. This further improves the directivity and increases the ability to differentiate a "wanted" signal in background noise. Unfortunately, the price paid for this differentiation is an overall decrease in the input signal to the hearing aid. This means that the internal noise generated by the hearing aid may become noticeable to the point of being objectional.

In application, it must be understood that the diffraction caused by the human head will significantly alter the directional properties compared to those of the bare aid. In early fittings of directional hearing aids, acousticians lost sight of this effect, with the result that the performance of the aid with the directional microphone was disappointing. Even when properly used in practical application, the improvement in signal-to-noise ratio was "only" 3 to 4 dB. This may not seem dramatic but, in practice, for noisy situations such as the cocktail party, a few decibels improvement may be sufficient to make an unintelligible conversation understandable. As a matter of fact, the "cocktail party effect" is caused by the multitude of speakers adjusting the SPL of their voices until it can just barely be heard above competing conversations. This causes an upward spiral of voices. As it turns out, people with normal hearing in both ears have an advantage of several decibels over most hearing aid users in their ability to understand speech in noise, and it is just this "edge" that allows those with normal hearing to understand at a cocktail party while the hearing impaired are left bewildered.

Directional microphones were very popular in the 1970s. Unfortunately, some hearing aid manufacturers had difficulty designing directional hearing aids. This resulted in the perception that the effectiveness of directional microphones was questionable. Other means of noise reduction using signal processing have been developed. As with the directional microphone, the effectiveness of these signal-processing schemes has also been questioned.

Until recently, no sophisticated coupling of a directional microphone with a signal processor has been attempted. A patent by Zlatan Ribic (Ribic, 1993), appears to attempt such a union. As the directional microphone addresses the problem of understanding a conversation while in a crowd, its resurgence would be welcomed.

### Passive Versus Active Devices

Early hearing aids performed the process of converting an acoustic input to an electrical signal, followed by amplification and filtering of that electrical signal and the conversion of the electrical signal back to an acoustic signal using the microphone, amplifier, and receiver. The telecoil that converted a radiated electromagnetic field to an electrical signal could be used to replace the microphone in special situations. However, all amplification of the input signal was performed by the amplifier as a separate entity.

However, conditions have changed in that signal processing, including amplification and filtering, has become more complex. As the functional requirements of the amplifier increased, it became useful in some circumstances to transfer some of the functions of the amplifier onto the transducer. Actually, these functions were joined with the transducer and incorporated into a single housing. It is currently possible to use microphones, telecoils, and receivers with each containing its own amplifier. The requirements for these amplifiers are characterized by the transducer to which it is joined.

Microphone technology has changed over the years. The current technology is based upon the use of the diaphragm as the moving plate of a capacitor. As such, the diaphragm displacement is very small, on the order of the diameter of molecules for the lowest amplitude measurable signal. Unfortunately, such small displacements generate extremely small currents. These currents are so small that wire leads of any appreciable length directly attached to the transducer will pick up stray electromagnetic signals that will produce currents of similar magnitude. Therefore, it is necessary to reduce lead length as much as possible and to shield both the leads and the structure. Once the current has been amplified, the problem is greatly reduced. An obvious, but possibly not practical, solution is to place an amplifier within the microphone housing.

It required the advent of the transistor to make this approach possible. For over 25 years hearing aid microphones have been made that contain a miniature amplifier whose function is to amplify the current output of the microphone's transducer. A single *Field Effect Transistor* or *FET* is used along with other discrete components of subminiature size to perform this function.

Telecoils have been in use for many years. However, the trend has been towards smaller and smaller aids requiring smaller and smaller components. Unfortunately, telecoils suffer in signal level reduction as their size is reduced. Furthermore, there has been a reduction in the amplitude of the electromagnetic input signal with the result that, in most applications, the voltage level of the signal produced by the telecoil is significantly reduced below that of the microphone. To compensate for this, it was often necessary to provide an auxiliary amplifier for the telecoil in the hearing aid. This practice still occurs today, and such an auxiliary amplifier can be found on the Etymotic Research K-Amp™ as well as amplifiers made by the Gennum Corporation.

However, some hearing aid designers find it useful to have this amplification occur within the telecoil package itself. One reason is that not all hearing aids use telecoils, yet, if the amplifier is included as part of the main amplifier, all hearing applications would have to bear the cost of this feature's presence. Also, it is often necessary to shape the frequency response of the telecoil, which may require additional components if performed by the hearing aid designer. With a telecoil/amplifier combination in a single package, it is possible to have the frequency shaping adjusted by the telecoil manufacturer. The Tibbetts Industries *Powercoil*™ is a commercially available amplified telecoil. Its frequency response was previously shown as the upper curve on Figure 3–2. Both telecoil curves should be compared with the microphone curves in Figure 3–1.

The receiver can also benefit from its own internal amplifier. The use of a pulse width modulation, "Class D" amplifier has become popular. One advantage is that the amplitude of the drive voltage to the receiver can equal almost twice the DC power supply voltage. It also consumes very little power during quiet periods, as opposed to conventional Class A amplifiers. [Such amplifiers will be discussed elsewhere, but it is sufficient to know that switching Class D amplifiers produce higher signal levels than Class A amplifiers.] As with microphones, it is best to connect the amplifier with the receiver it is driving with as short as possible leads. As before, mounting the amplifier inside the receiver housing has some definite advantages.

In order of complexity, the internal amplifier of the microphone is the simplest, followed by the amplifier of the telecoil. The most complex is the Class D receiver amplifier. There is no particular reason why this need be so. The only problem with the integration of an amplifier with a transducer is that if the transducer fails, the amplifier is probably not salvageable. It is, therefore, important as the cost of the internal amplifier rises with complexity, that the component with which it is mated not fail.

## Transducer Limitations

There are different limitations on the microphone, telecoil, and receiver. However, most of the limitations are caused by three effects: (1) the desire to reduce the transducer to as small a size as possible to make the hearing aid as small as possible,

(2) the need to couple sound either into or out from the transducer, and (3) the need to place the aid over the ear or in the ear canal.

## Microphone Limitations

For microphones, the intent is to produce an electrical signal in response to an acoustic input. Unfortunately, microphones will also produce some output when shaken and even with no input at all! The electrical signal may be a distorted representation of the input acoustical signal. In addition, some unwanted filtering of the acoustical signal may occur. Finally, and perhaps most important, microphones cannot themselves differentiate between the "wanted" and "unwanted" acoustical signal.

The first limitation is that the microphone can produce an output signal when shaken. The microphone diaphragm acts as the heart of the transducer. Sound waves impinging on the diaphragm cause the diaphragm to move in tune with the oscillations of the acoustic wave. This movement then produces an electrical signal corresponding to the sound wave. However, it is possible that the microphone housing may be shaken, for example, when the hearing aid wearer is walking. If the microphone housing is moved, i.e., accelerated, the diaphragm may not follow directly this motion because of the diaphragm's mass. For the microphone, it doesn't matter if the diaphragm moves relative to the case in response to an acoustic input or the case moves relative to the diaphragm in response to when the case is shaken or vibrated. In either event, an output is produced.

This effect is very noticeable on piezoelectric microphones, as noted previously. Magnetic microphones have the same problem, because the moving elements are so massive. Even electret microphones, which have the least susceptibility to vibration, exhibit this problem. These effects can be minimized by reducing the mass of the diaphragm, usually by using thinner material. Some of the first electret microphones used diaphragms that were 1 mil thick, i.e., 0.001 inch or 0.00254 cm. Currently material of 0.00006 inch thickness (0.000152 cm) is routinely used. Some examples of trade names for such low mass devices are Zero G and Avibrometric.

Microphones, as with all types of sensors, produce their own output, i.e., noise, without an acoustic input. In general, such noise is a function of the size of the transducer and the craftsmanship of the microphone designer. It is not the noise itself that is a problem but, rather, the ratio of the microphone's sensitivity to its noise level that is important. For this reason, the noise level is often stated in terms of *equivalent sound pressure level*, or *equivalent SPL*. A value of 27 dB SPL for the equivalent noise is typical for the smaller hearing aid microphones, and 23 dB SPL is common for the next larger size. The lower the number, the easier it is to differentiate the true signal from the noise.

Microphones may also exhibit distortion. In this situation, the output electrical wave is not an accurate replica of the input acoustic signal. This usually occurs for high input sound pressure levels. For small displacements of the diaphragm (i.e., low input levels) there is a one-to-one (i.e., linear) correspondence with the electrical signal. For high input signal levels, the transducer or its internal amplifier may become nonlinear. In general, the transducer used in conventional electret microphones is fairly linear to very high sound pressure levels (i.e., levels so high they produce pain). However, the amplifier is limited by the power supply range, possibly as low as 0.9 volt. Signal inputs of 110 SPL may be enough to produce electrical signals whose peak-to-peak value would approach 0.9 volts and, therefore, distortion occurs. Such distortion will produce additional frequencies beyond those present at the input. These additional frequencies are related in that they are multiples of the applied frequencies.

The microphone also modifies the input signal due to its variation in sensitivity with frequency. Often, this is a desired effect and does not need to be viewed as a limitation. Often, the hearing aid wearer has a greater hearing loss at the higher frequencies and the microphone will have an attenuation of the low frequencies.

There is usually an upper frequency range where the frequency response of the microphone peaks and, beyond that point, its sensitivity to sound decreases precipitously. Most hearing aid microphones today peak between 4000 and 6000 Hz. At this point, acousticians differ as to the desired frequency range for a microphone. Some believe that the frequency response of the microphones should extend as far as 20,000 Hz. Others feel that 4000 Hz is a practical upper limit and that the trade-offs necessary for higher frequencies are not worth the additional range.

There is a further problem with microphones whose frequency response extends beyond 4000 Hz. Surveillance equipment often uses ultrasonic signals. These signals are high in level but at a frequency beyond the range of human hearing. Unfortunately, they may not be beyond the frequency range of the microphone, with the result that the microphone or the amplifier may overload and temporarily stop functioning. An apparently intermittent hearing aid that passes inspection by the manufacturer may be a symptom of this problem.

The issue of the desired upper frequency range of a microphone may ultimately depend on the hearing aid wearer. Patients interested in high-fidelity listening might approve of the attempt to restore a semblance of normal hearing, particularly if they have a mild to moderate hearing loss. Patients with a severe hearing loss, or a loss that has continued for some time, may simply not be able to hear the higher frequencies no matter what the level of amplification. For these patients, making speech intelligible is a practical goal and band limiting may be the only solution. Band limiting may also be used because of feedback oscillation.

Feedback oscillation may be a fault of the microphone, the receiver, or design of the hearing aid. As will be discussed later, the output of a receivers may be coupled back to the microphone for various reasons. This may occur if the acoustic signal produced by the receiver leaks around the earmold back to the microphone. An alternate cause is the physical shaking of the hearing aid shell or case that a single receiver may cause in producing a sound wave. This may be picked up by the microphone, due to its diaphragm mass. Alternately, this shaking of the housing may cause sound waves to be produced at the same frequency as the receiver's output signal. The microphone would naturally pick this up by no fault of its own, and feedback could result. Feedback oscillations usually occur at the higher frequencies and, by limiting the response of the microphone, feedback can often be avoided.

Microphones will degrade and possibly fail for various other reasons. Poor workmanship obviously comes to mind. The transducers used in current hearing aids cost approximately $10, depending on their technology, degree of sophistication, and performance. Warranties of two or more years are common and result in direct replacement, usually at no cost. There is probably no other device of similar cost that carries such a warranty. Needless to say, with such a warranty the transducer manufacturer must be sure of the product.

Another limitation of microphones is related to the fact that they must perform under some very adverse conditions. Extreme temperatures can damage components. However, operation at different temperatures can also cause variations in the frequency response. Microphones rely on a stable balance of forces to set their initial conditions. With variations in heat, a mismatch in thermal coefficients of expansion can alter tensions and, therefore, alter performance. Modern microphones use materials with similar coefficients of expansion.

Most acousto/electric or electro/acoustic transducers use a diaphragm. Many materials have been used, but polyethylene terepthalate, also known as Mylar™, has been the most successful. For its mass, it is an extremely durable, compliant material, able to be formed in very thin sheets and commercially available. The last factor is critically important. Hearing aid transducers use very little of any one material in their construction and must, therefore, select material that is commercially available rather than have it made.

Mylar does have a drawback in that it is hygroscopic (i.e., it will absorb water and, as a result, change its physical properties). Mylar has a coefficient of expansion with humidity that will alter strains that are placed in the film. For a microphone, this will manifest as a change in sensitivity. If improperly designed, the diaphragm will even collapse. With exposure to both heat and humidity, the diaphragm will also hydolyze, becoming brittle, with more or less permanent changes in its properties.

The electret is also susceptible to heat and humidity. With high temperatures in a moist environment, the charge bound to the electret may slowly bleed off. This may take years or weeks, depending on the construction. If the charge were to entirely dissipate or significantly diminish, the microphone would fail.

### Telecoil Limitations

Telecoils have similar problems to microphones as they are also used as the input transducer. They may also produce a signal when shaken, not because of any normally moving element, but because of the presence of a static magnetic field. Telecoils pick up the variation in signal amplitude of an electromagnetic wave. A static magnetic field as, for example, that produced by a permanent magnet, would not affect the telecoil unless the field could be caused to change. Moving the telecoil in such a field will, however, cause a signal pickup. Fortunately, a telecoil is least sensitive to low frequencies and most sensitive to high frequencies so that relatively slow displacements are not an issue.

Telecoils have low sensitivity so that even low noise levels may be a problem. The first stage of amplification past the telecoil is important in setting the signal-to-noise ratio. It is often true that the amplifier's noise is greater than the telecoil's noise so that the proper selection of this amplifier is important. Although microphones have equivalent noise levels in the low to high 20 dB SPL range, telecoils with their first amplifier stage are often in the low 40 dB SPL range. The telecoils lower signal-to-noise ratio is the result of low electromagnetic signal levels, and the relatively high noise level is actually a fault of the amplifier in most applications. With the proper amplifier, telecoils could have a better signal-to-noise ratio than some microphones. Recent attempts to combine a telecoil with an attached pre-amp have improved the signal-to-noise ratio level somewhat, but there is still a need for improvement.

Telecoils can also produce a distorted signal when in the presence of an exceptionally high source field. This is less common now, as the fields from most telephones now in production are considerably lower than they have been in the past.

Telecoils, by their very nature, have a characteristic frequency response that rises at 6 dB/octave. That is, with every doubling of frequency there is a doubling of sensitivity. Some microphones have a similar frequency response and, therefore, no adjustment other than amplification is needed in switching from microphone to telecoil. On the other hand, most microphones have a more or less flat frequency response. It is, therefore, necessary to modify the frequency response of the telecoil to match that of the microphone. Unfortunately, many pieces of electrical equipment produce electromagnetic waves at line frequency (i.e., 60 Hz in the U.S. and 50 Hz in Europe) as well as harmonics of this frequency. These frequencies are low in the acoustic spectrum and can be alleviated with a low-frequency roll off. A compromise is a frequency response that rises at 6 dB/octave to 1000 Hz and is flat from 1000 to 6000 Hz.

Telecoils are fairly rugged and have a protective coating covering the wire coil. Unfortunately, when assembled into hearing aids they are often handled with tweezers, which can cut through this coating and damage the wire. A new approach is to protect the telecoil with a nonferrous metal sheath.

The two most common uses for telecoils in hearing aids is for telephone pickup and the input transducer for an assistive listening (loop system) device. In the United States, the use for telephone pickup is much more common than for use as an assistive listening device; the converse is true in Europe. For telephone pickup, the coil should be mounted in the hearing aid shell or case so that the coil is horizontal with its axis parallel to a line between the two ears. For the loop system, the coil should be mounted vertically. Unfortunately, these two orientations, while increasing signal pickup for one application, degrade the performance for the other. In addition, because of space limitations, the telecoil is often mounted without regard for its intended application. What is needed is an omni-directional telecoil (i.e., one that works equally well with any orientation). Unfortunately, no such design has been presented. There is great interest in the problem, as some countries mandate the inclusion of a telecoil, where feasible, in all hearing aids. There is some indication that such a requirement will be in made in the United States in the near future.

### Receiver Limitations

The receiver has similar as well as different problems when compared to the microphone and telecoil. The differences come about because the receiver is an output transducer, and microphones and telecoils are input transducers. In general, the receiver does not add noise to the signal upon which it operates. There is little data on the output of a receiver when shaken, so apparently it is not a problem. The receiver does produce distortion. This is mainly because the receiver must handle much more power than the microphone or telecoil because it is an output rather than an input transducer. The more profound the hearing loss, the greater the output signal the receiver must supply.

In general, the larger the receiver, the larger the output signal it can supply. However, because of cosmetic reasons, most users of hearing aids prefer as small a hearing aid as is possible. This may mean forcing the receiver to tax its limits of output capability. A receiver produces sound by using a varying electrical signal to modulate the total force on a metal armature exposed to a magnetic field supplied by one or more magnets. In response to the time-varying force, the armature undergoes displacement. The armature is, in turn, connected to a diaphragm that, therefore, also undergoes displacement. The diaphragm then produces an acoustic wave that is ultimately picked up by the wearer's ear. The greater the displacement of the armature, the greater the sound pressure level. Almost all energy systems are linear for low input signals but the larger the displacement, the more nonlinear receivers become. Eventually, the armature can be forced to the limits of its travel.

It often happens that the receiver is blamed for more distortion than it actually causes. For sufficiently high signal levels, the amplifier may not be able to supply either enough current or enough voltage to maintain a nondistorted signal to the receiver.

Receivers are designed in families so that for a given family with the same power supplied to the receiver, the same acoustic signal level will be produced. What is changed is the impedance of the receiver. As the impedance of the receiver increases, a higher input voltage but lower input current is required for the same acoustic output, with the product of current and voltage, i.e., the power, held constant. Therefore, either the amplifier must be selected to match the receiver or, more commonly, the receiver must be chosen to match the amplifier. If a mismatch occurs in the hearing aid design, there is a limitation on maximum acoustic output that can be produced without noticeable distortion.

Receivers also have other problems that may cause them to degrade or fail in performance. If a receiver or the aid in which it is mounted is dropped onto a hard surface, the armature in the receiver may be shocked into a new position. The receiver manufacturer choses the original position to maintain linearity of the device with the extremes of signal input, and the new position is likely to be less than optimum. Distortion is the likely result at output levels that were originally distortion free.

Finally, the receiver outlet is usually open to the ear canal. The ear canal secretes cerumen, a waxy material, as a cleaning agent to trap material foreign to the ear. This material works its way from the inner to the outer portion of the ear canal. It is, therefore, possible upon inserting the hearing aid into the ear, that cerumen will work its way into whatever tubing connects the receiver to the hearing aid sound outlet. It may also work its way further, into the receiver itself. If the tubing or receiver outlet is partially plugged, then the frequency response of the hearing aid may be affected. If either is plugged, then there may be no output at all.

This problem with cerumen affects even BTE hearing aids, by plugging the earmold or the tubing leading to it from the hearing aid. The receiver is relatively remote and, therefore, less likely to be damaged. It is essential for the hearing aid wearer to clean the earmold and the tubing. If not, the local supplier generally is capable of cleaning the earmold and/or tubing.

With the advent of ITE, ITC, and CIC hearing aids, the amount of tubing past the receiver has declined to the point where some devices have no tubing at all. It has, therefore, become more likely that the receiver will become contaminated by cerumen. Most receivers cannot be cleaned, either by the user or the audiologist. Fully 40% of hearing aids in the United States are returned within the first year due to the presence of cerumen in the receiver. Often, the receiver must be discarded and a new receiver put in its place. The cost of this repair is quite high to the hearing aid manufacturer, not to mention the inconvenience to the hearing aid user.

Some approaches to correct this problem have involved the use of removable wax guards or shields, whose purpose is to trap wax in their structure. They can then be removed and cleaned or replaced. The Knowles OV receiver uses this approach.

An alternate idea has been to design a receiver that is very rugged and essentially has no restriction on the sound outlet. Cerumen could accumulate on the diaphragm of the receiver, but a periodic cleaning by the user would prevent sufficient accumulation to appreciably reduce performance. Such a device has been patented by Tibbetts Industries (Tibbetts and Madaffari, 1993).

Receivers can also be the source of other problems. As noted when discussing the microphone, feedback involves all components of the hearing aid, but is normally due to a signal from the receiver finding its way back to the microphone. The signal may be acoustic due to sound leakage around the shell or case of the hearing aid, or the signal can pass through the vent of the earmold or shell. However, the most common form of feedback is due to the physical vibrations of the shell or case of the hearing aid caused by the receiver.

As mentioned earlier, the receiver armature and diaphragm move in response to an electrical signal to produce an acoustic signal. As Newton's third law states, for every action there is an equal and opposite reaction. If the armature and diaphragm move in one direction, then the rest of the receiver and shell or case of the hearing aid will move in the opposite direction. Suitable mounting of the receiver can often reduce these vibrations and, as reported earlier, a microphone is fairly insensitive to these vibrations. However, the gain of the hearing aid may be so great that even the most minor agitation may be picked up by the microphone, amplified, and fed to the receiver where the vibration becomes reinforced. The receiver vibrations may even produce an acoustic signal, as the shell or case of the hearing aid acts as a sound board, producing an acoustic signal in the vicinity of the microphone.

To minimize these effects, Victoreen (1978) developed a patent where two receivers are placed back to back, with their sound outlets coupled. [For two matched receivers, the vibrations cancel each other, yet the output sound reinforces.] It is then possible to mount the receiver directly to the shell or case of the hearing aid without the need for shock mounting. The Tibbetts 163 dual receiver is licensed under Victoreen's (1978) patent.

Receivers have a characteristic frequency responses that can alter the acoustic output unless compensation is applied. In general, there is a resonant peak in the frequency response due to the mechanical structure of the moving armature and another resonant peak caused by the length and diameter of the sound outlet. If appreciable tubing is used with the receiver, as in a BTE aid, there may be one or more resonances due to the tubing itself.

The presence of these resonances is not necessarily a problem. The human ear canal, when unimpeded, naturally resonates at about 2800 Hz (Shaw, 1974). With the hearing aid in place, the canal is often occluded. By shifting one of the receiver peaks to 2800 Hz, the natural resonance can be restored.

## The Future of Transducers

Any experienced transducer designer will report that transducers are always getting smaller. Whether there is a practical limit to reduced size is hard to say, because one manufacturer's claim for the smallest transducer has always been superseded by another manufacturer in a short period of time.

One approach that some feel is very promising is the *silicon microphone*. This is an electret microphone manufactured with the same process used to construct integrated circuits (Sprenkels and Bergveld, 1990). In fact, an *Integrated Circuit* (IC) might be formed at the same time as the microphone is fabricated. Because of the micro-machining capability of this process, extremely small microphones, perhaps as small as 1-mm square may be possible. To date, there have been limitations in signal level, noise level, and thermal variations, but this is a new technology that has not yet had its chance to come to the forefront.

With the introduction of new transducer designs, it appears almost unavoidable that performance will decrease along with the size reductions. However, sometimes the benefits of reduced size more than compensate for reduced performance. A case in point is the output of receivers, which seem to follow a predictable decline in maximum output as size decreases. However, the smaller size allows them to be placed ever closer to the ear drum. With the reduction in enclosed volume comes a higher efficiency in delivering sound to the ear drum, that is, compensating for the reduced power capability.

Advances may come in the way transducers are used. A recent patent shows the ear drum being driven mechanically rather than acoustically (Perkins and Shennib, 1993). The force driving the ear drum is derived from an electromagnetic field so that no physical connection is necessary. Electromechanical drivers further down the human auditory system have also been suggested (Lenkauskas, 1994). Finally, there is the direct electrical stimulation of the auditory nerve. As you proceed further down the auditory network, the methods used become more intrusive and experimental but, in the end, may hold the most promise.

## *Options*

An attempt will be made in this section to integrate the information discussed as to the options available for transducers. Please keep in mind the following divisions among manufacturers of hearing aids, as well as designers within these companies. One group, probably those whose expertise is strongest in amplifier design and application, feels that the amplifier alone is all that is required to drive the performance of the hearing aid. The microphone and receiver should have as flat, or at least monotonic, a frequency response as possible, with the response shaping controlled by the amplifier. Any transducer that deviates from a flat response must first become compensated by the amplifier before true response shaping can occur. For this group, it might be said that a single model of a microphone, receiver, and telecoil is sufficient.

A second group may feel that it is best to modify the frequency response via the transducer. In this way, whole families of hearing aids can be based on families of transducers. The same amplifier could be used throughout with a "pick and choose" method used to define the final hearing aid.

In practice, it has been difficult to strictly follow either of these two approaches. In the end, the manufacturer willing to combine both of these two viewpoints will probably end up with the most versatile product line.

When selecting a transducer, whether it be a microphone, telecoil, or receiver, several factors can be used to sort among the various options for a particular application. First, is the application for a patient with a mild, moderate, or severe hearing loss? Second, what frequency response is necessary based on the magnitude and configuration of the hearing loss? Third, are there cosmetic or cost concerns? Fourth, is there a particular need or problem in understanding speech when contending with background conversations or other noise?

### Magnitude of Hearing Loss

For a severe hearing loss, the first concern is to deliver sufficient gain and output so that the amplified signal is audible and free of feedback. For this application, a receiver capable of the highest output is necessary without regard to size. To provide high output, and to prevent feedback due to mechanical vibration from the receiver, a dual receiver might be considered. Class D or switching Class B amplifiers will somewhat overcome the limitations in level of the power supply, with the Class D possibly incorporated in the receiver itself.

It might seem that the microphone selection is unimportant in obtaining high gain and output, but amplifiers do have limits on the amplification available. Some of the larger microphones have greater output than the smaller microphones and would present less strain (i.e., distortion) on the amplifier to achieve the same output level. However, some of the larger, but older, microphones are actually poorer than their newer and smaller descendants. For high gain and output power, choose the microphone for high output rather than for size. An internally amplified microphone might be preferred, but only if it is relatively immune to feedback problems and distortion.

For a telecoil, for maximum output, it is probably true that the larger telecoil is the better unless the telecoil contains its own amplifier. Again, the intent is to have as large an input signal level to the amplifier as is possible.

In general, the size of the transducer is probably not as great a problem as the output level without the result of feedback. This presence of feedback may preclude an ITE hearing aid and require a BTE or even body-worn aid. For moderate to mild gain hearing aids, the remaining concerns can be more easily addressed.

### Frequency Response

For frequency response, there are many options that can be created by the transducer. In general, the various microphone response shapes are available for even the smallest microphones. Telecoils with different frequency responses are available in the smaller sizes. Receivers have more of a limitation, not because their size precludes frequency response shaping, but because a good portion of receiver modification is performed via tubing that may not be practical for ITC or CIC applications. In this instance, the BTE hearing aid has an advantage.

### Cosmetic Concerns

If the hearing loss is mild to moderate, cosmetic concerns may dominate the application. In this circumstance, the smaller the better is probably true. The smallest transducers possible, regardless of performance, may be needed. If CIC or ITC fitting is attempted, some protection from cerumen occlusion would probably be best.

### Conversation in Background Noise

Finally, for those who complain that their hearing aid works fine in quiet, but speech is impossible to understand with background competition, perhaps a directional microphone might be appropriate. ITE applications of directional microphones is a new approach to an old problem. Only time will tell if it is a good solution.

## *Conclusion*

The authors of this chapter are transducer designers, not hearing aid designers or audiologists. It would be difficult for them to objectively differentiate between their own products and transducers offered by competitors. As noted earlier, most transducer manufacturers maintain a complete product line with generic equivalents of size, shape, and performance. In addition, any attempt to present a complete listing of available transducers will be obsolete before it is printed. The only way for a hearing aid designer or audiologist to be aware of the state of the art is to be in constant contact with transducer manufacturers. To this end, Table 3–1 is provided with the name, address, and phone numbers of the larger transducer manufacturers.

Transducers have been designed to fill a need, and hearing aid transducers were designed to fill the need of the hearing impaired. Unfortunately, the transducer designer is most proficient in the design and less proficient in the application of

**Table 3–1.**   Transducer Manufacturers

Knowles Electronics, Inc.
  1151 Maplewood Dr.
  Itasca, IL 60143
  Phone (708) 250-5100 Fax (708) 250-0575
  Microphone, Receivers

Lectret S.A.
  25 Pr. des Champs-Frechets
  1217 Meyrin, Geneva, Switzerland
  Phone 022 782 38 82 Fax 022 782 10 63
  Microphones

PI-AC
  Siemens Nederland N.V. Audiological Components
  Zekeringstraat 9, NL 1014 BM Amsterdam, The Netherlands
  P.O. Box 61200, NL 1005 HE Amsterdam, The Netherlands
  Phone +31 20-606.8100 Fax +31 20-684.2381
  Microphones, Receivers

Tibbetts Industries, Inc.
  Box 1096 Colcord Ave.
  Camden, ME 04843
  Phone (207) 236-3301 Fax (207) 236-3303
  Microphones, Telecoils, Receivers

Microtronics A/S
  12-14, Byleddet
  4000 Roskilde, Denmark
  Phone 45 42 36 56 91 Fax 45 46 32 00 54
  Telecoils

these designs to the needs of the hearing impaired. It is the responsibility of the audiologist not only to diagnose the needs of the hearing impaired, but also to request and, if necessary, demand improvements in transducer technology. These demands must be specific, and attempts at satisfying these needs must not only be verified experimentally but, if successful, they should be supported.

## References

ANSI S3.7-1973. *Method for Coupler Calibration for Earphones.* New York: National Standards Institute.

Bauer BB. (1948). Magnetic translating device. United States Patent Number 2,454,425.

Bauer BB. (1953). A miniature microphone for transistorized amplifiers. *J Acoust Soc Am* 25:867–869.

Carlson EV. (1963). Electro-mechanical transducer. United States Patent Number 3,111,563.

Carlson EV, Cross FW, Killion MC. (1971). Miniature acoustic transducer of improved construction. United States Patent Number 3,588,383.

Carlson EV, Killion MC. (1972). Acoustic transducer having diaphragm pivoted in its surround. United States Patent Number 3,701,865.

Carlson EV, Killion MC. (1973). Diaphragm assembly for electret transducer. United States Patent Number 3,740,496.

Carlson EV, Madaffari PL (1988). Acoustic transducer with improved electrode spacing. United States Patent Number 4,730,283.

Egolf DP, Carlson EV, Mostardo AF. (1989). Design evolution of miniature electroacoustic transducers. The 118th Meeting of the Acoustical Society of America. St. Louis, MO.

Fener H. (1963) Hearing-aid sound transducer. United States Patent Number 3,076,062.

Flint WT, Tibbetts GC. (1972). Transducer having piezoelectric struts. United States Patent Number 3,967,790.

Fraim FW, Murphy PV. (1974). Electret transducer cartridge and case. United States Patent Number 3,816,671.

Hodgson WR, Skinner PH. (1977). Hearing Aid Assessment and Use in Audiologic Rehabilitation. Baltimore: Williams & Wilkins Co.

Hunt FV. (1982). *Electroacoustics, the Analysis of Transduction and its Historical Background.* Cambridge: Harvard University Press.

Killion MC. (1984). Microphone with stepped response. United States Patent Number 4,450,930.

Knowles HS, Plice WA. (1959). Electro-mechanical transducing device. United States Patent Number 2,912,522.

Knowles HS, Mullen. (1959). Electroacoustic transducer. United States Patent Number 2,912,523.

Lenkauskas E. (1994). Private communication.

Madaffari PL. (1974). Pressure response about the ear. The 88th meeting of the Acoustical Society of America. St. Louis, MO.

Marshall BF. (1992). *Telecoils: State of the Art.* ASHA Annual Convention, San Antonio, TX.

Perkins RC, Shennib AA. (1993). Contact transducer assembly for hearing devices. United States Patent Number 5,259,032.

Ribic Z. (1993). Hearing aid for persons with a hearing impaired faculty. United States Patent Number 5,214,709.

Schmitt TA. (1973). Backplate construction for electret transducer. United States Patent Number 3,772,133.

Sessler GM, West JE. (1973). Electret transducers: A review. *J Acoust Soc Am* 53:1589–1600.

Shaw EAG. (1974). Wave properties of the human external ear and various physical models of the ear. The 88th Meeting of the Acoustical Society of America.

Sprenkels AJ, Bergveld P. (1990). Electroacoustic transducer of the so called "electret" type, and a method of making such a transducer. United States Patent Number 4,908,805.

Stanley WK. (1977). The transducer—The last dinosaur. *Hear Aid J* 6:10–53.

Stanley WK, Tibbetts GC. (1985). Transducer with translationally adjustable armature. United States Patent Number 4,518,811

Tibbetts RW. (1945). Piezoelectric device. United States Patent Number 2,386,279

Tibbetts GC. (1946). Piezoelectric device. United States Patent Number 2,403,692.

Tibbetts RW, Tibbetts GC. (1961). Magnetic translating device. United States Patent Number 2,994,016.

Tibbetts GC. (1970). Magnetic translating device. United States Patent Number 3,515,818.

Tibbetts RW, Sawyer JA. (1971). Magnetic reed type acoustic transducer with improved armature. United States Patent Number 3,617,653.

Tibbetts GC. (1983). Transducer with adjustable armature yoke and method of adjustment. United States Patent Number 4,410,769.

Tibbetts GC, Madaffari PL. (1993). Hearing-aid sound transducer. United States Patent Number 5,220,612.

Tibbetts GC. (1994). Balanced armature transducers with transverse gap. United States Patent Number 5,299,176.

Victoreen JA. (1978). Hearing aid transducer with plural transducers. United States Patent Number 4,109,116.

Whitney A. (1973). The diabow microphone. *Hear Dealer* 4:8–9.

# 4

# Amplifiers and Circuit Algorithms of Contemporary Hearing Aids

## TODD FORTUNE

## Introduction

In recent years, the hearing aid industry has undergone a technological transformation that is unprecedented in its history. Advances in hearing aid design, manufacturing, and miniaturization have led to the creation of products that, until recently, existed only as concepts in the minds of engineers, researchers, and audiologists. The rate at which new products are introduced has also increased dramatically, making the task of selecting appropriate amplification for the hearing-impaired listener increasingly complicated.

This chapter is intended to help clarify some of the complex and often confusing issues associated with amplifiers and circuit designs that are currently available or may soon be available in hearing aids. This discussion has been written not by a hearing aid engineer or circuit designer, but by an audiologist employed by a hearing aid manufacturer. As such, the writer represents a link between those who design and ultimately create new products, and those who dispense and adjust these devices to assist the hearing impaired. Rather than discuss the characteristics or features of specific products, the approach of this chapter will be to illustrate principles that apply to product performance. These principles will apply long after current products have disappeared from the marketplace, and may be used to evaluate new products as they become available. If successful, this chapter will help convince the reader that, despite the vast array of technical hearing aid specifications that now exist both within and across manufacturers, informed decisions about amplification *can* be made and appropriately applied to the needs of the hearing-impaired client.

This chapter is organized around three topics. The first topic describes three types of amplifiers that are currently used in hearing aids. Although there has been much discussion about class A, class B, and class D amplifiers, relatively little has

157

been said about how these amplifiers function, how they differ, and what the advantages or disadvantages of these three types of amplifiers may be.

The second topic is devoted to linear and nonlinear amplification, topics that could fill a book by themselves. This discussion will address basic concepts associated with linear amplification, illustrate principles that differentiate various nonlinear circuit algorithms, and provide examples of recently implemented signal-processing strategies. This section will also provide evidence from the scientific literature that addresses the benefits, limitations, and unanswered questions pertaining to both linear and nonlinear amplification for the hearing-impaired listener, and will offer basic guidelines and considerations that should be made when selecting and fitting these devices.

The chapter will conclude with a discussion of current and future directions in hearing aid technology. Numerous advances in analog and digital technology are reshaping the way hearing aids are designed, and soon circuit algorithms may provide benefits to the hearing impaired that are not currently possible. This section will describe some of the new technologies and signal processing strategies currently under development.

### *Hearing Aid Amplifiers: In a Class by Themselves*

A hearing aid amplifier consists primarily of small transistors that are built into an integrated circuit. Transistors provide current sources, govern switching networks, and serve a variety of other purposes essential to the operation of electronic circuits. The primary function of transistors in hearing aids, however, is to increase the power of an electrical signal, i.e. to provide amplification. Most hearing aids require hundreds of transistors to function, a potential problem were it not for the fact that transistors are incredibly small in size, and likely to become smaller in the future. As they do, it will become possible to build increasingly complex circuits into smaller and smaller hearing aids, an outcome that will likely appeal to many hearing aid wearers.

Hearing aids typically have two or more stages of amplification. The electrical signal provided by a hearing aid microphone is first amplified by an input stage amplifier, also known as a preamplifier. Usually, the amount of gain provided by a preamplifier is relatively low, with the majority of amplification supplied by the output stage or power amplifier. Between stages of amplification the signal may be filtered or in other ways processed, but the final signal generally requires an output stage amplifier to provide appropriate gain.

The class or type of output stage amplifier used in modern hearing aids has been a widely discussed topic in recent years, frequently addressed in literature provided by manufacturers that promotes one particular amplifier type or another. The most common amplifiers referred to are class A, class B, and class D. These amplifiers are distinguished from one another by the manner in which electrical signals are processed and by the efficiency in which battery current is utilized. Although the three amplifier classes listed above are those most commonly used in hearing aids, they are, in fact, part of a larger family of amplifier types that are used in a variety of electronics applications. Class A, B, and D amplifiers are quite distinct, and each type has characteristics that make it appropriate for use in hearing aids. The true advantage of one type of amplifier over another depends primarily on the gain and output sound pressure level (SPL) needed to fit a particular hearing loss, the amount of physical space available within the hearing aid shell, and, to some extent, the personal preference of the dispenser.

## The Class A Amplifier

The class A amplifier has been used in hearing aids longer and more extensively than any other amplifier class. The success of the class A may be attributed to a variety of characteristics that make it attractive for hearing aid use. First, the class A amplifier can be quite small in physical size and, as such, will fit in even the smallest hearing aids. The class A is reliable, requires little circuitry to operate, and is inexpensive to build. These characteristics make the class A amplifier appealing to those who prefer inexpensive, "no frills" amplification.

The class A amplifier, however, also has undesirable characteristics. Its greatest limitation may be that it continuously draws battery current, even in the absence of a signal. The inefficient use of battery current can lead to excessively low battery life unless the amplifier has been specifically designed for low current drain. In doing so, the SSPL90 (ANSI S3.22-1987) of the hearing aid will be relatively low. When designed in this way, the class A amplifier does not have the capability to generate high-level output signals without also generating significant saturation-induced distortion. This is illustrated in Figure 4–1, which shows the amplification of three hypothetical sinusoids that differ in amplitude. These signals could represent three input levels, three gain settings, or perhaps three combinations of input and gain. The two lower amplitude sinusoids have been amplified without distortion, as indicated by their smooth sinusoidal patterns. These tones would probably sound "clean" to a listener. The strongest signal, however, has been asymmetrically "clipped," as indicated by the squared-off peaks that occur during one phase of the waveform. Clipping occurs when the combination of input and gain exceeds the output capability of the power amplifier or some other component of the circuit, such as the preamplifier or receiver. The asymmetrical clipping associated with class A amplifiers generates distortion that consists of both even and odd order harmonics of the input signal, which can be quite detrimental to the sound quality of the hearing aid (Gioannini and Franzen, 1978). The class A *can* be built to produce less distorted high-level output, but only by raising the quiescent current drain and, therefore, the rate at which batteries are consumed. To avoid this, class A amplifiers are typically "starved for current," which results in practical battery life at the expense of low SSPL90. The link between quiescent current drain and maximum power output leads to a situation that has been referred to as a lack of "headroom," a term that describes the difference between the SSPL90 of the hearing aid and the sum of input plus gain (Preves and Newton, 1989). When high gain is applied to an input signal of even moderate intensity, the SSPL90 of the typical class A instrument is easily reached, resulting in saturation-induced distortion and an inevitable decrease in sound quality for the listener. For this reason, the class A amplifier is most appropriate for hearing aids requiring low gain and low output SPL, unless the user is willing to accept high battery consumption.

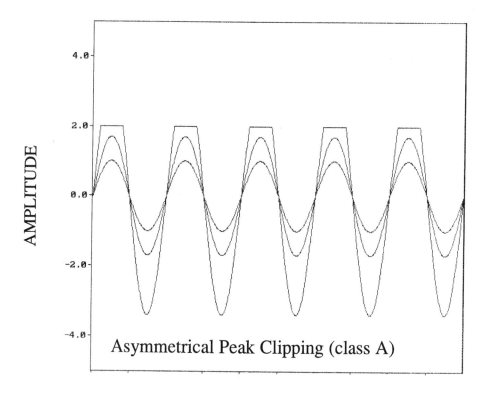

TIME

**Figure 4–1.** Hypothetical amplification of three sinusoids by a class A amplifier, illustrating asymmetrical peak clipping.

### The Class B Amplifier

The class B amplifier was designed in part to overcome the limitations of the class A. The class B amplifier (more properly referred to as class AB, to be described shortly) consists of two amplifiers, one acting on the positive phase of an incoming signal, the other on the negative phase. This design has earned the class B the title of "push-pull" amplifier. Each amplifier has minimal current drain when idle, but can generate high current and high output SPLs when required. These characteristics give the class B amplifier a higher SSPL90 and more headroom than is possible with a typical class A amplifier. Figure 4–2 illustrates class B processing of the same three signals shown in Figure 4–1, as well as a fourth signal that illustrates peak clipping. The upper panel illustrates the activity of two amplifiers, which respond alternately, depending on the phase of the input signal. The lower panel shows the combined outputs of the two hypothetical amplifiers. The three original waveforms from Figure 4–1 have been amplified without being clipped, a result that would be consistent with the greater headroom of the class B amplifier. At high input or gain, however, peak clipping will, in fact, occur, but will affect both phases of the waveform equally. Symmetrical clipping, as this is

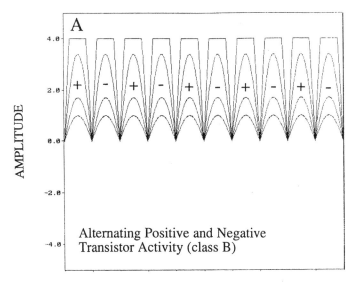

TIME

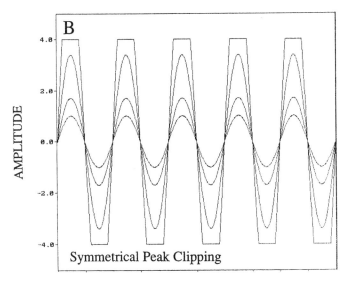

TIME

**Figure 4–2.** Hypothetical amplification of 3 sinusoids by a class B amplifier. (A) Alternating positive- and negative-phase transistor activity. (B) Amplified waveforms, illustrating symmetrical peak clipping at high levels.

called, generates primarily odd order harmonics of the input signal, which can also reduce sound quality (Kates and Kozma Spytek, 1994). Although formal research has yet to be conducted comparing the effects of symmetrical versus asymmetrical clipping on sound quality, symmetrical clipping has been reported to be less objectionable (Dirks, 1994; Hawkins, 1994). Thus, not only is the class B amplifier less prone to saturate than the class A, but the distortion produced by a class B amplifier at saturation may be less objectionable than that associated with a class A.

A true class B amplifier has zero current drain in quiet, and is completely off during that phase of a signal to which it does not respond. A true class B, however, has its own disadvantages, most notably a phenomenon known as crossover distortion. Crossover distortion occurs at the transition between activation and deactivation of the two amplifiers. If the positive-phase amplifier is not activated at the precise moment that the negative-phase amplifier is turned off (or vice versa), the transition between phases of amplification is imperfect, and crossover distortion occurs. Crossover distortion can become audible and can reduce sound quality. It is prevented by applying a small amount of current to both amplifiers at all times, which prevents the amplifiers from completely shutting off. Technically called a class AB design, an amplifier of this type helps guarantee a smooth transition between amplified signal phases. The class AB amplifier (which will be referred to as class B for the remainder of this chapter) has significant advantages over the class A amplifier, but it is also more complex and requires more components to function. In the past, the physical size of the class B amplifier has limited its use to larger hearing aids. In recent years, however, this situation has improved (Johnson and Killion, 1994), making the class B feasible for use in a variety of hearing aid styles, including canal aids.

### The Class D Amplifier

The class D output stage amplifier represents a further refinement in signal processing efficiency, and operates in a manner that is distinct from class A and class B amplifiers (Carlson, 1988). The essential elements of the class D amplifier are illustrated in Figure 4–3. The class D amplifier generates an inaudible, very high-frequency (typically 100 kHz) electrical signal called a carrier (panel A). This carrier is present whenever the amplifier is turned on. When an acoustic signal, such as that represented in panel B, is presented to the hearing aid, the electrical carrier is modulated by the acoustic input signal. This combined waveform, illustrated in panel C, serves as the input to a comparator circuit. The function of the comparator is to control the duration of an electrical pulse that governs the average current provided to the hearing aid receiver coil. This current, in turn, drives the receiver diaphragm that provides the amplified acoustic signal. The comparator switches between a high and a low state, depending on whether its input is above or below a fixed trigger threshold. When the input level exceeds the comparator's trigger threshold, the comparator switches to a high state, starting the electrical pulse. When the input drops below the trigger threshold, the comparator switches to a low state, which ends the electrical pulse. The duration (or "width") of each pulse is thus determined by the length of time the comparator's trigger threshold is exceeded, a process known as pulse width modulation. This process is illustrated in panel D, which shows a series of pulses that correspond to the waveform segment highlighted in panel C. It can be seen that the duration of each pulse varies with the instantaneous amplitude of the signal. Longer duration pulses (like those toward the left and right sides of the figure) cause the average current applied to the receiver coil to increase, while shorter duration

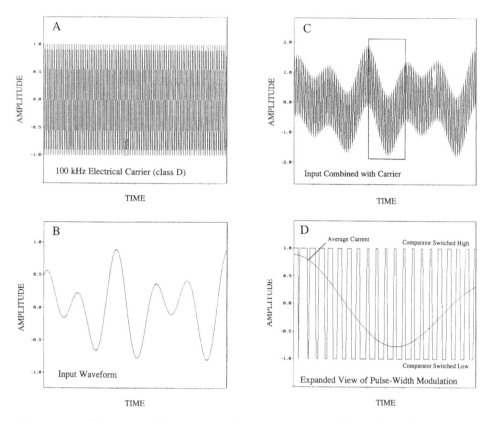

**Figure 4–3.** Class D signal processing. (A) Representation of a 100 kHz class D carrier signal. (B) Acoustic waveform serving as input to the hearing aid. (C) Waveform representing the sum of the input and carrier signals. (D) Pulse-width modulation of the summed waveform, also showing changing average current applied to the receiver coil, which faithfully represents the input waveform.

pulses (in the middle of the figure) cause the average current applied to the coil to decrease. The coil does not respond to the extremely high-frequency carrier, but does respond to the fluctuating average current, which faithfully follows the original input signal. The result is an amplified acoustic signal that is generated with very efficient use of battery current. The class D amplifier is also a high-headroom device, generates symmetrical clipping upon saturation, and is built *within* the receiver casing (Knowles Electronics), conserving space and allowing use of the device in very small hearing aids.

## Which Class is Really Best?

Much of the professional discussion of amplifier classes has maligned the class A amplifier (with good reason) in favor of the class D amplifier (also with good reason). Indeed, recent research has indicated that both sound quality and aided loudness discomfort levels (LDLs) are higher for class D amplification than for comparable class A amplification, probably due to the influence of headroom. The effect of headroom on sound quality has been examined by Palmer, Killion, Wilber, and Ballad (in press). In this investigation, sound quality judgments were obtained from both normal-hearing and hearing-impaired subjects who compared class D and class A linear hearing aids at input levels ranging from 70–100 dB SPL. Their results, shown in Figure 4–4, indicated that both normal-hearing (panel A) and hearing-impaired (panel B) listeners found the class D hearing aid superior to the class A in sound quality at each level tested. Equally important, the difference in sound quality between the two hearing aids increased with signal presentation level, a result that the authors attributed to the high distortion associated with the class A amplifier. Similar results were reported by

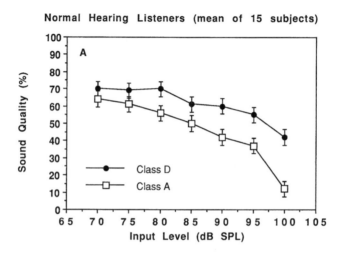

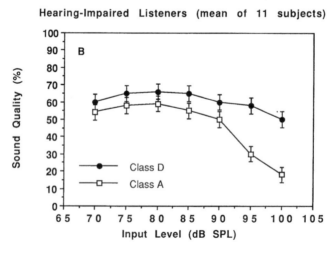

**Figure 4–4.** Sound quality ratings as a function of input level for class D and class A amplifiers for (A) normal-hearing and (B) hearing-impaired listeners (from Palmer et al., 1995, reprinted with permission).

Potts, Valente, Agnew, and Goebel (1994). These data suggest a strong relationship between the amount of saturation-induced distortion and the sound quality
of hearing aids. They imply that minimizing distortion should increase user
satisfaction.

Fortune and Preves (1992) obtained aided LDLs from a group of five hearing-
impaired subjects who listened extensively to continuous discourse through class
D and comparable class A linear hearing aids. The results of this study, shown in
Figure 4–5, indicated that the mean aided LDL (panel A) associated with the
class D hearing aid was 6 dB higher than that associated with the class A device.
Coherence measurements (panel B, see Chapter 1) obtained at the time of testing
indicated that saturation-induced distortion was considerably lower at LDL for
the class D hearing aid than was true for the class A device. These data suggest
that saturation-induced distortion may contribute to the sensation of loudness
(thus lowering the aided LDL unnecessarily) and also suggest that a high-level

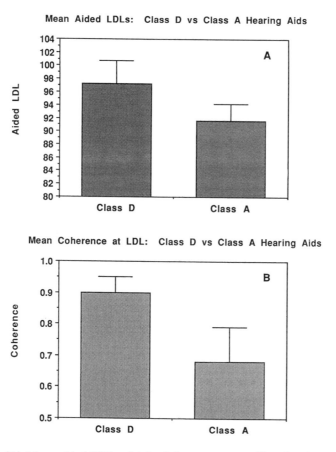

**Figure 4–5.** (A) Mean aided LDLs obtained from a group of hearing-impaired listeners
wearing Class D and comparable Class A hearing aids. (B) Mean coherence obtained at
LDL for the same group of listeners.

"clean" signal will likely be found more tolerable than a high-level distorted signal.

In comparing amplifier types, one should not overlook the merits of the class B output stage, which is comparable in many respects to the class D (Johnson and Killion, 1994). From an electroacoustic standpoint, both the class D and class B amplifiers are superior to the class A for high-fidelity hearing aid applications but, unfortunately, behavioral research comparing the class B with either the class D or class A amplifier is almost nonexistent. In the only such study that the author is aware of, Perreault (1994) presented sentences representing class B and class D signal processing to a group of normal-hearing listeners. Using a three-alternative forced-choice paradigm, a three-interval test block was created in which two intervals represented one type of amplifier (either class B or D), and the third interval represented the other amplifier type. Listeners were asked simply to identify which of the three listening intervals was different from the other two. Results indicated that at recording levels of 60, 75, and 85 dB SPL, subjects were unable to identify the odd intervals at levels above chance performance, which suggests that sound processed by class B and class D amplifiers may be quite comparable.

Class B and class D amplifiers are also comparable electroacoustically. Similar gain and SSPL90 values may be produced with either output stage. In fact, the only distinguishing feature between class B and class D amplifiers may be current drain, as illustrated in Table 4–1. The table shows typical current drain per ANSI S3.22 (1987) and expected battery life for high-powered class B, class D and class A hearing aids with similar HFA full-on gain and HFA SSPL90 values. Current drain for the class D hearing aid is the lowest overall, followed closely by the class B instrument. The class A hearing aid has the highest drain overall. By dividing the milliamp hours associated with a given battery type by the current drain of the hearing aid, an estimate of battery life may be obtained. For both types of battery shown (#13 and #312), the expected battery life is highest for the class D device, followed closely by the class B device. Both types show considerably higher expected battery life than the class A hearing aid. It is for this reason that class A amplifiers are typically designed for maximum battery life rather than high gain and output.

Due to its small size and low cost, the class A amplifier will likely continue to be used prominently within the industry, despite its limitations. The advantages of class B and class D amplifiers, however, far outweigh the fact that they may be slightly larger or slightly more expensive than the class A.

**Table 4–1.**    Expected Battery Life for Representative High-Powered Class D, Class B, and Class A Linear Hearing Aids

| Output Stage Type | HFA Full On Gain (dB) | HFA SSPL90 (dB SPL) | Current Drain (mA) | Expected Battery Life (#13 Battery) | Expected Battery Life (#312 Battery) |
|---|---|---|---|---|---|
| Class D | 52 | 123 | .59 | 390 hours | 204 hours |
| Class B | 50 | 121 | .63 | 365 hours | 190 hours |
| Class A | 52 | 116 | .75 | 307 hours | 160 hours |

## *Linear Amplification*

Perhaps the greatest distinction between hearing aid circuit designs, regardless of the class of amplifier used, is whether the circuit is "linear" or "nonlinear." In one sense, the two circuit types are not mutually exclusive; all linear algorithms become nonlinear at saturation, while most nonlinear algorithms operate linearly over at least some part of their operating range. For practical purposes, a linear hearing aid is one that maintains a 1:1 input/output (I/O) function across its unsaturated operating range. That is, for a given amount of gain, a linear hearing aid will produce a 10 dB change in output for each 10 dB change in input until the onset of saturation. Linear amplification represents the most common type of hearing aid fitting in use today (Cranmer, 1992).

A linear hearing aid may be designed with a class A, a class B, or a class D output stage, and the type of output stage used will affect the performance of the instrument. Those individuals with low gain requirements make good candidates for class A amplifiers, but most hearing-impaired individuals are more appropriately fit with either class B or class D amplifiers, due to the efficient use of battery current and the greater gain and output SPLs typically associated with these devices. A word of caution is warranted, however, when fitting stronger hearing aids. The preceding discussion may have suggested to the reader that a high SSPL is always preferable to a low SSPL, because the likelihood of saturation is reduced when the instrument is capable of generating higher output SPLs. Although true to a degree, this statement must be tempered by the fact that under certain circumstances loudness discomfort can occur if the SSPL of a hearing aid is too high. In reality, a tradeoff exists between preventing excessive distortion (by keeping the SSPL high) and preventing loudness discomfort (often assumed to be accomplished by keeping the SSPL low). As discussed earlier, however, saturation-induced distortion has been shown to *contribute* to the sensation of loudness (Fortune and Preves, 1992), which means that a report of loudness discomfort will not necessarily be solved by reducing the SSPL of a hearing aid. The decision to limit the output of a hearing aid at a given level should be based on avoiding excessive distortion as well as preventing loudness discomfort for the hearing aid wearer.

### The Problem With Peak Clipping

As stated above, one purpose of output limitation is to prevent the output sound pressure level of a hearing aid from exceeding a hearing-impaired listener's level of discomfort. The method used to achieve output limitation determines the amount and type of distortion generated at saturation. Peak clipping is the most frequently used method of output limiting in the United States (Hawkins and Naidoo, 1993). As previously discussed, peak clipping occurs when an electrical signal exceeds the maximum output of some component of the hearing aid circuit, which causes numerous forms of distortion. The amount of distortion increases as the input to the hearing aid or hearing aid gain increases beyond the clipping threshold, and distortion caused by peak clipping has been shown to reduce the intelligibility and subjective quality of speech (Gioannini and Franzen, 1978).

Kates and Kozma-Spytek (1994) also examined the relationship between peak clipping and the sound quality of speech, and provided convincing evidence of the detrimental effects of peak clipping. In this investigation, normal-hearing subjects were asked to listen to sentences peak clipped at 0, 4, 8, and 12 dB above a 75 dB SPL presentation level and to provide their impressions of sound quality. The results, reproduced as Figure 4–6, showed that for each of three distinct frequency responses, sound quality ratings improved as the peak clipping threshold increased. Severely clipped speech (0, 4 dB conditions) was associated with much lower sound quality ratings than speech that was less severely clipped (8, 12 dB conditions). These results clearly suggest that distortion due to peak clipping has a negative effect on speech quality in hearing aids. Fortunately, peak clipping is not the only method of output limitation available in hearing aids. As will be discussed in a following section, compression is superior to peak clipping as a means of output limitation, and is recommended for all but the most severe hearing losses.

## Summary

The acoustic performance and potential benefits of linear amplification are clearly affected by the amount of distortion present in the amplified signal. The low

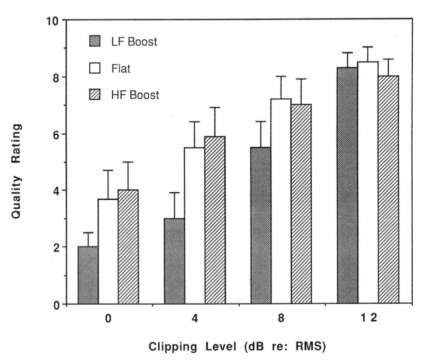

**Figure 4–6.** Sound quality ratings as a function of clipping level for hearing aids adjusted to three frequency responses (from Kates and Kozma-Spytek, 1994, reprinted with permission).

SSPL associated with the typical class A linear amplifier can lead to unsatisfactory sound quality due to the presence of high distortion. Higher headroom class B and class D amplifiers are less likely to distort, and more likely to maintain high sound quality. Regardless of output stage type, linear algorithms that peak clip upon saturation will likely be found unsatisfactory when clipping occurs, particularly if clipping is asymmetrical (as in class A devices). The highly negative consequences of saturation-induced distortion has, in part, prompted the development of nonlinear algorithms, which also serve a variety of other purposes.

## Nonlinear Amplification

Nonlinear amplification can take a wide variety of forms, but common among nonlinear hearing aids is some type of level-dependent signal processing, such as a change in gain or frequency response with input level variations. Most nonlinear hearing aids reduce gain as input or output levels increase and, therefore, generate an I/O function with a slope of less than 1.0 over some part of their operating range. The "amount" of nonlinear processing, the factors that trigger it, and the range of frequencies affected by it depend on the objectives of the signal processing strategy. Like linear hearing aids, nonlinear hearing aid algorithms are designed to perform two basic functions. First, they should amplify a wide variety of environmental sounds so that they become audible to the hearing-impaired listener without being uncomfortably loud. As one might expect, this can be difficult when the listener's dynamic range is small, particularly for linear amplifiers. The second function of nonlinear amplification is to minimize saturation, an objective that can also be difficult to achieve with linear amplification. By adjusting gain in a level-dependent manner, nonlinear hearing aids are more likely to provide comfortable amplification and less likely to generate saturation-induced distortion than comparable linear hearing aids.

The following section is devoted to three of the most common types of nonlinear amplification; algorithms that provide compression, bass increases at low levels (BILL), and treble increases at low levels (TILL). These algorithms are not mutually exclusive, in that both BILL- and TILL-type processing (Killion, Staab, and Preves, 1990) may be accomplished with *multiband* compression circuits, but each of these signal-processing schemes is based on a unique set of assumptions about how best to accomplish the objectives of amplification. For this reason, these three types of nonlinear amplification will be discussed separately.

## Compression

Loudness recruitment is perhaps the greatest reason for the use of compression in hearing aids. Loudness recruitment refers to an abnormally rapid growth of loudness that often accompanies hearing loss. It is experienced by those who have elevated thresholds but normal LDLs, and, therefore, an abnormally small dynamic range of hearing. It has long been known that linear hearing aids are not well suited to those with recruitment, because linear amplification cannot compensate for a reduced dynamic range. In a quiet environment, the listener wearing a linear instrument will often adjust the gain (volume) control to a reasonably high setting, in order to hear speech as clearly as possible. In doing so, a sudden impulsive sound may easily cause loudness discomfort. In a noisy environment, the listener often adjusts the gain control downward, which increases the risk that speech will be misunderstood due to insufficient gain. This scenario can easily lead to frustration on the part of the listener, who may stop using the device for lack of sufficient benefit.

Compression amplifiers are designed to prevent some of the problems associated with linear amplification. Depending on the design, compression amplifiers reduce gain when either the input to the device or the output from the device exceeds a predetermined level. This process tends to result in comfortable amplification for the hearing aid wearer and tends to prevent the hearing aid from saturating. When properly selected and properly fit, a compression hearing aid can help ensure that components of speech essential to intelligibility will be audible, that less essential speech components will not disrupt speech recognition, and that impulsive or high-level sounds will not cause discomfort. To date, no one type of compression hearing aid has been shown to accomplish each of these objectives for all hearing-impaired listeners. Perhaps as a result, variations in compression amplification are many, a fact that can lead to confusion on the part of those selecting and fitting the devices. Although the number of types of compression systems commercially available today is high, each may be described by properties that may be measured. Before discussing various types of compression, a discussion of principles that apply to compression amplifiers is necessary. These principles help to differentiate the various types of compression that are used in hearing aids, but as it will be shown, the precise description or quantification of compression characteristics is not always a straightforward process.

### Static and Dynamic Properties of Compression Hearing Aids

Compression hearing aids are distinguished from one another by their static characteristics, such as compression threshold and compression ratio, and their dynamic or time-dependent characteristics, such as attack and release times. The static properties of a compression hearing aid are illustrated in Figure 4–7, which shows an I/O function that might be observed when testing a compression hearing aid on a 2-cc coupler. In the example, the function has a linear slope at input levels between 50 and 65 dB SPL. At 65 dB SPL, the slope of the function changes, indicating that compression has begun. As defined by ANSI S3.22 (1987), the *compression threshold* is the input level corresponding to the point where the I/O function departs from a linear slope by 2 dB. The compression threshold in the example is approximately 68 dB SPL. The *compression ratio* is the ratio of the change in output SPL corresponding to a given change in input SPL, i.e., the change in input level divided by the change in output level. In the example, the compression ratio is 2:1, because a 10 dB increase in input level (above the compression threshold) results in only a 5 dB increase in output level.

The definitions of compression threshold and compression ratio, although appropriate for many compression amplifiers, do not provide an adequate description of all compression circuits. When compression is used as a form of output limiting, for example, the compression threshold is based on output SPL

## Input/Output Function

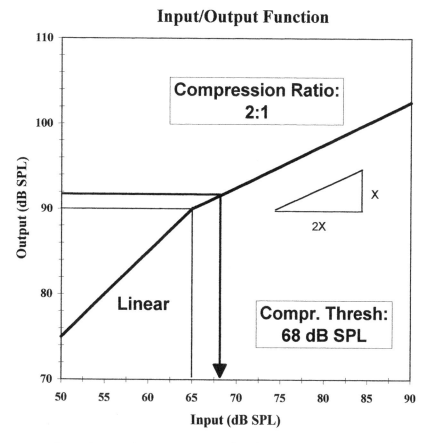

**Figure 4–7.**  Input/output function associated with an input compression hearing aid with a 68 dB SPL compression threshold and a 2:1 compression ratio.

rather than input SPL, and the compression ratio is often high enough that the 2 dB criterion used in the definition of threshold cannot be applied. Similarly, complex compression algorithms are often not adequately described by a single compression threshold or ratio. Figure 4–8A shows an I/O function associated with another compression hearing aid, which shows a linear slope at low input levels, a region of 2:1 compression at moderate input levels, and a region of 10:1 compression at high input levels. This circuit, therefore, has two compression thresholds and two compression ratios. Figure 4–8B shows an I/O function demonstrating "curvilinear" compression (3M MemoryMate). This I/O function changes continuously over the entire input range, making it somewhat difficult to describe either the compression threshold or the compression ratio. The compression threshold is approximately 60 dB SPL, although the function lacks a well-defined linear segment on which to base the calculation. The compression ratio increases with input level and is, therefore, dependent on the input level range used in the calculation. When calculated between input levels of 50 and 70 dB SPL, the compression ratio is approximately 1.4:1, but when calculated between input levels of 70 and 90 dB SPL, the compression ratio is approximately 5.7:1.

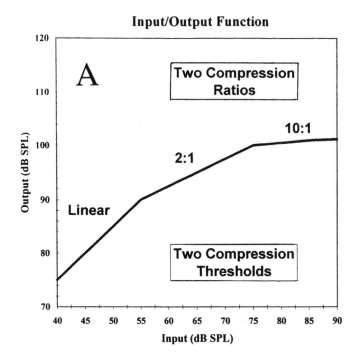

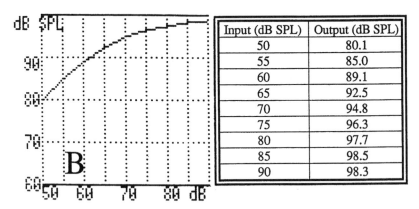

| Input (dB SPL) | Output (dB SPL) |
|---|---|
| 50 | 80.1 |
| 55 | 85.0 |
| 60 | 89.1 |
| 65 | 92.5 |
| 70 | 94.8 |
| 75 | 96.3 |
| 80 | 97.7 |
| 85 | 98.5 |
| 90 | 98.3 |

**Figure 4–8.** (A) Input/output function associated with a compression hearing aid with two compression thresholds and two compression ratios. (B) Input/output function associated with curvilinear compression (3M MemoryMate).

The static properties of compression amplification have been shown to affect user satisfaction. For example, Neuman, Bakke, Hellman, and Levitt (1994) obtained listener preference data for a digitally simulated hearing aid with a compression threshold of 65 dB SPL and a compression ratio that was variable between 1:1 and 10:1. A portion of their results, shown in Figure 4–9, indicated that subjects with both small (panel A) and large (panel B) dynamic ranges preferred

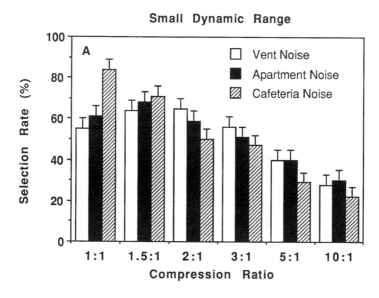

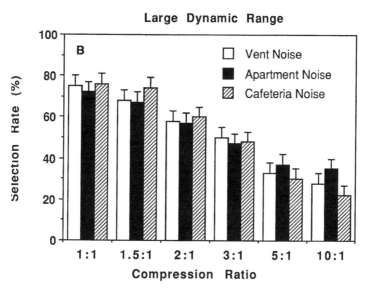

**Figure 4–9.** Circuit selection rates as a function of compression ratio for listeners with (A) small and (B) large dynamic ranges (from Neuman et al., 1994, reprinted with permission).

lower compression ratios when listening to speech mixed with noise. As the compression ratio increased above 1.5:1, selection rates decreased. The authors concluded that compression ratios greater than 3:1 may not be appropriate for hearing-impaired listeners when combined with low compression thresholds.

The dynamic properties (attack and release times) of compression hearing aids are determined by measuring the output of the hearing aid as the input level of a test signal (typically a 2000 Hz tone) is abruptly changed between 55 and 80 dB

SPL. As illustrated in Figure 4–10, *attack time* is the time required for the output of the hearing aid to stabilize to within 2 dB of its steady-state value once the input level is abruptly increased from 55 to 80 dB SPL. *Release time* is similarly defined as the time required for the hearing aid output to stabilize to within 2 dB of steady state after the input level is returned from 80 to 55 dB SPL. Although straightforward under most circumstances, attack and release time measurements as specified by ANSI S3.22 (1987) do not adequately describe the characteristics of compression amplifiers with dual-attack or variable release times, such as those with Adaptive Compression™ (Telex). For example, the K-Amp™ (Etymotic Research), which utilizes the Telex circuit, has both a very fast and a much slower attack time, as described in Chapter 1. This can make attack time estimates misleading. Adaptive compression circuits also have release times that vary with stimulus duration. For circuits such as these, release time measurements are more appropriately made using both long- and short-duration test signals, an option available with some hearing aid analyzers (e.g., Frye Electronics).

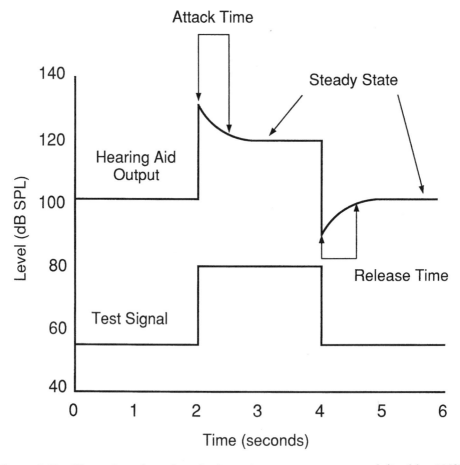

**Figure 4–10.**    Illustration of attack and release time measurements, as defined by ANSI S3.22-1987.

Given the variety and complexity of modern compression hearing aids, the ANSI committee is currently revising the S3.22 standard to better reflect product characteristics. The reader should be aware, however, that standardized tests provide only some of the information needed to quantify product performance.

### Three Classes of Compression Amplifiers

Compression hearing aids have often been classified according to their static and dynamic properties (Walker and Dillon, 1982; Johnson, 1993; Hickson, 1994). Unfortunately, these properties do not fall into distinct categories, and it is difficult, if not impossible, to categorize all compression hearing aids into nonoverlapping types. Be that as it may, general patterns in compression thresholds, compression ratios, and attack/release times may be found that tend to separate compression circuits into three broad categories, which have been described as automatic gain control (AGC), syllabic compression, and compression limiting. Based on a review of the literature and numerous lively discussions, the general characteristics of single-band compression hearing aids have been identified and are presented in Table 4–2.

AUTOMATIC GAIN CONTROL (AGC)

As its name implies, an AGC amplifier is designed to eliminate the need to adjust gain manually as the listening environment changes. Hearing aids with AGC typically have a low compression threshold, a high compression ratio, a relatively fast attack time, and a very long release time. Due to a release time that can be as long as 1 or 2 seconds, the output of an AGC hearing aid remains relatively stable despite input level variations. The advantage of AGC would likely be apparent to a listener who encounters listening environments that frequently vary in level; such an individual might find gain control adjustments unnecessary most of the time. One disadvantage of AGC is that weak elements of speech can be lost if the gain reduced by compression is not restored quickly enough to amplify these sounds to audibility. Another possible problem is that sound quality may deteriorate if the AGC compression ratio is too high (Neuman et al., 1994).

Some studies have indicated improvement in speech recognition using AGC relative to linear amplification (Laurence, Moore, and Glasberg, 1983; Moore, Laurence, and Wright, 1985), while others have indicated either no difference or poorer performance with AGC (Lippmann, Braida, and Durlach, 1981; Boothroyd, Springer, Smith, and Schulman, 1988). In what may be described as a "typical"

**Table 4–2.**  Common Static and Dynamic Characteristics of Single-Band Compression Hearing Aids

| Hearing Aid Type | Compression Threshold (dB SPL) | Compression Ratio | Attack Time (msec) | Release Time (msec) |
|---|---|---|---|---|
| AGC | <65 | >5 | 10–50 | 150–2000 |
| Syllabic Compression | <60 | <5 | <5 | 10–100 |
| Compression Limiting | >80 | >5 | <5 | 50–100 |

finding, Peterson, Feeney, and Yantis (1990) reported that AGC significantly improved speech perception in quiet for listeners with narrow dynamic ranges. This advantage, however, was not found when testing was conducted in a noise background. If sound quality is evaluated instead of speech recognition, AGC has also been shown to offer some benefits. King and Martin (1984) reported that hearing-impaired listeners preferred the sound quality of AGC over linear amplification at high listening levels, in quiet *and* in noise. Thus, the benefits associated with AGC (in fact, any type of amplification) are dependent upon how those benefits are defined. AGC may have certain advantages over linear amplification in quiet listening environments or at high listening levels, but does not appear to improve speech recognition in noise.

WHOLE RANGE SYLLABIC COMPRESSION

Syllabic compression circuits are designed to follow the temporal pattern of speech and to reduce the dynamic range of individual speech components so that they fall within the dynamic range of the listener's hearing. Hearing aids with syllabic compression are, in general, characterized by low compression thresholds, low compression ratios, and fast attack and release times. A low-compression threshold ensures that many elements of speech will trigger compression. Fast attack and release times are designed so that high-amplitude vowels are compressed, while low-amplitude consonants (that often follow vowels) are not. In addition to compressing speech, syllabic compression circuits may also provide better protection against transient sounds than do AGC circuits. The primary problem associated with syllabic compressors is an audible artifact sometimes described as "pumping," a phenomenon that is caused by rapid gain fluctuations. This problem can usually be prevented by increasing the release time of the amplifier, either at the factory or by way of an external control. The duration-dependent release time of Adaptive Compression™ circuits is also designed to prevent pumping.

Studies of the effects of syllabic compression on speech recognition have been largely inconclusive. Dreschler (1988) reported compression to be superior to linear amplification for phoneme perception in quiet. Dreschler (1989) furthered this conclusion by reporting that the perception of plosive sounds was improved as a result of syllabic compression. Dreschler, Eberhardt, and Melk (1984) and Tyler and Kuk (1989), however, reported little or no advantage of syllabic compression over linear amplification when testing was conducted in a background of noise. In addition to the problems associated with background noise, speech recognition has also been shown to be affected by the release time of the compression amplifier, which, when longer than about 300 milliseconds, can adversely affect performance (Schweitzer and Causey, 1977). Like AGC circuits, some evidence exists to support the use of syllabic compression in hearing aids, although difficulties remain, particularly with regard to improving speech recognition in noise.

COMPRESSION LIMITING

Compression limiting provides a method of output limitation that is often used as an alternative to peak clipping. Compression limiters are described by their high compression thresholds, high compression ratios, and very fast attack times. As discussed previously, the primary purpose of compression limiting is to prevent loudness discomfort, and to do so without generating significant saturation-induced distortion. In its simplest form, a hearing aid with compression-limiting functions as a linear device across most of its operating range, but at some relatively high output SPL (generally above 80 dB) compression acts to prevent excessively high levels from reaching the ear. Compression-limiting devices are less prone to saturate, and generate much less distortion at high levels than comparable peak clipping instruments (Walker and Dillon, 1982). Compression limiting can be used in conjunction with AGC or syllabic compression to accomplish more than one objective.

In an effort to establish whether peak clipping or compression limiting provides superior output limitation, Hawkins and Naidoo (1993) obtained sound quality data from a group of 12 hearing-impaired subjects with mild to moderate losses. These subjects listened to connected discourse and music through hearing aids with either peak clipping or compression limiting as the method of output limitation. Testing was conducted at input levels 12 dB below circuit saturation, 5 dB above saturation, and 20 dB above saturation, and subjects were asked to indicate which of the two hearing aids they preferred for each of the three conditions. Results indicated not only that subjects preferred compression limiting over peak clipping for each of the three conditions, but also that the *strength* of the preference increased with the amount of saturation. These data suggest that compression limiting may be superior to peak clipping not only below saturation but also well above the saturation threshold. An exception to this finding may exist for listeners with severe or profound losses, who have been shown to prefer peak clipping circuits simply because of their higher output level capabilities (Dawson, Dillon, and Battaglia, 1991).

### Input Versus Output Compression

Compression hearing aids are often described as either input or output controlled. The difference is determined by where the compressor's level detector and control circuitry are located in relation to the gain control. An input compressor's level detector is positioned prior to the gain control, as illustrated in Figure 4–11A. Compression is determined by the input level seen by the device, regardless of how the gain control is adjusted. Panel B shows a family of output curves and the I/O function associated with a single-channel input compression device with a fairly low compression threshold (about 55 dB SPL) and a 2:1 compression ratio. This type of device is representative of syllabic compressors. At input levels above the compression threshold, each 10 dB increase in input level produced a 5 dB increase in output level. Compression produced a corresponding reduction in gain with increasing input levels, as shown in panel C.

When the compressor's level detector is positioned after the gain control (Fig. 4–12A), compression is governed by output rather than input level. This configuration is typical of compression-limiting devices. In this case, compression is determined in part by the adjustment of the gain control. The output and gain curves shown in panels B and C of Figure 4–12 reflect a compression threshold of

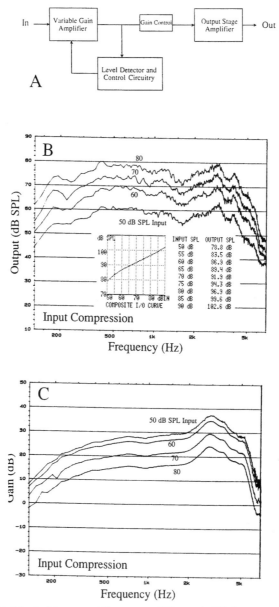

**Figure 4–11.**    (A) Block diagram, (B) output SPL, and (C) frequency–response curves associated with a single-band input compression hearing aid with a 55 dB SPL compression threshold and a 2:1 compression ratio.

approximately 100 dB output SPL and a compression ratio of about 5:1. It should be noted that although the output and gain curves shown in Figures 4–11 and 4–12 differ between figures, the compression characteristics provided by input versus output compression are not necessarily different. Both are determined by the static and dynamic properties of the compression amplifier, which vary with the intended purpose of the device.

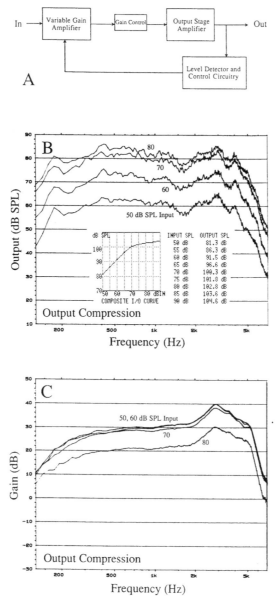

**Figure 4–12.** (A) Block diagram, (B) output SPL, and (C) frequency–response curves associated with a single-band output compression hearing aid with a 100 dB SPL compression threshold and a 5:1 compression ratio.

As mentioned earlier, one practical distinction between input and output compression is the effect of gain control adjustment on the output of the aid. Figure 4–13A shows three I/O curves representing an input-controlled device, and illustrates the effect of gain control adjustment on the output of the hearing aid. Each of the three I/O functions shows a "knee point" at 60 dB input SPL, a compression

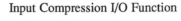

Input Compression I/O Function

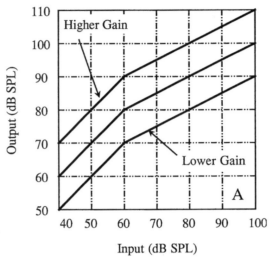

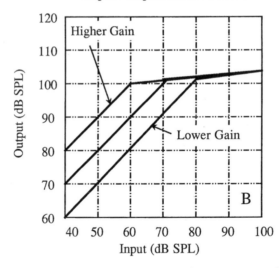

Output Compression I/O Function

**Figure 4–13.** Input/output functions representing three gain control positions for an (A) input compression and (B) output compression device.

threshold at about 62 dB SPL, and a compression ratio of 2:1. As gain is increased, output is also increased, both below and above the compression threshold. Fixed compression thresholds and parallel shifts of gain and output SPL are characteristics of input compressors that help to identify the circuit type of hearing aids of unknown design. Panel B shows comparable data representing an output-controlled instrument. In this case, adjustment of the gain control changes gain with minimal effect upon maximum output SPL. At the highest gain control setting, the compression threshold of slightly above 100 dB SPL corresponds to an input level of about 60 dB SPL. At the lowest gain setting, this output is not reached until the input level has reached 80 dB SPL. By examining I/O functions obtained at different volume control settings, it is possible to determine whether a compression hearing aid is input or output controlled.

Recent innovations go beyond simple input- or output-based compression. For example, Johnson (1993) described a circuit whose compression characteristics are governed not before or after the gain control, but actually *by* the gain control (Fig. 4–14). This circuit provides a linear response at low gain settings, and increasing amounts of compression as gain is raised, allowing the listener to adjust gain and compression ratio simultaneously. As innovations such as these continue, more and more hearing aids will deviate from the traditional pattern of simple input- or output-based compression.

## Multiband Compression

Most early compression hearing aids consisted of a single band of nonlinear signal processing. These devices were and are appropriate for individuals with a narrow dynamic range across a wide range of frequencies. Some individuals, however, such as those with sloping high-frequency hearing losses, typically have a normal dynamic range at lower frequencies, but a restricted dynamic range at higher frequencies. In these cases, compression is only necessary in the higher frequencies, a fact that has prompted the development of circuits with more than one compression band. In principle, multiband compression hearing aids should allow the appropriate manipulation of gain within a specific frequency region without affecting signal processing (linear or otherwise) in adjacent fre-

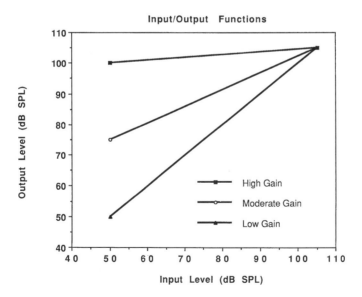

**Figure 4–14.** Input/output functions representing three gain control positions for a gain-controlled compression circuit (from Johnson, 1993, reprinted with permission).

quency regions. Single-band BILL- and TILL-type circuits are based on a similar rationale, and are also designed to provide level-dependent signal processing only where it is needed.

Early experiments (Villchur, 1973; Yanick, 1976) in multiband compression revealed encouraging results, and prompted further research that examined the effects of a wide variety of compression characteristics and an assortment of multiband configurations (Braida et al., 1979; Walker, Byrne, and Dillon, 1984; DeGennaro, Braida, and Durlach, 1986). These experiments, however, failed to show consistent benefits of multiband compression, forcing an examination of the factors that might have contributed to the negative results. One argument, proposed by Plomp (1988), was that fast-acting wide dynamic range compression amplifiers distorted the natural temporal characteristics of speech, leading to degraded speech recognition. Villchur (1989), however, challenged Plomp's argument, claiming that significant distortion would only occur when compression was applied to a large number of frequency bands. Indeed, research by Leek, Dorman, and Summerfield (1987) indicated that the benefits of compression may be reduced if more than two or three bands of compression are used, because each band of multiband compression tends to reduce both spectral and temporal contrasts that naturally exist in speech and other complex sounds. For listeners with impaired frequency and temporal resolution, the contamination of speech caused by large numbers of compression bands can be particularly detrimental.

Multiband compression hearing aids of today come in a wide variety of forms. Some combine linear processing in one frequency band with compression of one form or another in an adjacent band. Others provide different types of compression in each band. Often, it is possible to adjust compression characteristics in at least one frequency band, and some circuits allow the crossover frequency between bands to be adjusted. Moore (1993) provided an example of how multiband compression circuits can be designed to accomplish multiple objectives. The circuit he described consists of a slow-acting AGC amplifier that controls overall gain, a fast-acting compression limiter that takes over when brief impulsive-type sounds occur, and a syllabic compressor that functions only in the high-frequency band of the two-band circuit. In principle, this type of device should compensate for a reduced dynamic range and also protect against loudness discomfort when transient sounds occur. Circuit algorithms such as these may have advantages over single-band designs and will likely continue to be developed and evaluated.

### Expansion ("Reverse Compression")

Expansion is a nonlinear circuit algorithm that functions in a manner directly opposite that of compression. The effect of single-channel expansion on the output and gain of a hearing aid is illustrated in Figure 4–15. Unlike compression, expansion generates an I/O function with a slope that is *greater* than 1.0. That is, for a 5 dB increase in input level, the output of the device will increase by *more* than 5 dB. This effect is evident in both the I/O function and the output curves shown in panel A of the figure. As input level increases, so does the amount of gain, as shown in panel B. Intuitively, expansion would not appear to be useful

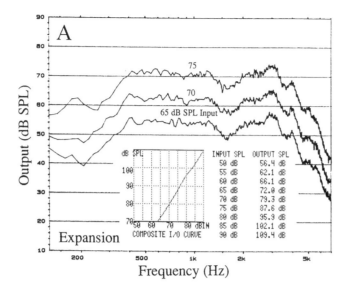

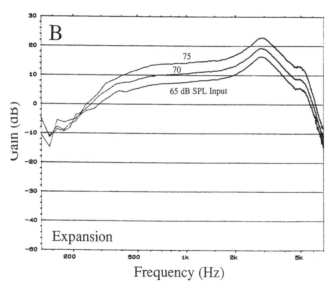

**Figure 4–15.**  (A) Output SPL and (B) frequency–response curves associated with an expansion circuit.

in hearing aids. Not only would expansion seem inappropriate for those with loudness recruitment, but rapid increases in gain can easily result in acoustic feedback. Indeed, expansion has rarely been used in hearing aids, primarily for these reasons. However, expansion can serve a variety of purposes when carefully controlled. For example, expansion may be used in conjunction with high-pass filtering to attenuate low-frequency vowels but emphasize high-frequency consonants, an appropriate amplification scheme for many types of hearing loss.

Expansion may also be applied in multichannel devices to provide extra gain within narrow frequency regions. Although the benefits of expansion are far from established, this type of algorithm does have a place within hearing aid circuit designs.

## Summary

The preceding discussion has shown that compression amplification can exist in a wide variety of forms, making the classification of compression hearing aids a complex task. Compression amplifiers may be input, output, or gain controlled, depending on the manner in which the circuit is designed. They may be described as automatic gain controls, syllabic compressors, or compression limiters, depending on the circuit's static and dynamic characteristics. The acoustic properties of compression hearing aids will vary with each of these factors, but the measurement of these characteristics is not always straightforward. The suitability of one particular type of compression over another depends on a variety of factors, including the dynamic range and loudness discomfort levels of the listener, which often vary with frequency. As a result, the selection of compression characteristics requires a thorough documentation of an individual's audiometric profile as well as a thorough understanding of the effects of compression on complex sounds such as speech.

## Bass Increases at Low Levels (BILL)

BILL-type hearing aids provide a level-dependent frequency response in which low-frequency gain varies with input level. While BILL-type characteristics can be produced with multiband compression, they are most often associated with adaptive high-pass filtering (Iwasaki, 1981; Kates, 1986). A block diagram of a hearing aid with adaptive high-pass filtering (Argosy Manhattan II™) is illustrated in Figure 4–16A. Essential to the circuit are the blocks representing the rectifier and the voltage-controlled high-pass filter, which form a feedback loop. The signal level at the output of the high-pass filter is detected by the rectifier, which governs the voltage supplied to the filter and, therefore, the filter cutoff frequency. As the signal level increases, so does the high-pass cutoff frequency, which reduces low-frequency gain. The frequency response shown as the uppermost curve of Figure 4–16B was obtained with a 50 dB SPL speech-shaped noise input and is associated with a low filter cutoff frequency. At higher input levels, the cutoff frequency of the high-pass filter is raised, which reduces low-frequency and, to a lesser extent, high-frequency gain. Although this type of circuit, indeed, provides a bass increase at low levels, it is perhaps better described as a bass decrease at high levels, which is, in fact, the motivation for the design.

The rationale behind BILL-type hearing aids is based upon several elements. First, many types of environmental noise are dominated by low-frequency energy (Ono, Kanzaki, and Mizoi, 1983). A device that reduces low-frequency energy when high signal levels are present should reduce noise levels for the wearer. Second, some hearing-impaired individuals have been shown to demonstrate greater upward spread of masking than those with normal hearing (Trees and Turner, 1986; Gagne, 1988). Upward spread of masking refers to the fact that

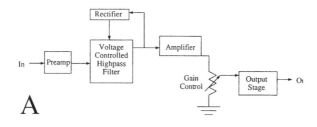

A

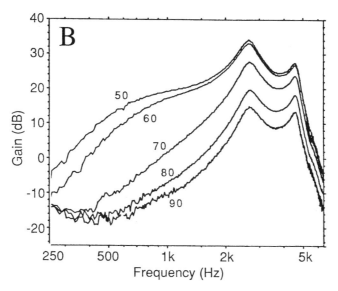

**Figure 4–16.** (A) Block diagram and (B) frequency–response curves associated with a BILL-type hearing aid with an adaptive high-pass filter.

low-frequency sounds, such as vowels, can often interfere with the perception of high-frequency sounds, such as consonants, due to the mechanical properties of the cochlea. If low frequencies are attenuated by a BILL-type amplifier, upward spread of masking might be reduced, possibly increasing speech recognition. Third, BILL-type algorithms might increase the consonant-to-vowel intensity ratio (CVR). Because vowels contain significant low-frequency energy but contribute little to intelligibility, an increase in the CVR may help to improve speech recognition (Freyman and Nerbonne, 1989). Fourth, the input level necessary to cause saturation-induced distortion in a BILL-type circuit is high, relative to a comparable linear amplifier (Killion, 1991). A BILL-type circuit is, therefore, more likely to retain good sound quality over a greater range of input/gain levels than a comparable linear aid. Finally, the *presence* of low frequencies has been shown to be associated with favorable impressions of sound quality (Punch, Montgomery, Schwartz, Walden, Porsek, and Howard, 1980; Punch and Beck, 1986). In a relatively quiet environment, the presence of low-frequency gain might serve to enhance sound quality for the listener.

The validity of some of these assumptions has been empirically addressed. Rankovic, Freyman, and Zurek (1992) examined the effects of frequency selective versus wide-band attenuation of maskers on the recognition of nonsense syllables. Nonsense syllables presented at 68 dB SPL were mixed with 95 dB SPL octave-wide maskers centered at 500, 1000, and 2000 Hz. These signals were subjected to both wide-band and frequency-selective attenuation to determine which approach would provide greater speech recognition. Results showed that frequency selective attenuation of either the low (500 Hz) or the midfrequency (1000 Hz) noise bands resulted in score improvements of nearly 50%, while wideband attenuation resulted in much smaller improvements. The improvements in recognition coincided with decreases in upward spread of masking, exhibited by masking patterns obtained during testing. These results suggest that varying the frequency-gain response of a hearing aid to eliminate low-frequency noise has the potential of improving speech recognition in noise by reducing the upward spread of masking. Similar results were reported by Fabry, Leek, and Walden (1990).

Although numerous investigators have shown improvements in speech recognition with BILL-type algorithms (Stein and Dempesey-Hart, 1984; Wolinski, 1986; Van Tasell, Larsen, and Fabry, 1988), others have failed to do so. Fabry and Van Tasell (1990) reported no significant differences in speech intelligibility ratings for maximum versus minimum adaptive filtering conditions in a group of 12 hearing-impaired listeners. The authors attributed their findings to the fact that adaptive filtering reduces signal and noise levels simultaneously, *without changing* the signal-to-noise ratio. Thus, improvements in speech recognition associated with high-pass filtering may be due to a release from masking or a "release from distortion," rather than an improvement in the signal-to-noise ratio. It may also be true that adaptive high-pass filtering simply improves listening comfort in noisy situations (Kuk and Tyler, 1990).

Any advantages of BILL-type signal processing could easily change with the electroacoustic characteristics of the circuit. For example, Figure 4–17 shows three temporal waveforms of the syllable /ish/. The waveform in panel A was obtained unaided from a real ear, and shows a CVR of –8.9 dB, indicating that the consonant was about 9 dB weaker the vowel preceding it. Panel B shows an aided real-ear recording of the same syllable, as processed by a BILL-type circuit (HPF1). The aided syllable had a CVR of –2.7 dB, an increase in consonant energy relative to the vowel of 6.2 dB brought about by adaptive high-pass filtering. Panel C represents amplification by a BILL circuit (HPF2) that responded more quickly to low-frequency energy than HPF1. The faster response time of HPF2 resulted in greater attenuation of the low-frequency vowel and a further increase in the CVR. This effect occurred across a variety of syllables, as shown in Figure 4–18A. These data represent mean real-ear recordings obtained from a group of four hearing-impaired listeners. When these listeners were tested for syllable recognition, HPF2 was also associated with the fewest number of response errors, as shown in panel B. Because these hearing aids differed only in their response times, it is possible that amplifier sensitivity may have contributed to the results. Although the factors affecting speech recognition are obviously complex, these data suggest that behavioral performance may be affected by even small differences in

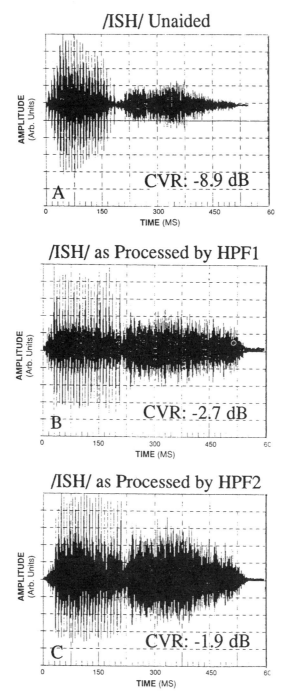

**Figure 4–17.** Temporal waveforms and associated consonant-to-vowel ratios (CVRs) for the syllable /ish/, obtained (A) unaided, (B) as processed by a BILL-type hearing aid, and (C) as processed by a BILL-type hearing aid with a faster response time.

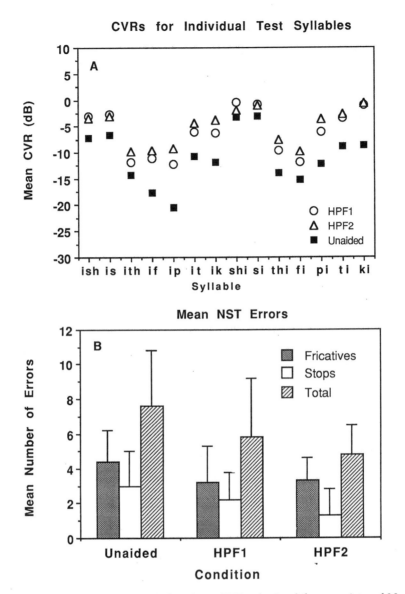

**Figure 4–18.** (A) Unaided and aided real-ear CVRs obtained for a variety of Nonsense Syllable Test (NST) syllables. Hearing aids represented two BILL-type algorithms differing in response time. (B) Mean NST errors associated with the three conditions represented in panel A.

hearing aid circuit characteristics, an issue that could easily apply to all types of hearing aids.

### Treble Increases at Low Levels (TILL)

A TILL-type algorithm, exemplified by the K-Amp™ (Etymotic Research), is based on assumptions that differ from those associated with BILL-type instruments (Killion, 1993). The K-Amp rationale assumes that most hearing-impaired listeners have greater hearing loss in the high frequencies than in the low frequencies and, therefore, require high-frequency emphasis amplification. The rationale also assumes that maximum high-frequency gain is required for low-level sounds, and that less gain is necessary when input levels increase. These assumptions are applied in a level-dependent frequency response illustrated in Figure 4–19. Although technically a single-band compressor, the algorithm provides significant high-frequency gain at low input levels and progressively less high-frequency gain as input levels increase. The treble increase at low levels is intended to provide or improve the audibility of weak high-frequency consonants. As the input level is raised, decreasing high-frequency gain serves to prevent loudness discomfort, minimize hearing aid saturation, and possibly compensate for abnormal loudness growth. The K-Amp circuit also applies Adaptive Compression™ (Telex), and has recently been designed with an adjustable compression ratio.

To date, the assumptions underlying TILL-type circuits such as the K-Amp have not been thoroughly evaluated. Skinner (1980) measured word recognition scores for hearing-impaired listeners with sloping high-frequency hearing losses and reported that performance improved as the amount of high-frequency emphasis amplification increased. In a subsequent investigation, Skinner, Karstaedt, and Miller (1982) reported that word recognition performance of 2 hearing-impaired listeners increased with the overall bandwidth of the test material. The bandwidth associated with typical hearing aids of the time was associated with generally poor performance. Killion and Tillman (1982) reported that experimental hearing aids built with high-fidelity microphones and receivers similar to those now used in the K-Amp were associated with subjective fidelity ratings

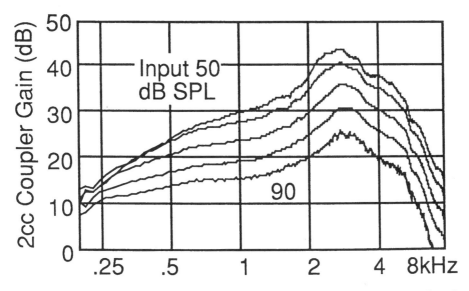

**Figure 4–19.** Representative family of frequency–response curves associated with a TILL-type hearing aid.

that were comparable to those associated with high-fidelity loudspeakers. These results, however, were based on the impressions of normal-hearing listeners. These investigations support the rationale for the K-Amp circuit, although all were conducted before the K-Amp was introduced. To date, empirical investigations of the K-Amp have yet to be reported, although numerous reports have indicated that the circuit is being used successfully in the field (Knight, 1992; Kruger and Kruger, 1993). After formal research on the K-Amp has been completed, it should become possible to determine the true benefits and limitations of the algorithm.

Although the contrasts between BILL and TILL algorithms appear substantial, they exist primarily for low-level inputs. When appropriate venting and frequency response shaping are used to accommodate typical high-frequency hearing losses, BILL and TILL algorithms provide similar amplification, particularly at moderate input levels (Fabry, 1991). Both types of amplification help to prevent saturation-induced distortion (Killion, 1991), a characteristic that could largely account for the success of both algorithms in the field. In addition to single-band designs, both BILL and TILL-type circuits are also commercially available in multiband configurations.

## Programmable Hearing Aids

The previous discussion has described 3 broad types of nonlinear amplification that are currently used in hearing aids. Compression, BILL-, and TILL-type circuits are each complex, and performance will vary, depending on how it is internally configured and externally controlled. Most modern hearing aids have many types of external potentiometers available for use, including those that adjust gain, SSPL, frequency response, and compression characteristics. This makes it difficult not only to keep track of the multitude of control functions available, but also to decide which controls are *most* needed for a particular hearing aid wearer, who often insists on the smallest hearing aid possible. The complexity and flexibility of many modern hearing aids has necessitated a way to simplify their use, and this need has in part prompted the development of programmability. Programmable devices often have features that are unavailable with conventional instruments. Some programmable hearing aids have multiple memories and remote controls that allow the user to change circuit characteristics as the listening environment changes. Others have automatic fitting capabilities that simplify the fitting process. One currently available product (Phonak) provides four types of output limiting, while another (3M) automatically records the amount of time individual programs are used. Equally important, programmability allows the audiologist more control over the device, because the programming of all adjustable parameters is accomplished without the need for external potentiometers. Although the features associated with programmable hearing aids do not make fittings more likely to succeed, they do provide more options and more control over the fitting process than would otherwise be possible.

At the time of this writing, there were no fewer than 18 programmable hearing aids on the market (Skafte and Strom, 1994), and this number will likely increase in the future. All of the programmable products currently available incorporate some form of compression. Most programmable instruments are currently single band, but several two- and three-band devices have been developed. Currently, the number of programs available in programmable products ranges from one to eight. As the complexity of hearing aids continues to increase, it is likely that the number and variety of programmable products will also increase. The challenge that lies ahead, however, will not be to decide which programmable system is superior, but to define, distinguish, and maximize those factors most likely to contribute to a successful hearing aid fitting.

## Circuit Selection and Adjustment Considerations

The selection of a hearing aid to best match the needs of a hearing-impaired listener is by no means a simple task. Not only are the 4 major circuit types discussed in this chapter (linear, compression, BILL, TILL) different from one another, but many variations of these circuit types exist across manufacturers. Any confusion that arises when comparing products will not necessarily end with the selection of a circuit, because the electroacoustic performance of most hearing aids may be varied greatly. If the factors necessary for optimal hearing aid benefit were known, the selection and adjustment of a hearing aid would be a straightforward process. Unfortunately, this is not the case, particularly with regard to maximizing speech recognition. Despite this state of affairs, informed decisions can be made, and appropriate adjustments of circuit characteristics can help to provide the best possible benefit to the hearing aid user. The discussion that follows provides some of the basic considerations regarding amplifier and circuit characteristics that should be addressed during the selection and fitting of a hearing aid. These considerations are based on the psychophysical effects of hearing loss and the effects that the alteration of speech caused by hearing aids may have on speech recognition. A more detailed review of this topic may be found in Van Tasell (1993).

### Psychophysical Correlates of Hearing Impairment

Hearing loss can be classified into two broad physiological categories, based on the severity of the impairment. Hearing loss up to approximately 60 dB is associated with the loss of outer hair cells within the cochlea, while more severe losses are associated with the loss of both inner and outer hair cells (Patuzzi, Yates, and Johnstone, 1989). The loss of outer hair cells causes a decrease in auditory sensitivity, which in turn, causes two psychophysical effects. First, the bandwidths of auditory filters become abnormally broad, due to the elevated signal levels necessary for signal detection. When processed through broadly tuned auditory filters, some of the spectral detail of speech is lost, which may disrupt speech recognition in noise (Van Tasell, 1993). Second, sensitivity loss results in a restricted dynamic range, because loudness discomfort levels are often normal despite the elevation of hearing thresholds. An abnormally rapid growth of loudness disrupts the normal loudness relationships that exist among components of speech. The disruption of cochlear function becomes even more complicated as the hearing loss becomes more severe. Although less well understood, the loss of inner hair cells associated with severe hearing losses may impair the ability to resolve temporal as well as spectral information. To the extent that these factors affect the recognition of speech, each must be overcome by a hearing aid if auditory communication is to succeed. Because hearing loss often varies with frequency, the deficits associated with hearing impairment are often frequency dependent, and the task of maximizing speech recognition through electronic amplification becomes all the more challenging.

### Hearing Impairment and Speech Recognition

Poor sensitivity, broadly tuned filters, upward spread of masking, loudness recruitment, and loss of temporal resolution are potential barriers to effective speech recognition for hearing-impaired listeners. But how important are they? Although the impairments associated with hearing loss are many, they do not always cause a communication handicap. Information provided by contextual cues often makes auditory communication possible even when participants are significantly hearing impaired. This may explain why speech recognition in quiet is often good even in listeners with broadly tuned auditory filters (Dreschler and Plomp, 1985). In favorable listening environments, sensitivity loss may often be the only significant barrier to communication, a barrier that can be overcome with amplification that simply provides audibility. If the signal-to-noise ratio is poor, however, communication can easily deteriorate, regardless of the hearing loss or the type of hearing aid worn.

THE ARTICULATION INDEX (AI)

The importance of audibility to speech recognition is reflected in the Articulation Index (AI) (French and Steinberg, 1947), which provides a good prediction of speech recognition performance in listeners with mild to moderate hearing loss. The AI is based on estimates of the audibility of speech within specific frequency bands, with each estimate weighted by the importance of the information carried within each band. Higher frequency bands are weighted more heavily than lower frequency bands, because high-frequency consonants contribute much more to speech intelligibility than low-frequency vowels. AI research has shown that audibility alone can account for speech recognition in quiet without the need for adjustments based on abnormally wide auditory filters, loudness recruitment, or the loss of temporal resolution. This suggests that if amplification can provide audibility without discomfort across as wide a frequency range as possible, speech recognition in quiet should be maximized. In noise, though, poor frequency resolution can affect speech recognition in a manner that differs from a loss of sensitivity. To date, no hearing aid has been shown to solve the dilemma of improving speech recognition in noise that often plagues hearing aid wearers, although some algorithms (Rankovic et al., 1992) have been shown to reduce the upward spread of masking.

LOUDNESS

The effect of loudness recruitment on speech recognition is currently under much discussion. The restoration of normal loudness growth has become an objective of several programmable and nonprogrammable hearing instruments, although no published reports have indicated that doing so will offer any advantages to the hearing impaired. In fact, differences of opinion regarding this topic abound. Some researchers (Villchur, 1973; Skinner, Pascoe, Miller, and Popelka, 1982b) have concluded that components of speech should be heard with the same loudness relationships as those heard by normal-hearing listeners. Others (Byrne and Dillon, 1986) have proposed that elements of speech should be equally loud across the entire spectrum, a somewhat different conclusion. Although it is generally accepted that the prevention of loudness *discomfort* is very important to a successful hearing aid fitting, the relationship between the loudness of individual speech sounds and recognition when speech falls within the listener's dynamic range remains unclear. What is clear is that if portions of speech fall below threshold or above the level of discomfort, they will not contribute to recognition and may detract from it.

TEMPORAL CUES

Unlike the loss of spectral information, the loss of temporal cues appears to cause minimal impairment in speech recognition. The relative importance of spectral versus temporal cues may be determined by comparing the results of studies in which either spectral or temporal cues have been selectively removed from the speech stimulus. Van Tasell, Soli, Kirby, and Widin (1987) found that the removal of spectral cues from speech drastically reduced its intelligibility, even though temporal information was available to their listeners. In contrast, the complete loss of temporal information via infinite peak clipping does not drastically reduce speech recognition (Licklider and Pollack, 1948). Although it is clear that the spectral characteristics of speech carry more information than do temporal envelope cues, the information contained in the speech envelope does provide manner and voicing cues that may be important when spectral information is unavailable (Freyman, Nerbonne, and Cote, 1991; Van Tasell, Greenfield, Logeman, and Nelson, 1992).

## Summary

Most available evidence suggests that the primary goal of a hearing aid fitting should be to provide audibility without discomfort across as wide a frequency range as possible. In doing so, the recognition of speech presented in quiet should be maximized. In noise, recognition may be compromised if the signal-to-noise ratio becomes poor, and emphasis should be placed not only on maintaining the audibility of the signal of interest, but also on improving the signal-to-noise ratio whenever possible. In some cases, listening comfort in noise or reduced upward spread of masking may be achieved via nonlinear signal processing. In all cases, however, the counseling of realistic expectations to patients should be a significant part of the hearing rehabilitation process.

## *The Selection and Fitting of Linear and Nonlinear Hearing Aids*

The selection and adjustment of a hearing aid can be a complicated task, and no universally accepted guidelines exist to simplify the process. Although a consensus has yet to be reached on how best to fit hearing aids, certain considerations should be made both before and during the fitting process. Because hearing aid fitting strategies go beyond the scope of this chapter, the following discussion is intended merely to provide an overview of considerations that should be made during the process of fitting a hearing aid.

### Linear Hearing Aids

Although linear amplification has certain limitations, it is also widely used, and provides benefit to individuals representing a variety of types of hearing loss. Linear amplification is particularly appropriate for those with mild hearing losses who require only small amounts of gain. Low-gain linear hearing aids are less likely to saturate than high-gain linear hearing aids with similar SSPLs, and should have good sound quality most of the time. At the opposite extreme, linear hearing aids are also appropriate for those with severe to profound hearing losses, particularly in those cases for which adequate gain or output cannot be achieved with nonlinear devices. Individuals with quite severe losses often prefer linear amplification despite the presence of distortion, simply because the aid provides audibility, whereas nonlinear devices may not. Finally, some evidence suggests that many listeners who are *accustomed* to linear hearing aids make good candidates for continued use of linear amplification. Whether appropriate or not, this suggests that acclimatization plays a significant role in hearing aid use and preference. Thus, although linear amplification is not ideally suited to all individuals, it can be quite beneficial when used selectively.

Before a linear hearing aid is chosen, the dynamic range of the listener should be carefully considered. When the listener's dynamic range is less than 30 dB, it may not be possible to adjust gain and frequency response in such a way as to provide audibility without discomfort. For example, a gain control can be used to compensate for changes in the *average* level of speech, but it cannot compensate for the fact that the peak-to-valley intensity ratio of speech can be as high as 30 dB. If gain is adjusted so that the average level of speech is comfortably loud, the peaks of speech may cause discomfort, while the weakest elements of speech may not be heard. For this reason, individuals with dynamic ranges of less than about 30 dB may not make suitable candidates for linear amplification.

When fitting linear hearing aids, every effort should be made to minimize saturation-induced distortion. This can be accomplished by use of the class B or class D output stage, the cautious use of output limiting potentiometers, and the use of compression limiting rather than peak clipping as the method of output limitation. By minimizing saturation-induced distortion, sound quality should be maximized and aided LDLs should be higher than if distortion is frequently present. The gain and frequency response of linear hearing aids should be adjusted with audibility in mind. Virtually all prescriptive approaches to hearing aid fitting (e.g., NAL, POGO, etc.) are intended to overcome a loss of sensitivity, and any of these prescriptive approaches may be used when fitting a linear hearing aid. Although it has often been noted that different prescriptive formulas can generate different targets for the same hearing loss, it has yet to be demonstrated that any one prescriptive approach is superior to the others. Until this issue is resolved, it is reasonable to assume that as long as a target match is achieved, most sounds should be audible to the listener most of the time, regardless of the prescription used to generate the target curve.

Achieving a match to a prescriptive target is no longer as difficult as it once was. Although older generation linear hearing aids were characterized by single-band circuit designs, poor receiver frequency response, and limited filtering capabilities, modern linear devices are often multiband, have better quality receivers, and are much more flexible in terms of frequency–response shaping. For example, Figure 4–20 shows three families of frequency–response curves, each generated by a modern three-band linear hearing aid (Argosy 3-Channel Clock™). This device allows low-frequency (panel A), midfrequency (panel B), and high-frequency (panel C) gain to be precisely adjusted, and also allows the crossover frequencies between bands to be varied. Designs such as these make it possible to match prescriptive targets with much more precision than was previously possible (Sammeth, Preves, Bratt, Peek, and Bess, 1993) and also allow the audiologist more flexibility when fitting the instrument and more opportunities to correct problems when they arise. Although all hearing aids are not the same, the state of technology today is such that frequency response shaping is no longer a factor limiting hearing aid candidacy. This statement is true of both linear and nonlinear hearing aids that utilize the latest technology.

## Compression

Although the objectives of a compression fitting are similar to those of a linear fitting, the method used to accomplish these objectives can be much more complicated. If the factors critical to speech recognition in impaired listeners were known, it might be possible to adjust circuit characteristics to optimize these factors. Unfortunately, the effects of hearing impairment on speech recognition are not well understood, and the audiologist is often faced with a "seat of the pants" fitting strategy, particularly when working with nonlinear multiband or programmable hearing aids. Until more is known, the strategy used to fit compression hearing aids should include flexibility and common sense, and should strive to provide audibility without discomfort for the hearing-impaired listener.

Before fitting a compression hearing aid, the reasons for doing so should be clear, so the appropriate type of circuit can be selected and the appropriate adjustments made. If an individual has an adequately large dynamic range (>30 dB) and compression is needed primarily to prevent loudness discomfort, compression limiting is an appropriate choice. The compression circuit should have a relatively high compression threshold, a high compression ratio, and fast time constants, either by design or by external controls. If the person to be fit is frequently exposed to changing sound levels but is not disturbed by occasional impulsive-type sounds, an AGC instrument might be the circuit of choice. The compression circuit should have a low compression threshold, a fairly high compression ratio, and a long release time. An AGC instrument will not cause appreciable spectral or temporal distortion of speech as long as signal processing is limited to only a few processing bands, and should have acceptable sound quality as long as the compression ratio is not too high. Finally, an individual with a

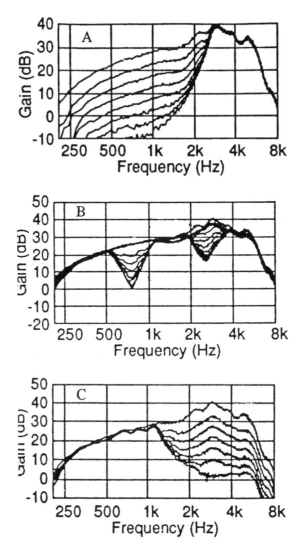

**Figure 4–20.** Examples of (A) low-frequency, (B) mid-frequency, and (C) high-frequency gain adjustments possible with a 3-band linear hearing aid.

narrow dynamic range (<30 dB) might benefit most from an instrument with syllabic compression. When syllabic compression is necessary, however, it should only be used in a hearing aid with no more than three processing bands. The instrument should have a low compression threshold and relatively fast time constants. The compression ratio should be adjusted to provide only as much compression as is needed for the individual; a compression ratio of 3:1 should probably be avoided if a ratio of 2:1 provides satisfactory amplification.

Most prescriptive methods for adjusting gain and frequency response are not well suited to the fitting of compression hearing aids, because they do not provide a way to evaluate level-dependent signal processing. Real ear testing, for example, is typically conducted at only one test level and, although this might provide appropriate gain and frequency response for the testing level used, it does not ensure that response characteristics will be optimal at input levels higher or lower than that used during testing. Cornelisse, Seewald, and Jamieson (1994), however, describe an alternative prescriptive approach that may be quite appropriate for fitting compression hearing aids. The Desired Sensation Level (DSL) approach that they have developed prescribes the desired output of the hearing aid at each of *several* input levels. The method generates a desired I/O function that is based on the dynamic range of the listener at a particular frequency. A similar approach, based on the loudness of speech, is currently under development by the Independent Hearing Aid Fitting Forum (IHAFF (Mueller, 1994)). Methods, such as these that employ multiple testing levels, are necessary when fitting nonlinear hearing aids, because they provide much more information about how these devices will function in a realistic environment. They also provide a rationale for setting specific compression characteristics, such as the compression threshold or compression ratio. Alternative prescriptive methods such as these will likely become more common as the use of nonlinear amplification proliferates.

## BILL/TILL

The considerations that apply to compression fittings also apply to algorithms that apply BILL- or TILL-type signal processing. Research discussed earlier suggested that a reduction of low-frequency gain at high input levels might be appropriate for individuals frequently exposed to environmental noise, which is typically low-frequency weighted. If a prescriptive method is used to fit a BILL-type device, testing should be conducted at a level that is high enough to partially activate the nonlinear circuitry, and appropriate gain and frequency response adjustments should be made at this level. Testing should then be conducted at higher and lower levels to assess the circuit's level-dependent characteristics. When adjusted in this way, some low frequency gain will be provided for soft sounds, which should enhance sound quality, but little or no low-frequency gain will be provided for loud sounds. Whenever possible, control over the amount of signal processing should be available, so that the needs of those preferring less adaptive filtering (or low-frequency compression) can be met. This is important for both single and multiband circuit designs.

   TILL-type hearing aids are appropriate for many individuals with sloping high-frequency hearing losses who require appreciable high-frequency gain in quiet environments but minimal gain in high level environments. When testing by prescriptive means, TILL-type hearing aids should be adjusted to provide appropriate gain and frequency response for moderate-level input signals, and should also be evaluated at more than one input level. When properly adjusted, a TILL-type hearing aid should have acceptable sound quality without feedback in quiet environments, and should not sound uncomfortably loud in high level environments. In some cases, the response shaping capabilities of TILL-type hearing aids is limited (e.g., the K-Amp™ has a maximum 6 dB/octave rising response slope), making it more difficult to fit steeply sloping and precipitous hearing losses than to fit gradually sloping losses. This difficulty can, at times, be overcome by the use of microphones with steeply rising slopes. As is true of all hearing aids, as much control over circuit characteristics as possible should be available.

## Current Developments in Hearing Instrument Technology

In recent years, tremendous strides have been made in both the technical sophistication and component miniaturization of hearing aids. As advances in signal processing continue, the benefits associated with amplification are likely to increase. Unfortunately, although many new signal processing algorithms have been developed, none has been shown to offer consistent benefit to the hearing impaired. Despite this frustrating set of circumstances, numerous analog and digital algorithms have shown a degree of promise in improving the signal-to-noise ratio for the hearing-impaired listener. Improving the signal-to-noise ratio, either by reducing noise or enhancing speech, is by far the most sought after outcome of these new technologies. Although technological changes occurring within hearing-related industries are too numerous to describe in detail here, this chapter would not be complete without a summary of some recent and innovative developments in technology that may soon be available in hearing aids.

### Multiple Microphone Approaches to Noise Reduction

Most approaches to noise reduction, both analog and digital, subject the output of a single microphone to a particular noise reduction algorithm. Although some single microphone algorithms are effective under certain conditions, the improvement in signal-to-noise ratio brought about by a noise reduction algorithm can be increased if more than one microphone is used, particularly when microphones can be spatially separated to record either signal plus noise or noise alone. When configured in such a way, microphone outputs can be constructively combined for signals originating from one direction but destructively combined for signals coming from other directions. An array consisting of 2 or more microphones can greatly increase directional sensitivity, often increasing the signal-to-noise ratio.

In a multimicrophone array, directional sensitivity is increased by subjecting the outputs of two or more spatially separated microphones to a combination of filtering, time delay, and amplitude weighting. As these parameters are varied, directional selectivity is affected, as illustrated in Figure 4–21. The directivity patterns shown represent the strength of the combined microphone outputs as a function of the direction of the signal source. Panel A illustrates a directivity pattern representative of a two-microphone array. The pattern shows that a signal originating at zero degrees (the target direction) is transduced at unity gain, whereas a signal originating at 120 degrees is attenuated by 20 dB. The location of this null can be moved to any angle by altering the manner in which the two microphone signals are processed. Thus, for unchanging signal and noise sources, the directional pattern can easily be modified to maximize the signal-to-noise ratio. The addition of a third microphone introduces a second null, which can be used to attenuate a second fixed noise source, as illustrated in panel B. Once again, the positions of these nulls can be altered by changing the manner in

**Directional Sensitivity Pattern:  Two Microphone Array**

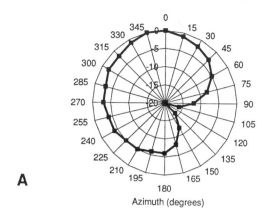

A

Azimuth (degrees)

**Directional Sensitivity Pattern:  Three Microphone Array**

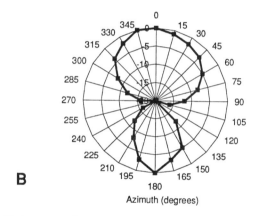

B

Azimuth (degrees)

**Figure 4–21.**  (A) Directional sensitivity pattern representing a two-microphone array, showing a distinct null at 120 degrees. (B) Directional sensitivity pattern representing a three-microphone array, showing nulls at 120° and 255°.

which microphone outputs are combined. Each additional microphone added to the array further modifies the directivity pattern, and as long as the signal and noise sources never vary, directional sensitivity can be adjusted to provide the best possible listening environment.

Figure 4–22 (from Hoffman, Trine, Buckley, and Van Tassell, 1994) provides an example of how multiple microphone arrays can help improve the signal-to-noise ratio. Hoffman, Trine, Buckley, and Van Tasell (1994) measured speech reception thresholds (SRTs) in noise for a group of normal-hearing listeners wearing one, three, and seven microphone arrays in three types of reverberant environments. The figure shows that, for each environment, the SRT in noise

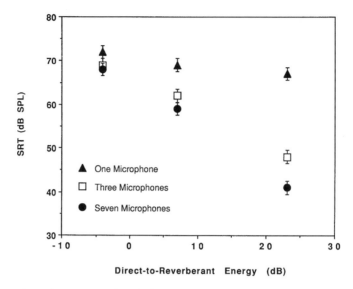

**Figure 4–22.**   Speech reception thresholds in noise as a function of reverberation for subjects wearing one, three, and seven microphone noise reduction arrays (from Hoffman et al., 1994, reprinted with permission).

decreased (improved) as the number of microphones in the array increased. In a nonreverberant environment (right-hand column) the SRTs associated with the three- and seven-microphone arrays were 19 and 26 dB lower than that found in the single (omnidirectional)-microphone condition. In environments designed to simulate a typical living room (middle column) and a reverberant conference room (left-hand column), these improvements became progressively smaller, but continued to show an advantage of multimicrophone arrays over single microphones. Encouraging as these results may be, these data also clearly show that, regardless of the number of microphones, the performance of multimicrophone arrays can be greatly reduced by reverberation.

One question that may be asked regarding multimicrophone arrays is whether they offer any advantages over single, *directional* microphones. Indeed, depending on how they are constructed, directional microphones can generate directivity patterns similar to those shown in Figure 4–21, and may provide noise reduction comparable to two- and perhaps three-microphone arrays. The true advantage of multimicrophone arrays over directional microphones becomes apparent as the number of microphones in the array is further increased. For example, Soede, Bilsen, and Berkhout (1993) measured the SRT in noise for 45 hearing-impaired subjects, using omnidirectional, directional, and two types of five-microphone arrays. Results indicated that SRTs associated with the five-microphone arrays were 7 dB and 4.5 dB lower than those associated with omnidirectional and directional microphones, respectively. These results suggest that multiple microphone arrays can be quite effective in improving the signal-to-noise ratio for hearing-impaired listeners, and can offer advantages over single directional microphones.

Recent multimicrophone algorithms have been further advanced, and are designed to adjust to *varying* acoustic conditions (Greenberg and Zurek, 1993). As the characteristics and source directions of noise vary, these adaptive algorithms continuously adjust the way in which microphone outputs are combined, in an ongoing attempt to minimize noise power. In doing so, the positions of nulls in the directivity pattern are constantly modified as the acoustic environment changes. Although adaptive algorithms such as these offer great promise for future hearing aid applications, they, like their nonadaptive predecessors, tend to lose effectiveness in reverberant environments (Peterson, Durlack, Rabinowitz, and Zurek, 1987; Schwander and Levitt, 1987).

In addition to the detrimental effects of reverberation, both fixed and adaptive multimicrophone algorithms are also affected by array imperfections such as "misteering," which occurs when the listener does not directly face the target signal, and array misalignment, which exists when individual microphones are not precisely positioned within the array. These variables degrade the effectiveness of the algorithm, and can result in a loss of signal as well as ineffective noise cancellation. "Robustness" refers to the degree to which an algorithm is affected by variables such as these, and recent research (Hoffman et al., 1994) has shown that robust processing can partially compensate not only for array imperfections, but also head shadow and reverberation, resulting in realistically achievable benefits. At the time of this writing, multiple microphone hearing aids are becoming commercially available and, as processing refinements and packaging improvements are made, it is likely that multiple microphone hearing aids will become more common.

## Sinusoidal Modeling

Sinusoidal modeling (McAulay and Quatieri, 1986; Quatieri and McAulay, 1986; Kates, 1991, 1994) is another signal processing technique that offers promise for improving the signal-to-noise ratio. This algorithm divides a sample of speech into a series of discrete time segments and determines the most intense sinusoidal components of each segment. Once determined, sine waves with frequency, amplitude, and phase characteristics corresponding to the strongest elements of the original waveform are synthesized and summed to produce a speech-like signal with temporal characteristics and sound quality similar to the original speech sample. Intelligible speech can be represented by a synthesized signal consisting of only a small number of sinusoids. The sinusoidal modeling technique is based on the assumption that speech will generally be more intense than background noise. When this is true, sinusoidal modeling should eliminate background noise, because components of the noise spectrum would not be reproduced.

In a pilot study, Kates (1991) reported that speech intelligibility ratings for sentences modeled with 16 sinusoids were similar between normal-hearing and hearing-impaired listeners. At a +5 dB signal-to-noise ratio, three of six hearing-impaired subjects found the 16-component speech more intelligible than unprocessed speech. Given these results, a second experiment (Kates, 1994) was conducted to determine more clearly whether sinusoidal modeling could be used as an effective noise reduction technique. Five normal-hearing subjects were tested on a consonant recognition task in quiet and in a background of competing

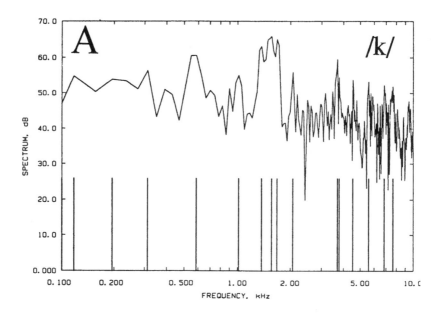

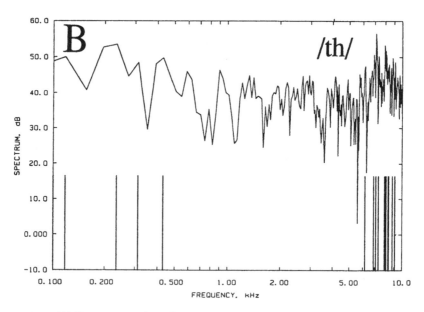

**Figure 4–23.** (A) Spectrum and 16 dominant sinusoidal components of the /k/ in "ka." (B) Comparable data for the /th/ in "tha" (from Kates, 1994, reprinted with permission).

speech babble. Test materials were synthesized using both 8 and 16 sinusoids. Results indicated that processed speech was somewhat *less* intelligible than unprocessed speech in both quiet and noise, but speech intelligibility was also found to increase with the number of sinusoids used to model the signal. One subject (the investigator) performed particularly well for all conditions, suggesting that listening experience and acclimatization may contribute to the effectiveness of the algorithm.

Although the overall results of this study were inconclusive, numerous patterns emerged from the data. For example, the technique was found to be most effective for signals with pronounced, well-defined spectra, such as vowels and stop consonants, and least effective for signals with broad, diffuse spectra, such as unvoiced fricatives. The contrast is illustrated in Figure 4–23 (from Kates, 1994). The upper panel shows the spectrum of the consonant /k/ in "ka" together with the 16 dominant sinusoidal components used to model the signal. For this consonant, primary components were present across the entire spectrum, and subjects tended to perform well in perceiving the consonant in noise. In contrast, the lower panel shows the spectrum and dominant sinusoids for the /th/ in "tha." In this case, no strong sinusoidal components were present between 500 and 6000 Hz, and subjects tended to perform poorly in recognizing the consonant in noise. This suggests that low-amplitude spectral components of speech contain information necessary for intelligibility, and that eliminating them may be equivalent to masking them by noise. Thus, although sinusoidal modeling may hold promise for future circuit designs, further research is necessary to determine the factors essential for speech recognition.

### Binaural Cue Enhancement

Several circuit algorithms, both analog and digital, have been developed with the intention of either preserving or restoring the acoustic cues associated with binaural hearing. It is well known that interaural time and intensity cues provide information that listeners use to localize sounds. These cues may also help to improve speech recognition in noise, particularly when the signal and noise come from different directions. One approach is offered by Kollmeier and Koch (1993), whose technique is to analyze interaural intensity and phase cues to identify the presence of noise. To accomplish this, a reference condition is first created by comparing the envelopes of signals recorded at both ears for a pulse-like stimulus presented from directly in front of a listener. Similar recordings of signals originating at other angles around the head reveal interaural intensity and phase differences that deviate from those obtained at the 0° reference condition. Deviations from baseline that exceed specified values are interpreted as noise and attenuated. This algorithm was found to improve sentence intelligibility re: unprocessed signals for normal-hearing listeners tested with both real and simulated speech maskers, a variety of noise source positions, and several signal-to-noise ratios. Perhaps more importantly, the algorithm also improved speech recognition performance under reverberant conditions.

Nilsson and Soli (1994) examined the effects of interaural time and intensity, as well as head shadow effects on the perception of speech in noise for hearing-impaired listeners. Head-related transfer functions were derived by measuring head shadow effects for signals presented at various angles around the head. By manipulating these transfer functions, it was possible to simulate masking noises presented at various locations and to determine the separate contributions of binaural magnitude and phase cues to the perception of speech mixed with noise.

Results indicated that both magnitude and phase cues were important for speech perception in noise, although significantly more benefit was found when both cues were available than if only one was present. These results suggest that any disruption of normal binaural amplitude or phase cues caused by hearing aids could have detrimental effects on speech perception in noise. This issue could have an important influence on the design of future hearing aids.

### Automatic Speech Recognition (ASR)

One form of digital signal processing that could conceivably eliminate noise is automatic speech recognition (Levitt, Bakke, Kates, Neuman, and Weiss, 1993), a technology that has been advancing rapidly and may one day be available for use in hearing aids. Levitt, Bakke, Kates, Neuman, and Weiss (1993) describe an ASR system that has been successfully tested on a small number of ears. The system amplifies and digitizes incoming speech and subjects it to an ASR algorithm that is capable of identifying over 25,000 words. Once identified, the speech is synthesized, amplified, and presented to a listener. The potential advantage of this technique is that if the algorithm can successfully identify individual words in the presence of background noise, the signal of interest could be synthesized without the interfering noise. The ASR system described by Levitt and his colleagues has a hit rate for speech in quiet of over 95%; 80% system recognition has been achieved when speech is mixed with noise at a +5 dB signal-to-noise ratio. Future refinements of the algorithm, together with improved synthesis techniques designed specifically to enhance speech recognition for hearing-impaired listeners, should lead to great improvements in signal-to-noise ratios and better understanding of digitally processed speech.

### Signal Processing Based on Loudness Growth

There has been increasing interest in suprathreshold tests of hearing aid benefit such as those based on estimates of loudness. The restoration of normal loudness growth is an objective of at least two programmable hearing instruments (ReSound, Oticon) and serves as the basis for a hearing aid fitting protocol described by IHAFF.

Loudness growth analysis is also being used in algorithms such as that described by Dillier and Frohlich (1993). The object of the method described by Dillier and Frohlich is to restore normal loudness perception by spectrally analyzing an input signal and modifying the amplitude spectrum by a series of pre-programmed gain tables derived from a listener's loudness growth functions. This algorithm was evaluated on a group of 21 hearing-impaired subjects who were tested on consonant and vowel recognition tasks. Overall results showed that scores associated with the test device were significantly higher than those obtained with conventional instruments, especially at low signal levels and low signal-to-noise ratios. Although other factors, such as the characteristics of the subject's own hearing aids, need to be considered when interpreting data such as these, the results suggest that digital signal processing based on estimates of loudness growth may represent a viable approach to hearing aid fitting.

## Spectral Subtraction

Another method of noise reduction subtracts an estimate of noise from a spectrum consisting of both signal and noise (Hochberg, Boothroyd, Weiss, and Hellman, 1992). A block diagram of the algorithm is shown in Figure 4–24. To accomplish noise reduction, an input signal is spectrally analyzed, and magnitude and phase components of the signal are separated. Phase information is temporarily stored while the magnitude spectrum is converted back into the temporal domain. The intensity and periodic structure of the transformed waveform is used to determine whether the input stimulus consists of both speech and noise or of noise alone. When the input signal is determined to consist solely of noise, a running average of its spectrum is initiated, allowing the intensity and spectral distribution of the noise to be monitored. This continuously updated noise measurement provides the noise function that is subtracted from signals determined to contain both speech and noise. After noise has been subtracted, the original phase information is restored and the final temporal waveform is presented to the listener.

The spectral subtraction technique has been evaluated in both normal-hearing and hearing-impaired listeners. In general, the method has not been shown to provide significant improvements in speech recognition, but it has been found to be quite effective for cochlear implant users. Hochberg, Boothroyd, Weiss, and Hellman (1992) examined the effects of processing in 10 implant users tested with consonant-vowel-consonant words mixed with speech-shaped noise. Processed signals were associated with significantly higher phoneme recognition scores than unprocessed signals at signal-to-noise ratios ranging from +15 to –5 dB. Overall results showed that processing provided an increase in the signal-to-noise ratio of about 5 dB, a result that suggested that spectral subtraction could increase the range of environmental conditions in which the implant would provide benefit to the user. Although similar improvements were not found in normal-hearing listeners, these results suggest that spectral subtraction may be beneficial in select populations.

## Simplicity at its Finest

Although the trend in hearing aid design has been toward increased complexity, some improvements can be achieved by relatively simple means. It has recently

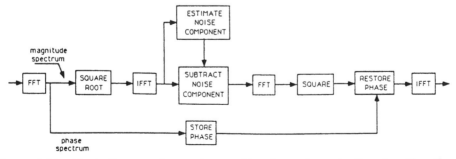

**Figure 4–24.** Block diagram of a spectrum subtraction noise reduction algorithm (from Hochberg et al., 1992, reprinted with permission).

been shown that hearing aids that simply fit deeply within the ear canal are associated with greater sound pressure levels at the eardrum, greater high-frequency response, less perception of occlusion, and less amplification of wind noise than comparable hearing aids that are not worn as deeply. The acoustic benefits of "deep canal fittings" are thought to be due to a combination of reduced residual ear canal volume and deep placement of the hearing aid microphone (Fortune and Preves, 1994; Preves, 1994), and the reduced feeling of occlusion is thought to be due to contact of the hearing aid shell with the bony portion of the ear canal wall (Killion, Wilbur, and Gudmundsen, 1988; Staab and Finlay, 1991). By constructing the hearing aid with a long canal and a deeply placed microphone, appropriate gain and output can often be achieved, and a variety of problems associated with hearing aid use can often be minimized. Although completely-in-the-canal hearing aids cannot specifically improve the signal-to-noise ratio, they appear to provide a variety of benefits without the need for highly complex circuitry.

## Summary

The signal processing algorithms that have been described above represent only a sample of a wide variety of techniques that may soon be incorporated into modern hearing aids. Other methods, both analog and digital, are being designed to further enhance the consonant-to-vowel ratio, the spectral contrasts of speech, and characteristics of the temporal speech envelope. These evolving technologies have shown potential in providing benefit to hearing-impaired listeners, but it is clear that much work remains to be done. Although complete success has yet to be achieved, significant progress in our understanding of hearing impairment and the factors that contribute to speech intelligibility have been made. This understanding, together with further advances in hearing instrument technology and more sophisticated validation methods, will ultimately lead to greater benefits for the hearing impaired.

## Acknowledgments

The author would like to acknowledge James Newton, Brian Woodruff, Chris Stephenson, Jay Jendersee, Charles Witt, and David Preves of Argosy Electronics, who not only assisted in the preparation of this manuscript, but who also strive for that elusive better mousetrap. The author is also grateful for the contributions of Jerry Yanz, Michael Valente, and William Johnson, who provided many insightful comments on an earlier version of this work.

## *References*

American National Standards Institute (1987). Specification of hearing aid characteristics. (ANSI S3.22-1987). New York: ANSI.

Boothroyd A, Springer S, Smith L, Schulman J. (1988). Amplitude compression and profound hearing loss. *J Speech Hear Res* 31:362–376.

Braida LD, Durlach NI, Lippman RP, Hicks BL, Rabinowitz WM, Reed CM. (1979). *Hearing aids—A review of past research of linear amplification, amplitude compression and frequency lowering. (ASHA Monograph No. 19).* American Speech-Language-Hearing Association, Rockville, MD.

Byrne D, Dillon H. (1986). The National Acoustic Laboratories (NAL) new procedure for selecting the gain and frequency response of a hearing aid. *Ear Hear* 7:257–265.

Carlson EV. (1988). An output amplifier whose time has come. *Hear Instrum* 39(10):31–32.

Cornelisse LE, Seewald RC, Jamieson DG. (1994). Wide-dynamic-range compression hearing aids: The DSL[i/o] approach. *Hear J* 47(10):23–29.

Cranmer KM. (1992). Hearing instruments dispenser survey results. *Hear Instrum* 43(6):8–15.

Dawson P, Dillon H, Battaglia J. (1991). Output limiting compression for the severe-profoundly deaf. *Aust J Audiol* 3:1–12.

DeGennaro SV, Braida LD, Durlach NI. (1986). Multichannel syllabic compression for severely impaired listeners. *J Rehab Res Dev* 23:17–24.

Dillier N, Frohlich T. (1993). Signal processing for the hearing impaired and audiological fitting strategies. In: Beilin JB, Jensen GR, eds. *Recent Developments in Hearing Instrument Technology, 15th Danavox Symposium.* Copenhagen: Stougaard Jensen, pp. 361–370.

Dirks D. (1994). Personal communication.

Dreschler WA. (1988). Dynamic range reduction by peak clipping or compression and its effects on phoneme perception in hearing-impaired listeners. *Scand Audiol* 17:45–51.

Dreschler WA. (1989). Phoneme perception via hearing aids with and without compression and the role of speech intelligibility. *Audiology* 28:49–60.

Dreschler WA, Eberhardt D, Melk PW. (1984). The use of single-channel compression for the improvement of speech intelligibility. *Scand Audiol* 13:231–236.

Dreschler W, Plomp R. (1985). Relations between psychophysical data and speech perception for hearing-impaired subjects. *J Acoust Soc Am* 78:1261–1270.

Fabry DA. (1991). Programmable and automatic noise reduction in existing hearing aids. In: Studebaker GA, Bess FH, and Beck, LB. eds. *Vanderbilt Hearing Aid Report II.* Parkton, MD: York Press, pp. 65–78.

Fabry D, Leek M, Walden B. (1990). Do "adaptive frequency response" (AFR) hearing aids reduce upward spread of masking? *J Acoust Soc Am* 87(Suppl 1):S87.

Fabry DA, Van Tasell DJ. (1990). Evaluation of an articulation-index based model for predicting the effects of adaptive frequency response hearing aids. *J Speech Hear Res* 33:676–689.

Fortune TW, Preves DA. (1992). Hearing aid saturation and aided loudness discomfort. *J Speech Hear Res* 35:175–185.

Fortune TW, Preves DA. (1994). The effects of ITE, ITC and CIC microphone placement on the amplification of wind noise. *Hear J* 47(9):23–27.

French NR, Steinberg JC. (1947). Factors governing the intelligibility of speech sounds. *J Acoust Soc Am* 19:90–119.

Freyman R, Nerbonne G. (1989). The importance of consonant–vowel intensity ratio in the intelligibility of voiceless consonants. *J Speech Hear Res* 32:524–535.

Freyman R, Nerbonne G, Cote H. (1991). Effect of consonant–vowel ratio modification on amplitude envelope cues for consonant recognition. *J Speech Hear Res* 34:415–426.

Gagne JP. (1988). Excess masking among listeners with a sensorineural hearing loss. *J Acoust Soc Am* 83:2311–2321.

Gioannini K, Franzen R. (1978). Comparison of the effects of hearing aid harmonic distortion on performance scores for the MRHT and PB-50 test. *J Aud Res* 18:203–208.

Greenberg JE, Zurek PM. (1993). Evaluation of an adaptive beamforming method for hearing aids. *J Acoust Soc Am* 91:1662–1676.

Hawkins DB. (1994). Personal communication.

Hawkins DB, Naidoo SV. (1993). Comparison of sound quality and clarity with asymmetrical peak clipping and output limiting compression. *J Am Acad Audiol* 4:221–237.

Hickson L. (1994). Compression amplification in hearing aids. *Am J Audiol* 3(3):51–65.

Hochberg I, Boothroyd A, Weiss M, Hellman S. (1992). Effects of noise and noise suppression on speech perception by cochlear implant users. *Ear Hear* 13:263–271.

Hoffman MW, Trine TD, Buckley KM, Van Tasell DJ. (1994). Robust adaptive microphone array processing for hearing aids: Realistic speech enhancement. *J Acoust Soc Am* 96:759–770.

Iwasaki S. (1981). Automatic noise suppression in hearing aids. *Hear Aid J* 13:10–11.

Johnson WA. (1993). Beyond AGC-O and AGC-I: Thoughts on a new default standard amplifier. *Hear J* 46(11):37–42.

Johnson WA, Killion MC. (1994). Amplification: Is class D better than class B? *Am J Audiol* 3(1):11–13.

Kates JM. (1986). Signal processing for hearing aids. *Hear Instrum* 37(2):19–22.

Kates JM. (1991). A simplified representation of speech for the hearing impaired. *J Acoust Soc Am* 89:1961.

Kates JM. (1994). Speech enhancement based on a sinusoidal model. *J Speech Hear Res* 37:449–462.

Kates JM, Kozma-Spytek L. (1994). Quality rating for frequency-shaped peak-clipped speech. *J Acoust Soc Am* 95:3586–3594.

Killion MC. (1991). The importance of overload distortion in hearing aids. *J Acoust Soc Am* 89:1931.

Killion MC. (1993). The K-Amp hearing aid: An attempt to present high fidelity for persons with impaired hearing. *Am J Audiol* 2(2):52–74.

Killion MC, Staab WJ, Preves DA. (1990). Classifying automatic signal processors. *Hear Instrum* 41(8):24–26.

Killion MC, Tillman TW. (1982). Evaluation of high-fidelity hearing aids. *J Speech Hear Res* 25:15–25.

Killion MC, Wilber LA, Gudmundsen GI. (1988). Zwislocki was right . . .. *Hear Instrum* 39(1):14–18.

King AB, Martin MC. (1984). Is AGC beneficial in hearing aids? *Br J Audiol* 18:31–38.

Knight JK. (1992). A subjective evaluation of K-Amp vs. linear hearing aids. *Hear Instrum* 43(10):8–11.

Kollmeier B, Koch R. (1993). Noise reduction for hearing aids employing binaural cues. In: Beilin JB, Jensen GR, eds. *Recent Developments in Hearing Instrument Technology, 15th Danavox Symposium.* Copenhagen: Stougaard Jensen, pp. 55–68.

Kruger B, Kruger FM. (1993). The K-Amp hearing aid: Clinical impressions with fittings. *Hear Instrum* 44(2):30–35.

Kuk FK, Tyler RS. (1990). Relationship between consonant recognition and subjective ratings of hearing aids. *Br J Audiol* 24:171–177.

Laurence RF, Moore BCJ, Glasberg BR. (1983). A comparison of behind-the-ear high fidelity linear hearing aids and two-channel compression aids, in the laboratory and in everyday life. *Br J Audiol* 17:31–48.

Leek MR, Dorman MF, Summerfield Q. (1987). Minimum spectral contrast for vowel identification by normal-hearing and hearing-impaired listeners. *J Acoust Soc Am* 81:148–154.

Levitt H, Bakke M, Kates J, Neuman A, Weiss M. (1993). Advanced signal processing hearing aids. In: Beilin JB, Jensen GR, eds. *Recent Developments in Hearing Instrument Technology, 15th Danavox Symposium.* Copenhagen: Stougaard Jensen, pp. 333–358.

Licklider J, Pollack I. (1948). Effects of differentiation, integration and infinite peak clipping upon the intelligibility of speech. *J Acoust Soc Am* 20:42–51.

Lippmann RP, Braida LD, Durlach NI. (1981). Study of multichannel amplitude compression and linear amplification for persons with sensorineural hearing loss. *J Acoust Soc Am* 69:525–534.

McAulay RJ, Quatieri TF. (1986). Speech analysis/synthesis based on a sinusoidal representation. *IEEE Trans Acoust Speech Signal Proc* 34:744–754.

Moore BCJ. (1993). Signal process to compensate for reduced dynamic range. In: Beilin JB, Jensen GR, eds. *Recent Developments in Hearing Instrument Technology, 15th Danavox Symposium.* Copenhagen: Stougaard Jensen, pp. 147–165.

Moore BCJ, Laurence RF, Wright D. (1985). Improvements in speech intelligibility in quiet and in noise produced by two-channel compression hearing aids. *Br J Audiol* 19:175–189.

Mueller HG. (1994). Getting ready for the IHAFF protocol. *Hear J* 47(6):10.

Neuman AC, Bakke MH, Hellman S, Levitt H. (1994). Effect of compression ratio in a slow-acting compression hearing aid: Paired-comparison judgments of quality. *J Acoust Soc Am* 96:1471–1478.

Nilsson MJ, Soli SD. (1994). *The separate contribution of interaural time and level differences and headshadow to directional hearing in normal and hearing-impaired listeners.* Paper presented at the annual meeting of the American Academy of Audiology, Richmond, VA.

Ono H, Kanzaki J, Mizoi K. (1983). Clinical results of hearing aid with noise-level-controlled selective amplification. *Audiology* 22:494–515.

Palmer CV, Killion MC, Wilber LA, Ballad, WJ. (1995). Comparison of two hearing aid receiver-amplifier combinations using sound quality judgments. *Ear Hear* (in press).

Patuzzi RB, Yates GK, Johnstone BM. (1989). Outer hair cell receptor current and sensorineural hearing loss. *Hear Res* 42:47–72.

Perreault JA. (1994). *A comparison of class B and class D hearing aid amplifiers.* Unpublished Masters thesis, University of Minnesota.

Peterson PM, Durlach NI, Rabinowitz WM, Zurek PM. (1987). Multimicrophone adaptive beamforming for interference reduction in hearing aids. *J Rehab Res Dev* 24:103–110.

Peterson ME, Feeney P, Yantis PA. (1990). The effect of automatic gain control in hearing-impaired listeners with different dynamic ranges. *Ear Hear* 11:185–194.

Plomp R. (1988). The negative effect of amplitude compression in multi-channel hearing aids in the light of the modulation-transfer function. *J Acoust Soc Am* 83:2322–2327.

Potts LG, Valente M, Agnew J, Goebel J. (1994). Sound quality judgments: Class A versus class D output stages. Poster presented at the Annual Meeting of the American Academy of Audiology, Richmond, VA.

Preves DA. (1994). Real-ear gain provided by CIC, ITC and ITE hearing instruments. *Hear Rev* 1(7):22–24.

Preves DA, Newton J. (1989). The headroom problem and hearing aid performance. *Hear J* 42(10):1–5.

Punch JL, Beck L. (1986). Relative effects of low frequency amplification on syllable recognition and speech quality. *Ear Hear* 7:57–62.

Punch JL, Montgomery AA, Schwartz DM, Walden BE, Prosek RA, Howard MT. (1980). Multidimensional scaling of quality judgments of speech signals processed by hearing aids. *J Acoust Soc Am* 68:458–466.

Quatieri TF, McAulay RJ. (1986). Speech transformations based on a sinusoidal model. *IEEE Trans Acoust Speech Signal Proc* 34:1449–1464.

Rankovic CM, Freyman RL, Zurek PM. (1992). Potential benefits of adaptive frequency-gain characteristics for speech reception in noise. *J Acoust Soc Am* 91(1):354–362.

Sammeth C, Preves DA, Bratt G, Peek B, Bess F. (1993). Achieving prescribed gain/frequency responses with advance in hearing aid technology. *J Rehab Res Dev* 30(1):1–7.

Schwander TJ, Levitt H. (1987). Effect of two-microphone noise reduction on speech recognition by normal-hearing listeners. *J Rehab Res Dev* 24:887–892.

Schweitzer H, Causey D. (1977). The relative importance of recovery time in compression hearing aids. *Audiology* 16:61–72.

Skafte MD, Strom KE. (1994). The hearing review programmable shopper. *Hear Rev* 1(5):21–27.

Skinner MW. (1980). Speech intelligibility in noise-induced hearing loss: Effects of high-frequency compensation. *J Acoust Soc Am* 67:306–317.

Skinner MW, Karstaedt MM, Miller JD. (1982a). Amplification bandwidth and speech intelligibility for two listeners with sensorineural hearing loss. *Audiology* 21:251–268.

Skinner MW, Pascoe DP, Miller JD, Popelka GR. (1982b). Measurements to determine the optimal placement of speech energy within the listener's auditory area: A basis for selecting amplification characteristics. In: Studebaker GA, Bess FH, eds. *The Vanderbilt Hearing Aid Report.* Upper Darby, PA: Monographs in Contemporary Audiology, pp. 161, 169.

Soede W, Bilsen FA, Berkhout AJ. (1993). Assessment of a directional microphone array for hearing-impaired listeners. *J Acoust Soc Am* 94:799–808.

Staab WJ, Finlay B. (1991). A fitting rationale for deep fitting canal hearing instruments. *Hear Instrum* 42(1):6–10.

Stein LK, Dempesey-Hart D. (1984). Listener-assessed intelligibility of a hearing aid self-adaptive noise filter. *Ear Hear* 5:199–204.

Trees DE, Turner CW. (1986). Spread of masking in normal subjects and in subjects with high-frequency hearing loss. *Audiology* 25:70–83.

Tyler RS, Kuk FK. (1989). The effects of "noise suppression" hearing aids on consonant recognition in speech-babble and low-frequency noise. *Ear Hear* 10:243–249.

Van Tasell DJ. (1993). Hearing loss, speech and hearing aids. *J Speech Hear Res* 36:228–244.

Van Tasell DJ, Greenfield DG, Logeman JJ, Nelson DA. (1992). Temporal cues for consonant recognition: Training, talker generalization, and use in evaluation of cochlear implants. *J Acoust Soc Am* 92:1247–1257.

Van Tasell DJ, Larsen SY, Fabry DA. (1988). Effects of an adaptive filter hearing aid on speech recognition in noise by hearing-impaired subjects. *Ear Hear* 9:15–21.

Van Tasell DJ, Soli SD, Kirby VM, Widin GP. (1987). Speech waveform envelope cues for consonant recognition. *J Acoust Soc Am* 82:1152–1161.

Villchur E. (1973). Signal processing to improve speech intelligibility in perceptive deafness. *J Acoust Soc Am* 53:1646–1657.

Villchur E. (1989). Comments on 'The negative effect of amplitide compression in multi-channel hearing aids in the light of the modulation transfer function. [*J Acoust Soc Am* 1988; 83:2322–2327.]. *J Acoust Soc Am* 86:425–427.

Walker G, Byrne D, Dillon H. (1984). The effects of multichannel compression/expansion amplification on the intelligibility of nonsense syllables in noise. *J Acoust Soc Am* 73:746–757.

Walker G, Dillon H. (1982). *Compression in Hearing Aids: An Analysis, a Review and Some Recommendations (NAL report No. 90).* Sydney, Australia: National Acoustic Laboratories.

Wolinski S. (1986). Clinical assessment of a self-adaptive noise filtering system. *Hear J* 39(2):29–32.

Yanick P. (1976). Effects of signal processing on intelligibility of speech in noise for persons with sensorineural hearing loss. *J Am Audiol Soc* 1:229–238.

# 5

## *Hearing Aid Adjustments Through Potentiometer and Switch Options*

### JEREMY AGNEW

### *Introduction*

This chapter is intended to provide the reader with insight into the numerous methods currently available to change various electroacoustic parameters of hearing aids. The following pages will describe the theory and practice behind the methods used to vary the characteristics of hearing aids, as well as details concerning the numerous options that are available to the audiologist.

There are at least two reasons for audiologists to need the flexibility of adjusting hearing aids: (1) to optimize the hearing aid fitting on the individual, and (2) to optimize listening in a particular environment.

The first category is to allow the measured frequency response to be set as close as possible to the prescribed frequency response. The second is to allow further adjustment of the hearing aid characteristics, so that the final setting comes closest to the user preference for the amplified sound, based on sound quality and speech intelligibility ratings.

### Optimization on the Individual

It is important to be able to change the electroacoustic characteristics when fitting hearing aids. For example, hearing aid prescriptive formulas, such as NAL-R (Byrne and Dillon, 1986) and POGO (McCandless and Lyregaard, 1983) are commonly used to provide an initial estimate of required gain, based upon audiometric thresholds, to allow average conversational speech to be comfortably loud. When an audiologist sends an order to a manufacturer for a custom hearing aid, the manufacturer enters the audiometric data into a computerized version of these fitting formulas, to determine the required electroacoustic characteristics (measured in a 2-cc coupler) necessary for the hearing aid to achieve the prescribed gain. Yet, large variations may occur between individuals that may not allow the audiologist to achieve the desired results. For example, manufacturers' fitting formulas typically use an average value for ear canal resonance. As reported in Chapter 2, the typical resonant peak of the ear canal for an adult is approximately 18 dB at 2700 Hz. However, for an individual patient, this value may vary by 12 dB, or more. Therefore, hearing aid prescriptive formulas should be viewed only as a first approximation to the hearing aid fitting. It is usually necessary to modify the initial prescribed gain and frequency response to provide the optimum match to the individual.

As another example, the ability to vary different frequency response filters provides a more precise adjustment of prescribed frequency response for the individual. This flexibility is important, because it is well known that careful matching of the hearing aid frequency response to the needs of the patient can produce a significant improvement in speech recognition (Pascoe, 1975).

## Optimization for the Environment

Though hearing aids may be optimized for speech recognition in quiet, it may be necessary to fine tune the hearing aids to provide better performance for the user's particular listening environment or environments.

It is well known that one set of electroacoustic characteristics will not be suitable for all listening environments (Kates, 1986; Libby and Sweetow, 1987). Thus, it may be necessary for the user to alter the electroacoustic characteristics of the hearing aids in different environments. For example, in noisy situations, a user may prefer a reduction of the low frequencies in order to make the amplified sound more pleasant and more tolerable. For music, many hearing aid users prefer a broader frequency response than that used for speech signals. Some listeners may prefer even a slight boost in the low frequency response when listening to music.

## Methods of Modifying the Electroacoustic Characteristics of Hearing Aids

There are at least six methods by which the electroacoustic characteristics of hearing aids may be adjusted.

These include: (1) modifications to the acoustic transmission line from the receiver to the tympanic membrane, with the appropriate selection of earhook, tubing, earmold, vent and damper; (2) switches; (3) potentiometer adjustments; (4) remote controls; (5) digitally controlled analog (DCA) hearing aids (commonly called programmable hearing aids); and (6) digital signal processing (DSP) hearing aids.

Acoustic modification is covered in greater detail in Chapter 6, and will not be discussed here further. The use of switches for various modifications will be described in the next part of this chapter. This will be followed by a description of the use of potentiometers, which is the most common method of modifying hearing aid performance. Subsequent sections will discuss hearing aids using remote controls, using programmability, which represents the current state of the art in circuit adjustability, and using digital signal processing, which is the future of hearing aid adjustability.

To fully understand the basis for hearing aid adjustments and to gain better insight into the information provided by manufacturers in their data sheets, it is useful to understand the physical and electrical basis for switches and potentiometers. Therefore, the next sections of this chapter will outline the electrical properties of switches and potentiometers. The reader is urged to pursue these short sections, because this will help with understanding the block diagrams presented later in this chapter.

**Circuit Symbols and Functions**

Whether a switch is used to turn a hearing aid on and off, to allow the audiologist to switch between microphone, telecoil, or direct audio input, or to change the frequency response of the hearing aid, the basic electrical and mechanical characteristics of the switch are similar.

Schematic symbols are shown in Figure 5–1 for switches and potentiometers commonly found in hearing aids. The switch symbol shown in Figure 5–1a is a simple off-on switch. This is also known as a SPST (single-pole, single-throw) switch. The name *single-pole* refers to a single contact operation, and *single-throw* indicates a simple off-on action. Switches with two contacts and simple off-on action may be referred to as DPST, or double-pole single-throw. Single contact switches with two switch actions may be referred to as SPDT (single-pole, double-throw), and so forth.

The symbol shown in Figure 5–1a is very similar to the way a switch physically works. When the center line segment is up, the electrical contact is broken, current does not flow, and the switch is *off*. When this segment is pivoted down, so

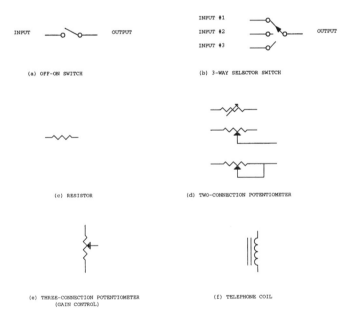

**Figure 5–1.** Schematic symbols for switches, resistors, and potentiometers.

that the line is bridging the circles, this symbolizes that electrical contact is made, current flows, and the switch is *on*. This on-off action is the simplest function of a switch and is exactly the same as an on-off light switch in the home.

Figure 5–1b symbolizes a 3-way selector switch. Similar to a 3-way lamp switch, which contacts different parts of the light bulb to create different brightness levels, a hearing aid function switch can be used to make contact to more than one circuit, depending on the switch position. In this way, a switch can be used to select from several inputs, such as switching between a microphone, a *telephone coil* (also often abbreviated to *telcoil* or *telecoil*), and a *direct audio input (DAI)*, as shown in Figure 5–2.

A DAI forms a connection to the hearing aid amplifier where the signal is directly wired to the input, instead of coupling through the microphone or telephone coil. When the input-select switch arm is up, it contacts the first input, which is the microphone. When it is in the center position, it contacts the second input, which is the telephone coil and, when it is in the down position, it connects to the third input, which is the direct audio input.

The schematic symbol in Figure 5–1c is the engineering circuit diagram symbol for a *resistor*, which is a device that "resists" the flow of current in an electronic circuit. Its function can be remembered by thinking that the zig-zag line of the symbol forms a longer pathway for electrical current to flow through than a straight line, thus "resisting" the flow of current. A resistor has a fixed resistance value, expressed in ohms. A *potentiometer*, also abbreviated as *pot*, is a resistor that is varied by some mechanical or electrical means.

A potentiometer performs the task of adjusting various parameters in a hearing aid as the audiologist adjusts a knob or screwdriver control. A potentiometer is usually described by various specific names that refer to its function in the circuit. Examples of adjustable functions include gain, SSPL90, frequency response, compression threshold (kneepoint), and compression ratio. The electrical circuit element used within the hearing aid to adjust all of these various functions is the same.

The symbol for a potentiometer or variable resistor is shown in Figures 5–1d and 5–1e. A potentiometer has a sliding electrical contact that touches different parts of an internal resistive element. The amount of resistance in the circuit is determined by the position of the sliding contact on the element. The upper symbol in Figure 5–1d is a resistor that has an arrow passing through the symbol to denote variability. The center symbol portrays a variable resistor where one connection is one end of the resistive element, and the other connection is the sliding element. The lower symbol in Figure 5–1d, which performs the same function, portrays one manner in which a variable resistor is constructed in practice. That is, connecting the sliding contact to one end of the resistive element.

Figure 5–1e is another symbol for a potentiometer that allows access to both ends of the resistive element, as well as the sliding contact that creates the variable resistance. Note that the lower symbol in Figure 5–1d is the same symbol as Figure 5–1e, but with one end of the resistor connected to the sliding contact. The symbol for a telephone coil is shown in Figure 5–1f.

When studying the rest of this chapter, the reader may wish to refer to Figure 5–2, which is a generic block diagram of a conventional *analog hearing aid* that

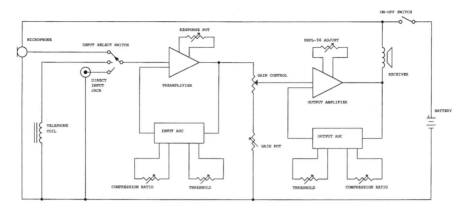

**Figure 5–2.** Generic block diagram of a hearing aid showing common switch and potentiometer options.

illustrates common switch and potentiometer options. An analog hearing aid is a hearing aid in which the signal processing takes places in a continuous fashion over time, as opposed to a *digital signal processing (DSP) hearing aid*, which is a hearing aid in which the signal path involves digital signal processing. Some of the functions shown and described in Figure 5–2 may not become clear until after reading the rest of this chapter.

The signal pathway in Figure 5–2 is through the top half of the diagram, from left to right. The signal source is either the microphone, the telephone coil, or the DAI, depending on the position of the input select switch. After the signal is routed through the switch, it is amplified by the preamplifier. The purpose of the preamplifier is to increase the signal level, though frequency response shaping is often also performed by this amplifier stage. If input AGC is present, it will be connected to this stage. Next, the signal goes through the gain control, where the appropriate loudness level is set by the listener. After this, the signal undergoes more amplification and is converted to a power signal that can drive the receiver to the appropriate acoustic levels. The output amplifier stage usually contains the output limiting control (either peak clipping or output AGC) and associated circuitry.

The diagram in Figure 5–2 is used only as a generic example. In practice, in-the-ear (ITE) or in-the-canal (ITC) custom hearing aids may only have one or two of these switches or potentiometers available when the hearing aids are ordered from the manufacturer. Usually, behind-the-ear (BTE) hearing aids have predetermined features when ordered from the manufacturer, and the functions controlled by the switches and potentiometers are standard for a particular BTE model.

## Switches

### Physical Construction of Switches

An *on-off* switch is mechanically constructed exactly as the schematic symbol shown in Figure 5–1a. The physical realization of an SPST switch consists of two electrical contacts mounted in a nonconductive housing. To turn the switch *on,* the contacts are physically pressed together so that the electrical circuit is complete. When the contacts are separated again, the circuit connection is broken and the circuit is *off.*

Another type of switch is what is referred to as a *solid-state switch.* This is a switch that has no moving parts, but uses the electrical properties of semiconductor action to make or break the circuit. The switching action is controlled by electrical impulses from a mechanical switch or from instructions programmed into the memory of a programmable hearing aid. This type of switch is commonly found in DCA and DSP hearing aids.

### Uses for Switches

There are three primary purposes for a switch on a hearing aid: (1) to turn the hearing aid on and off. The typical use for this switch is to power down the hearing aid at night, in order to extend the life of the battery. (2) To change the operation of the hearing aid from one function to another. An example of this change is to switch from a microphone input to a telecoil or DAI. (3) To change the acoustic characteristics of the hearing aid to another set of characteristics. An example of this is the use of a tone switch to change the frequency response of the hearing aid from a broad response to one in which the low-frequency region is attenuated. Another example is the use of a switch to change from one program to another in a multimemory programmable hearing aid.

ON-OFF SWITCHES

An on-off switch to remove the power from a hearing aid circuit may take one of several forms. In some hearing aids, the user simply opens the battery drawer to remove the connection between the battery and its contacts and, by doing so, uses it as an on-off switch. The battery drawer may have a slot or depression for the battery contact in its plastic housing, called a detent. To turn the hearing aid off, the door is opened to this detent. This action lifts the battery contact away from the battery and removes power from the circuit, but holds the battery drawer partially closed mechanically via the detent, so that the battery will not fall out.

Another design of on-off switch is one that is incorporated into the gain control. The gain control wheel is rotated to its lowest setting, and then rotated slightly more to a detent that is the on-off switch.

A third configuration of on-off switch is one that is a separate switch with a lever handle, similar to a wall-mounted light switch in the home. This type of switch is toggled back and forth to perform its on-off function, and, hence, is called a *toggle switch.* Toggle switches may be found on BTE or body-style hearing aids, with subminiature versions found on ITE or ITC hearing aids.

An on-off toggle switch may be combined with a telecoil switch. This switch is commonly labeled an *O-M-T* switch, denoting *off-microphone-telecoil* functions. In the *O* position, the hearing aid power is turned off. In the *M* position, the hearing aid is turned on and the microphone is connected. In the *T* position, the telecoil is activated.

A final version of the on-off switch that may be encountered is the *slide switch,* which slides back and forth to perform its function. The physical configuration of a hearing aid slide switch is a miniature version of the slide switches often found on electronic entertainment units or appliances. This may be configured as a 2-position switch, such as to switch between microphone and telecoil, or as a 3-position switch, such as the *O-M-T* switch described above. Sometimes a colored dot or a raised bump is used to indicate which position the switch is in.

TELECOIL SWITCHES

The function of a telephone switch is to change the hearing aid input from the microphone that is used for acoustic pickup, to a telecoil, which is used to provide direct electromagnetic pickup from a telephone, neck loop, or induction loop system. A loop system is one in which a room, or area of a room, has a loop of wire around its perimeter to transmit electromagnetic signals directly to the telephone coil. The purpose and advantage of a telecoil is that it allows direct amplification of sounds from the telephone or a loop-wired room system without amplification of potential interfering acoustic ambient noise. Telecoils have been covered in detail in Chapter 3.

The telephone coil function is schematically diagrammed in Figure 5–2. When the input selector switch is in the *microphone* position, only the microphone is connected to the input of the hearing aid. When the selector switch is in the *telephone* position, only the telephone coil is connected to the input of the hearing aid.

As its name and schematic symbol (Fig. 5–1f) imply, a telephone coil is a long length of fine wire wound in the shape of a spiral coil on a magnetic core. This coil picks up electromagnetic leakage from the telephone as an electrical signal, which is routed through the switch to the hearing aid amplifier and then to the user.

Another important reason for the use of a telephone coil with the telephone is to reduce the possibility of acoustic feedback. When a telephone receiver is placed close to the hearing aid microphone, the telephone earpiece forms an acoustic reflector that bounces sound waves back into the hearing aid microphone and initiates acoustic feedback. By using the telephone coil to amplify the electromagnetic leakage from the telephone, the possibility of acoustic feedback is removed and only the electromagnetic pathway is maintained.

There may be situations where the user may wish to hear conversation from the telephone, as well as conversation within the environment. This function may be achieved in the hearing aid via a switch position labeled *MT, M-T,* or *M/T,* with which both the microphone and the telephone coil are energized simultaneously. With this option, the user can hear on the telephone through the telecoil and yet still hear conversation within the surrounding environment through the microphone. When this function is active, the microphone output is usually attenuated in comparison to its normal acoustic output. This is to allow the telecoil to be the dominant signal source, and to reduce the likelihood of acoustic feedback due to the close proximity of the telephone receiver to the head.

Another telephone switch combination that may be seen on hearing aids is a 4-position switch labeled *O-T-MT-M.* This stands respectively for *off, telephone coil, microphone and telephone coil* (simultaneously), and *microphone* (only).

As well as picking up signals from the telephone, telecoils are useful for electromagnetically coupling the hearing aids to induction loop systems in rooms wired for the hearing impaired. As the name implies, an induction loop system is a loop of wire that is built into the perimeter of the room being used by the hearing-impaired listener. The signal comes from a microphone, public address system, theater sound system, or other desired source. This electrical signal is used to drive the room induction loop, and the loop transmits the desired signal via electromagnetic coupling through the telecoil to the hearing aid.

Large induction loop systems are commonly found in churches, theaters, classrooms, and other public gathering places (Ross, 1982; Marutake, Fukutome, and Inaba, 1983). Small loop systems are also available for individual use in seating areas, and for improved listening to the TV or radio (Leavitt and Hodgson, 1984). Methods of wiring these loops for personal use have been presented (Bunker, 1982; Smith, 1985).

Both large and small induction loop systems offer the advantage of directly transmitting the desired signal to the hearing aid wearer, while eliminating competing acoustic ambient noises and reverberation picked up by the hearing aid microphone (Pimental, 1980). In practice, this improves the *signal-to-noise ratio* (SNR) for the listener by effectively placing the hearing aid microphone closer to the talker (Gilmore and Lederman, 1989). This is particularly useful in acoustically reverberant environments, such as churches.

### Disadvantages of Telecoils

Along with the advantages of a telephone coil, there are several potential disadvantages. They include: (1) size; (2) directionality; (3) sensitivity; and (4) interfering electromagnetic fields.

SIZE

A telephone coil is a physically large component compared to the other components inside a hearing aid. Sometimes it becomes very difficult for a manufacturer to find sufficient space in an ITC or ITE hearing aid to mount the coil. The strength of the signal, the *electromagnetic sensitivity*, is proportional to the size of the magnetic core of the coil so, for reasonably sensitive operation, the coil has to be relatively large.

Also related to the issue of size is that there may not be enough room on the faceplate of a custom hearing instrument for the telephone switch. One solution to this problem is for the manufacturer to install an automatic telephone coil circuit. This circuit switches itself from microphone to telephone coil whenever it senses an electromagnetic field. This telephone option may also be useful for users who lack the dexterity to manipulate a telephone switch, or for users with frequent telephone needs. The disadvantage of this option is that the circuit cannot differentiate between a desired electromagnetic field and undesired spurious radiation, such as from fluorescent lighting; thus, the coil may occasionally energize itself on unwanted signals. Success with automatic telephone coil circuits has not been overwhelming, so it is recommended that this option should only be ordered when it is absolutely necessary.

DIRECTIONALITY

Another important issue related to size is directionality. For optimum pickup, the telephone coil should be oriented so that its magnetic axis points perpendicularly towards the telephone receiver. Due to the small size of many ITE and ITC hearing aids, the manufacturer is often obliged to mount the coil wherever he can, in whatever orientation that he can, just to be able to physically assemble the entire hearing aid circuit into the shell. It may be necessary to place the smallest coils in some hearing aids because of size constraints. Orientation and size issues may result in a reduction of optimum coupling, which is directly related to magnetic sensitivity and, thus, result in reduced electromagnetic pickup and a low telephone coil output. Often, the user has to move the bottom part of the telephone around the head to find the point of maximum pickup for a particular hearing aid. Sometimes it is necessary for the user to orient the telephone at awkward angles to the head to successfully achieve maximum coupling (ASHA, 1993). Further aspects of this variability have been reported by Gladstone (1985).

Currently, it is difficult to compare the performance of telecoils in different hearing aids under actual use conditions. Standard measurement conditions specify that the hearing aid be oriented for maximum acoustic output when measuring telecoil performance (ANSI, 1987). Although this measurement produces a useful figure for a comparison of maximum output values, the technique is not particularly useful for describing actual telephone or loop use, because the coil orientation within the hearing aid case may not be that for realistic or optimum use with the telephone or a loop system.

To further complicate the interpretation of these figures, the directions for optimum coupling for telephone and loop system use are different. Maximum sensitivity for use on the telephone requires orientation of the telecoil in the hearing aid case in a horizontal plane, whereas maximum sensitivity for loop use requires that the coil be vertically oriented. An expanded discussion of this problem is contained in Compton (1994) and is discussed in Chapter 1.

To provide more meaningful telephone coil sensitivity figures, measurement techniques have been proposed within the ANSI working group on hearing aid measurements that require specific orientations of the hearing aid within the electromagnetic measurement field, and specification of the output in those orientations. When a suitable technique is agreed upon, it will be incorporated into a future version of the standard for hearing aid measurement. This will allow a more realistic comparison among different hearing aid brands and models.

SENSITIVITY

Closely related to size and orientation of the coil is the issue of sensitivity. If the coil is mounted in the hearing aid at a less-than-optimum orientation, signal sensitivity decreases quite rapidly. This results in less amplification of the desired electromagnetic signal, greater amplification of undesired signals, and a poor signal-to-noise ratio.

Another sensitivity issue arises because the telephone coil output is typically lower than the microphone output to the hearing aid amplifier. In the past, this often led to a perceptible decrease in hearing aid output when the user switched from the microphone to the telephone coil (Rodriguez, Holmes, and Gerhardt, 1985). Current audiological fitting practices suggest that it is preferable for a hearing aid to have equivalent sensitivities when switching between microphone and telephone coil. The benefit of this is that the user does not have to adjust the gain control when switching between microphone and telecoil.

INTERFERENCE

Because a telephone coil is intentionally designed to pick up the electromagnetic field from a telephone, neck loop, or room loop when in use, it will also pick up any other strong stray electromagnetic fields in the vicinity. The most common interfering signal is 60 Hz radiation present in the environment from line-operated electrical devices, such as fluorescent lights. Other common sources of low-frequency interference are appliances that contain motors, such as drills and vacuum cleaners. To eliminate this troublesome interference, it would seem reasonable from a design standpoint to incorporate high-pass filtering in the hearing aid. However, even though interfering signals are often generated at the power line frequency of 60 Hz, harmonics occur all across the bandwidth of the hearing aid. This produces an irritating audible buzz that often interferes with hearing the desired speech signals.

One of the most severe interference problems occurs for users near, or using, digital mobile cellular personal telephones (Joyner, Wood, Burwood, Allison, and Strange, 1993). The GSM (Groupe Speciale Mobile) digital cellular telephone system has already been adopted in Europe and Canada, and its widespread use in those countries is causing concern among consumer groups. Electrical interference comes from bursts of noise radiated from the modulation method employed by these systems as the network polls the telephones during use. The GSM system switches between its receive and transmit modes at 2 millisecond intervals. This creates a square wave at 500 Hz, with many harmonics across the audible frequency range. The result is a very distracting buzzing sound in the output of the hearing aid (Hahn, Thorpe, and Fitch, 1993). Because of the broadband nature of this strong interference, simple shielding and filtering are not effective, and interference may be noted with both microphone and telecoil use. As of this writing, there has been no agreement between the telephone and hearing aid industries on a solution to the problem.

On the other end of the spectrum, telephone coils can also pick up and amplify interfering high-frequency signals from other electronic devices. A common source of high-frequency radiation is computer terminals and video display units, which typically radiate electromagnetic energy in the area of 14,000 to 20,000 Hz. Although this frequency region is above the audible bandwidth of most hearing aids, this interference is translated into the lower frequency regions and amplified by the hearing aid as audible intermodulation frequencies.

The electromagnetic sensitivity of a telephone coil generally increases with increasing frequency. Because the bandwidth of a telephone is restricted to frequencies between 300 Hz and 3000 Hz, it is possible to restrict the bandwidth of the hearing aid during telephone coil use to optimize this frequency span. Some manufacturers tune their coil circuits to produce a bandwidth that is approximately equivalent to the bandwidth of a telephone, to lower interfering signals and maximize sensitivity of the desired frequencies.

Another method to increase the sensitivity of the telephone coil without greatly increasing physical size is to use an *amplified telephone coil,* which is a type of telephone coil that contains its own preamplifier. This type of coil increases the electromagnetic sensitivity (Cranmer-Briskey, 1992). Though these coils amplify the desired signal they also equally amplify unwanted interference and, thus, do not improve the SNR for the user.

### Summary of Telephone Coil Use

Generally speaking, telephone coils are often not successful for ITE and ITC users because of the issues described above. The shells of ITC hearing aids typically do not provide sufficient room to include a telephone coil. In ITE hearing aids designed for very small ears, the use of a telephone coil may also be doubtful because of orientation issues.

Greater success is usually achieved when using telephone coils with BTE hearing aids, because the cases for BTE hearing aids are larger. This improves consistency of manufacture, and allows orientation of the coil to ensure optimum electromagnetic coupling. BTE hearing aids often have sufficient space to allow for additional amplifying circuitry, so that better telephone coil sensitivity can be achieved.

One alternative to telephone coils, in the appropriate fittings, is the use of low-gain ITC hearing aids or *completely-in-the-canal* (CIC) hearing aids. In these fittings, the microphone may be located deep enough within the ear canal to preclude feedback when the telephone receiver is close to the head. Thus, with these aids, it is often possible to acoustically use the telephone successfully without acoustic feedback.

Another switch-activated telephone option is the *telephone booster circuit.* This acoustic circuit uses a telephone switch, but does not include a telephone coil. When the circuit is activated, the circuit provides additional low-frequency gain and decreases high-frequency gain. The result provides a better match to the bandwidth of the telephone and reduces feedback.

Investigations are under way in several areas with magnetically sensitive solid-state devices. These are not coils, but are electronic semiconductor devices incorporated directly into integrated circuits. Though only in the early stages of development, this technology holds promise for providing smaller physical size in the future, as well as for better differentiation between amplification of desired and undesired input signals.

### Switches for Direct Audio Input (DAI)

Similar to changing the input of a hearing aid from a microphone to a telephone coil, some hearing aids incorporate a switch to change the hearing aid input from a microphone to a DAI. When using the DAI option, the microphone and telephone inputs are usually disconnected and the hearing aid amplifier electrical input is directly connected to the desired source. For this reason, DAI is sometimes also called a hard-wired system.

The advantage of a direct audio input is that the input signal bypasses the microphone or telephone coil and connects directly to the audio source. An analogy illustrating the effectiveness of DAI would be when trying to tape-record music from a television or radio. The effectiveness of DAI, and the resulting improved sound quality, is analogous to plugging the television electrical speaker output directly into the tape recorder auxiliary jack, rather than trying to hold the tape recorder close to the television and using the tape recorder microphone for acoustic pickup. The result is that interfering acoustic signals are eliminated and the recording is free from ambient interference.

The disadvantage of a DAI is that a direct-wired connection to the hearing aid must be used. This restricts user mobility to the length of the connecting input cable, unless a wireless link is used.

DAI is often used in combination with FM receivers for classroom auditory trainer use. However, other electrical inputs may also be used, including microphones, televisions, and radios (Pimental, 1984; Krutt, 1986).

Some hearing aids do not have a switch to activate the DAI, but incorporate circuitry to automatically activate the DAI circuit when the DAI connection is plugged in. On some BTE hearing aids, the direct audio input takes the form of a connection, called an *audio boot* or *audio shoe,* that fits over the back of the hearing aid and automatically connects the DAI when it is in place.

**Tone Control Switches**

Another generalized use for a switch is to change the basic hearing aid frequency response to a different frequency response. This provides the user the option of two frequency responses in one hearing aid. An example is a switch labeled *N-H.* In the *N,* or *normal,* position, the electroacoustic characteristics of the hearing aid are usually adjusted to provide the gain required for average conversational speech to be comfortable so that the measured response matches the audiologist-selected prescription fitting formula. In the *H,* or *high,* position, the amplification of the low frequencies is decreased, as shown in Figure 5–3, to theoretically provide a reduction of background noise. Low-frequency background noise may include traffic noise, machinery noise, or restaurant noise. Though this change in frequency response may not assist in speech recognition, the resulting reduction of low frequencies may be judged by the listener to be more pleasing.

A similar switch option may be labeled *N-L,* which stands for *normal* and *low.* In the *L* position, the high frequency gain is reduced. This may be useful for reducing the tendency toward acoustic feedback, for fitting reverse-slope audiograms, or for reducing annoying high-frequency noises in the environment.

A frequency response switch may be combined with the on-off switch on a BTE aid. It may be labeled as *M-S-O.* In this example, *M* is for microphone, *O* is for off, and *S* is for suppressor. In the *S* position, low-frequency gain is reduced, which provides some suppression of competing low frequencies. This is the same function as an *N-H* switch, with a different name. It can be seen that the lack of standardized terminology for switch settings and labeling can lead to confusion.

The idea of reducing gain in noisy situations is also found in *automatic signal processor (ASP)* circuits. In this case, the manual switching described above has

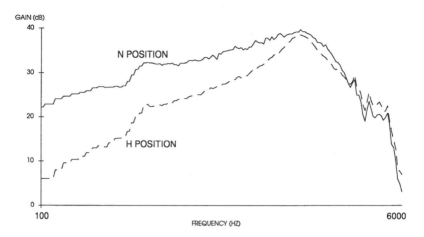

**Figure 5–3.** Typical response curves achieved with a N-H frequency response switch.

been changed to automatic switching. The term ASP has no engineering or audiological meaning, but is often used generically to describe hearing aids that modify their low-frequency amplification automatically, depending on the amount of low-frequency energy present in the input signal. This definition is not universally agreed upon, as some think that the term ASP applies to *BILL* (bass increase at low level) and *TILL* (treble increase at low level) hearing aids. Some even think that the term ASP applies generically to compression circuits. This type of circuit is also sometimes called *automatic noise suppressor (ANS)*, or *automatic noise reduction (ANR)*. Viewed in a simplistic sense, these circuits incorporate an input-activated low-cut frequency-response switch.

Multiposition switches may be used for the adjustment of frequency response, output, and other parameters on hearing aids. On BTE aids, this may be in the form of a small rotary switch located underneath a trapdoor on the top or bottom of the case. This type of switch looks like a potentiometer and is adjusted using a small screwdriver. However, unlike a potentiometer, these switches contain detents, so that the different switch positions have a positive feel, and click into each adjustment position. The difference between a switch-type of adjustment of hearing aid parameters and a potentiometer adjustment is that the switches only adjust the function in discrete steps, whereas a potentiometer adjusts the function in continuous form.

### Problems with Switches

Troubleshooting problems with switches is relatively straightforward. Switches that are not functioning properly either fail or become intermittent. Typically there is not much that can be done when a switch fails to function correctly and the hearing aid must be returned to the manufacturer or to an all-make repair facility.

As a temporary measure, it may be possible to use a *modest amount* of chemical switch cleaner lightly sprayed directly into the switch to clean it. Such cleaning agents are available in small pressurized spray cans at electronic wholesale stores. However, if a switch is intermittent, the chances are good that the problem has been caused by excessive mechanical wear, and that the problem will occur again in the near future. Replacing the switch is more reliable and is preferred.

## Potentiometers

A potentiometer is a variable resistor that is used to change a designated function of a hearing aid in a continuous fashion. Potentiometers are electrically the same as gain controls; however, there is a distinction made by function. The term *gain control* (often also called *volume control, VC* or *volume wheel*) is taken by common usage to refer to the large thumbwheel control available to the user to adjust the loudness output of the hearing aid. The term *potentiometer* generally refers to the small screwdriver trim controls manipulated by the audiologist while fitting the hearing aid, and are not intended to be adjusted by the user. Other common terms for a potentiometer are *pot* or *trimmer*. However, because the elements of a gain control and an adjustment potentiometer are identical, it is electrically possible to use the two interchangeably and, for example, to have a screwdriver-adjustable (also called screw-set) gain control.

### Physical Construction of Potentiometers

The variable resistive element shown in Figure 5–1e is often used for the gain control of a hearing aid. A gain control is a relatively large potentiometer with a thumbwheel than can be easily operated by the user. Sometimes the thumbwheel is mounted vertically with respect to the plane of the top of the case, in either BTE or ITE aids, and sometimes it is mounted horizontally. Similarly, a vertically mounted thumbwheel may be parallel or perpendicular to the axis of a BTE case. In any case, the mechanical and electrical functions are the same. The choice of horizontal or vertical mounting of the gain control is a matter of manufacturer preference, space limitations, and dispenser and user preferences.

Potentiometers used to adjust circuit function are usually smaller than gain controls, and have a slot in the top of the potentiometer for a screwdriver. Potentiometer adjustments are typically set only once to achieve the desired fitting parameters. Usually they are only readjusted if a change in the initial fitting is needed. For example, the patient may indicate that sounds are too loud. In this case, the audiologist may change the potentiometer setting to reduce the output or the compression kneepoint. In another example, the patient may report that the amplified sound is too tinny. In this case, the audiologist may increase the low-frequency gain and reduce the high-frequency gain.

Because screwdriver adjustments are not recommended for adjustment by the user, they are often located underneath a hinged or sliding door, or inside the battery compartment.

Figure 5–4 is a sketch of the typical mechanical construction of a potentiometer or gain control. The resistive element is deposited as a thin film on a nonconductive substrate with connections made to the 2 ends (Premanand and McLinn, 1984). A moveable arm, called the *wiper*, rotates around a pivot point and makes a sliding

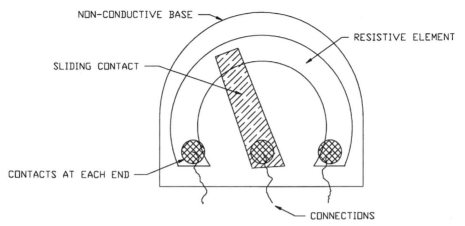

**Figure 5–4.** Typical mechanical assembly of a potentiometer.

contact to different parts of the element. Different resistive elements, consisting of different deposited resistance values and tapers, may be used for different circuit adjustments, depending on the specific design of the circuitry employed.

### Uses for Potentiometers

Potentiometers may be used for several different adjustment functions on a hearing aid. Commonly encountered potentiometer adjustments include: (1) gain, (2) frequency response, (3) maximum output (SSPL90), (4) compression threshold, (5) compression ratio, (6) compression release time, and (7) phase characteristics.

ITE hearing aids typically contain one or two potentiometers to provide these adjustments, but may contain as many as three or four. The number depends on the space available within the case of the hearing aid. BTE hearing aids typically contain one to four potentiometers. These commonly include overall gain, low-frequency adjustment, SSPL90, and compression threshold. The number and function of potentiometer adjustments may be allocated by the manufacturer or be ordered by the audiologist, depending on the particular style or model of hearing aid. The range of adjustments made by potentiometer controls varies widely from manufacturer to manufacturer, and from model to model within a manufacturer's offerings.

One highly flexible BTE hearing aid has been described that contains eight potentiometers for adjusting almost all the parameters discussed in this section (Brander and Briskey, 1988).

### Potentiometers for Gain Control

The terms *volume control* and *gain control,* though they have different meanings in other applications of electronics, are generally used interchangeably for hearing aids. Both names refer to the control by which the user adjusts the loudness of the hearing aid to a comfortable level. The term *volume control* has historical roots in the radio and television industry. The term *gain control* is more accurate for hearing aids, because its operation varies the amount of gain with different settings, and this term will be used consistently throughout this text.

As well as being used as standard gain controls, potentiometers have several other gain control uses in a hearing aid: (1) gain trimmer, (2) gain control for handicapped users, (3) gain control for inaccessible hearing aids, and (4) alternate volume control.

GAIN TRIMMER

Two gain controls may be present on one hearing aid. One is a gain control operated by the user. The other is an overall gain adjustment set by the audiologist. It should also be noted that some hearing aids do not have a gain control. Examples of this are those hearing aids in which the gain level may be preset to the user's MCL, or where the gain control is adjusted via a remote control.

If a gain control is designed to operate over the entire gain range of a hearing aid, the user may not have precise control over the loudness adjustment. This is due to the mechanical construction of gain controls, in which rotation is limited to 270°, or three-quarters of a turn. This limited rotation determines the resolution with which the gain control can make an adjustment. For example, a power hearing aid may be designed to provide 80 dB of overall gain. This gain range is so great that the limited three-quarters of a turn available on the gain control results in small adjustments of the gain control wheel producing a large variation in loudness for the user. In other words, the total gain range is so great that it may be difficult for the user to successfully set the loudness to precisely the desired level. Some of the problems of linearity of loudness with gain control settings have been discussed by Gold and Phipps-Davis (1990), and by Leidy (1984).

One way of overcoming this problem is to place two potentiometers in series. One potentiometer serves as a *coarse adjustment control*. The second potentiometer serves as a *fine adjustment control*. The coarse control is used by the audiologist to set the user's maximum gain control output level. The fine control then allows the user a finer, but more limited, range of adjustment within his general area of need. Typically, a range of 35 dB to 40 dB is the optimum adjustment range for a three-quarter turn mechanical gain control. The fine adjustment control then becomes the thumbwheel gain control, because it is adjusted more frequently by the user. The coarse control is a screwdriver adjustment potentiometer because it only needs to be set once during the initial fitting. This screwdriver control may also be called a *gain pot* (GP).

GAIN CONTROL FOR HANDICAPPED USERS

There are fittings where it may be desirable for the audiologist to adjust the initial gain control setting and not have the user change it at all. In this case, it is possible to have the gain control wheel replaced by a potentiometer that functions as a preset gain control. The audiologist sets the initial adjustment with a screwdriver and then the user does not alter the setting. This option is sometimes called a *screw-set gain control*.

Situations where this type of gain control may be useful are for geriatric or handicapped patients, who may be mentally incapable of manipulating the normal gain control wheel. Examples include patients with Down's syndrome or

Alzheimer's disease (Sweetow, 1990). This type of control may also be useful for very young children, or patients who are physically handicapped, such as an amputee. Another example may be a patient who has diminished mental capacity or physical skills following a stroke.

GAIN CONTROL FOR INACCESSIBLE HEARING AIDS

There are fittings where the hearing aid is so small that the gain control is inaccessible. An example is some CIC fittings, where the hearing aid is located deep in the ear canal and it is not possible for the user to manipulate the gain control. In this case, it is common to have a screw-set gain control. During fitting, the audiologist places the hearing aid in the ear canal and carefully inserts a small screwdriver into the potentiometer slot. The audiologist then adjusts the gain while the user is listening to samples of speech. Because this type of fitting normally requires less coupler gain than an equivalent ITE fitting, or incorporates some form of compression for limitation of gain, a one-time adjustment of the gain control is adequate. An alternative for gain control adjustment in these inaccessible situations is a hearing aid in which gain adjustments are made with a remote control. This option will be discussed in a later section of this chapter.

## Potentiometers for Frequency Response Changes

The most common use for a potentiometer is to manually adjust the frequency response of the hearing aid. Adjustment is often performed by using probe-microphone measurement equipment during the fitting procedure to monitor the frequency response of the hearing aid as it is being adjusted. As well as compensating for the user's hearing deficit, judicious setting of the hearing aid's frequency response characteristics can enhance sound quality and improve the recognition of speech in noise (Stearns, 1980).

Several different options are available for adjusting frequency response. These include: (1) *high-pass filtering*, which reduces low-frequency gain; (2) *low-pass filtering*, which reduces high-frequency gain; (3) *bandpass filtering*, which manipulates the peaks in the frequency response. Such peaks are often seen at the center of the frequency response for undamped BTE fittings; and (4) *notch filtering*, which decreases part of the frequency response.

Figure 5–5 illustrates examples of high-pass (Fig. 5–5a), low-pass (Fig. 5–5b), bandpass (Fig. 5–5c), and notch filtering (Fig. 5–5d).

High-pass and low-pass potentiometers are the most common adjustments found in hearing aids. Bandpass and notch filtering are more specialized controls for altering the frequency response. The latter two are not encountered as often, but will be discussed for completeness.

HIGH-PASS FILTERING

A high-pass filter is an electronic filter that restricts the range of amplified low frequencies. The effect of this filtering is to reduce low-frequency gain according to the adjustment of the potentiometer. This control is usually used to shape the

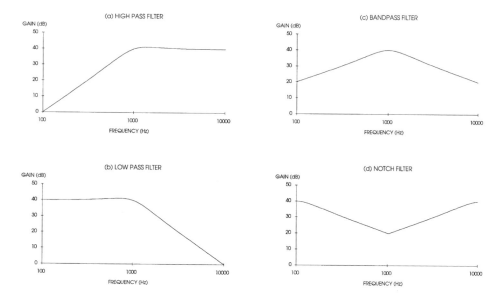

**Figure 5–5.**  Four filter functions used for frequency response adjustment.

magnitude of low-frequency amplification to achieve the prescribed response in the low frequencies. By reducing the low frequencies delivered to the listener, this control may also be used to improve word recognition in competing noise, to reduce user complaints of a tinny sound, or to produce what the user perceives as a more normal sound quality. An example of the range of adjustment in the low frequencies in a typical hearing aid response curve is shown in Figure 5–6a. This control may also be called a *variable low-cut pot*, a *frequency pot*, or a *Hertz (Hz) pot*.

Adjustment of this potentiometer is performed through a screwdriver slot in the case of the hearing aid. If there is space available, such as in a BTE aid, the hearing aid case may be labeled with *N* and *H* at the extremes of the potentiometer adjustment range. The *N* position usually stands for *normal*, or the broadest frequency response. The *H* position usually stands for *high*, or the minimum gain in the low frequencies. Alternately, this control may simply be labeled *L*, to indicate that it affects the *low frequencies*.

In some cases, the use of a frequency–response control is even more confusing. Normally, the gain control wheel is used to control the overall loudness of the hearing aid. However, hearing aids are available that do not have a gain control adjustment, and what would be the gain control wheel is actually a tone control that allows the user to change the magnitude of low-frequency amplification in different environments (Libby and Sweetow, 1987).

LOW-PASS FILTERING

A low-pass filter is an electronic filter that restricts the range of amplified high frequencies. A low-pass frequency control, if present, is used to shape the high

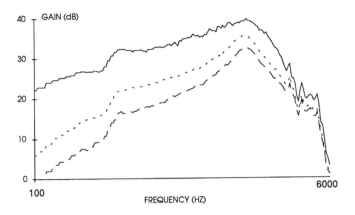

(a): EFFECTS OF HIGH PASS FILTERING

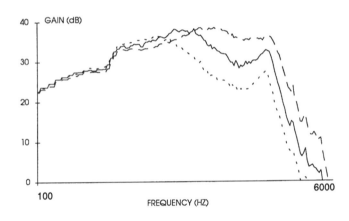

(b): EFFECTS OF LOW PASS FILTERING

**Figure 5–6.** The effects of low-pass and high-pass filtering on a typical hearing aid frequency response.

frequencies to decrease amplification at the upper end of the frequency response through low-pass filtering. This is shown in Figure 5–6b.

This type of control, if used judiciously, may also be used to decrease the high-frequency gain of the response curve to reduce acoustic feedback (Teder, 1992). By reducing high-frequency amplification, potential high-frequency feedback conditions are altered and any potential audible squeal is suppressed. However, it is important not to use a high-frequency control too aggressively or else amplification in the high frequencies may be reduced so much that the hearing aid becomes ineffective for correction of the user's hearing loss. This control may also be called a *variable high-cut (VHC) pot.*

Similar to the N-H potentiometer, the hearing aid case may be labeled with *N* and *L*. The *N* position stands for *normal*. *L* stands for maximum *high cut*, or the minimum high-frequency gain. This control may also simply be labeled *H*, to indicate that it affects the *high frequencies.*

## BANDPASS FILTERING

Some hearing aids incorporate circuitry that manipulates a particular region of the frequency response via a bandpass filter, which is an electronic filter that restricts the range of amplified frequencies. This control may be used to shift the peak of the frequency response, or to smooth a jagged frequency response. Other uses are to manipulate the frequency response in the high or low frequencies. The philosophy behind the ability to shift the peak of the frequency response is that, when the peak in the response curve coincides with the peak of the user's ear canal resonance, the resulting response will provide the user with the most satisfactory frequency response curve. This philosophy remains neither proven nor disproven, but the technology necessary to achieve this goal is available.

Another fitting strategy for wanting to adjust the peak in the response curve is to emulate the frequency response of a BTE hearing aid (which typically has a peak near 1600 Hz) for a new user of an ITE fitting who was a previous user of a BTE hearing aid. As the user becomes more comfortable with the ITE fitting, the peak may be shifted to a higher frequency that is closer to the user's own canal resonance. A peak shifting control may also be called a *resonant peak control (RPC)* or a *peak power filter (PPF) pot.* Powers and Sacca (1983) have discussed the use of an RPC control to reduce feedback.

As well as being present as a single filter in a hearing aid, high-pass, low-pass, and bandpass filtering may be combined in a single hearing aid. An example of this is the 3-channel clock circuit, which combines these filter functions to provide extremely flexible filtering of the frequency response (Preves, 1993).

## NOTCH FILTERING

As well as having the ability to adjust the peak of a frequency response, it is also possible to invert a bandpass filter and remove part of a peak in the frequency response. This is accomplished with an electronic filter that removes a range of frequencies from the hearing aid frequency response. This is called a *notch filter.* It removes a narrow part of the spectrum centered around the frequency of the filter. A notch filter is also known as a *band reject filter.*

This type of filtering has been used for control of acoustic feedback, where the notch is tuned to remove a narrow band of frequencies around the offending frequency (Agnew, 1993). Other suggestions for reducing feedback will be discussed in Chapter 6.

As well as for acoustic feedback control, this type of filtering can also be useful for frequency shaping. For example, if there is a troublesome resonant peak occurring at a particular frequency, a notch filter may be placed over it to smooth out the frequency response (Agnew, 1992). Various methods of acoustic damping to achieve the same goal are also discussed in Chapter 6.

## Potentiometers for Output Control by Peak Clipping

*SSPL90* (Saturation Sound Pressure Level for 90 dB input) is the output of a hearing aid for 90 dB SPL input, which is essentially the maximum output that a hearing aid can achieve. European standards refer to this quantity as *OSPL90* (Output Sound Pressure for 90 dB input). U.S. standards will probably adopt this designation in the future to harmonize the standards. *SPL* (Sound Pressure Level) is the fundamental measure of sound pressure, described in decibels referred to 20 µPascals.

A common use for a potentiometer is to set the SSPL90 of a hearing aid via peak clipping, so that the output does not exceed the user's measured *uncomfortable loudness level (UCL)*. Using this method of output limiting, the amplification provided by the output stage is truncated at the top and bottom of the amplified waveform, at a level that is predetermined by the SSPL90 control setting.

The effects of the SSPL90 control on the output are shown in Figure 5–7. The top (solid) curve is the maximum SSPL90 curve for the hearing aid, which is achieved with the potentiometer adjusted to the maximum output position. This curve indicates a maximum value of 110 dB at the peak. The lower 3 curves illustrate the reduction in SSPL90 obtained when the output potentiometer is rotated to reduce the output. It can be seen that the maximum SSPL90 is thereby reduced to approximately 105 dB, 100 dB, and then 90 dB, as the potentiometer is rotated. The upper curve may be appropriate for a patient with minimal loudness recruitment. The lower curves are appropriate for patients with a reduced degree of tolerance for loud sounds.

A potentiometer for peak clipping is typically labeled as an *SSPL90 control, output limiting control,* or *output control.* Other common names for this control include *output limit pot, limit pot,* or *PC (peak clipping) control.* Peak clipping output limiting should be differentiated from compression output limiting, which will be discussed below in the section on compression.

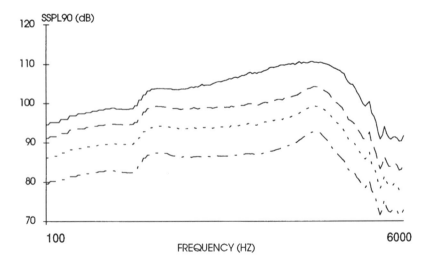

**Figure 5–7.**    The typical effect of an SSPL90 control on a hearing aid output.

Peak clipping, while simple and effective, leads to considerable distortion of the waveform, as shown in Figure 5–8a. This is not necessarily destructive for speech recognition, because distorted waveforms have been shown to be highly intelligible (Licklider, 1946). However, the quality of the sound delivered during peak clipping deteriorates significantly. Even though the fitting of compression circuitry (Fig. 5–8b) is a mature technique, Hawkins and Naidoo (1993) reported that 82% of the hearing aids dispensed in the United States used peak clipping as the method of output limiting.

A peak clipping control may be labeled with 0, –5, –10, and –15. This indicates the amount of SSPL90 reduction, in decibels, that is achieved at the indicated setting. Alternatively, the control may be labeled as 110, 120, and 130, to indicate the expected maximum SSPL90.

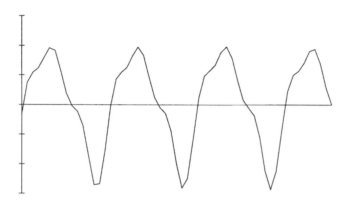

(a): PEAK CLIPPING, SHOWING HIGH DISTORTION

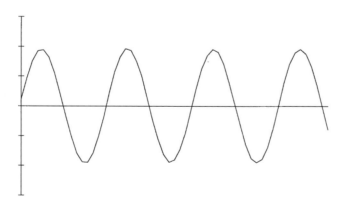

(b): COMPRESSION LIMITING, SHOWING LOW DISTORTION

**Figure 5–8.** A comparison of two methods of SSPL90 output limitation, showing the amount of distortion in the output waveform for a sine wave input.

## Potentiometers for Adjustment of Compression Characteristics

Compression is the amplification of the dynamic range of the input signal in a nonlinear fashion to produce a reduced range of output. With compression amplification, a change in input level always produces a lesser change in output level. This is contrasted to linear amplification, in which a specified change in input level produces the same amount of change in output level.

Though *compression* is used as a general term for *nonlinear amplification*, there are several types of compression function that are intended to provide different results. The uses, function, and philosophy of compression amplification have been discussed in greater detail in Chapter 4. In addition, the reader is directed to several comprehensive reviews by Hogg (1976), Braida and colleagues (1979), Schweitzer (1979), and Walker and Dillon (1982), for more specific information on compression in hearing aids. However, the basics of compression will be briefly discussed in this section, so that the reader can understand the uses of potentiometers to adjust the compression characteristics of hearing aids. It is hoped that this simplistic discussion will provide a different perspective for the reader than Chapter 4. It is intended primarily as an overview of compression controls and their settings.

For the purposes of this simplified discussion, compression hearing aids are usually categorized by manufacturers as either input compression or output compression. This difference divides the functions for clinical fittings: (1) *input compression* is intended to process the input signal in a nonlinear fashion as the signal passes through the amplifier. (2) *Output compression* is intended primarily as a means of output limitation.

These two types of compression are used clinically to achieve different results. In general, input compression is fitted on hearing-impaired users who have a severely reduced dynamic range, because it compresses the large dynamic range of the input signal into a smaller range of output signal.

Input compression may also have other uses. For example, input compression may be used to restrict the dynamic range of the preamplifier to prevent overload distortion. Generally, in these types of applications, the compression characteristics of the amplifier are not adjustable by the audiologist, so they will not be discussed here further.

Output compression is typically fitted on users who have a reduced tolerance for loud sounds. Output limitation reduces the maximum SSPL and thus limits the delivered SPL to below the user's uncomfortable loudness level (UCL). Some hearing aids contain both input and output compression. This requires the compression characteristics to be set for each method of compression. Readers wishing more than this simple explanation of input and output compression may wish to consult Hogg (1976), Braida et al. (1979), Schweitzer (1979), Walker and Dillon (1982), Dillon and Walker (1983), Herbst (1983), and Smriga (1985a, 1985b).

### Compression Controls

Compression controls commonly found on hearing aids are *compression ratio and compression threshold* potentiometers.

Though clinical usage of compression involves different fitting characteristics and goals, the operating controls are the same and can be discussed in general terms. The operation of these controls can be understood by referring to Figure 5–9, which is the input-output graph for a generic compression amplifier.

COMPRESSION RATIO

This is a number that denotes the amount of compression taking place above the threshold point. This number is calculated as a ratio of input signal change to output signal change, and then compared to 1. For example, if for every 10 dB of change in input SPL there is a change in output SPL of 5 dB, then the compression ratio is 10 divided by 5, or a 2 to 1 compression ratio (also written as 2:1). Similarly, a change in output SPL of 5 dB for a change in input SPL of 20 dB results in a compression ratio of 4:1. A compression ratio potentiometer adjusts the ratio over a specified range for a particular model of hearing aid, for example 2:1 up to 5:1.

*Linear amplification* may also be called a compression ratio of 1:1. That is, for every 1 dB increase in input SPL, there is a 1 dB increase in output SPL, up to the point where the SSPL90 is reached. Above this point, peak clipping or compression limiting will result.

COMPRESSION THRESHOLD

This is the input level at which amplification begins to deviate from linear amplification. The compression threshold potentiometer adjusts the setting of the *threshold kneepoint*. In Figure 5–9, this is seen as the point on the curve where the input-output function changes abruptly and starts to flatten into a more horizontal line. When the input level is below the compression threshold setting, amplification is linear. When the input level is above the compression threshold, the hearing aid output is compressed according to the compression ratio setting. Thus, in Figure 5–9, the line below the threshold is at 45°, or is a 1:1 compression ratio. Above the compression threshold, the line is at a slope of input level to output level that is the compression ratio.

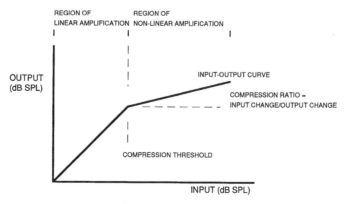

**Figure 5–9.** Generic input-output function for a compression hearing aid.

Sometimes the kneepoint of the threshold is not a well-defined transition between two line segments, but gradually curves from the linear region below the threshold into the compression region above the threshold. This is called *curvilinear compression.*

When the compression threshold control has a low setting, compression will begin for low input levels, typically 40 to 60 dB SPL. When the threshold control is set higher, the compression will begin at a higher input level and the hearing aid will be operating in a linear fashion for a wider range of input signals until the input signals are high, perhaps as high as 90 to 100 dB SPL.

Compression threshold is also called *compression kneepoint* or *breakpoint.* The threshold control is sometimes called a *threshold kneepoint (TK)* pot.

COMPRESSION CIRCUITS

Compression circuits operate, in general, by using a portion of the amplified signal to control the gain of certain parts of the hearing aid amplifier. This is shown in the diagrams in Figure 5–10 for both input (Fig. 5–10a) and output (Fig. 5–10b) compression amplifiers. In both instances, a control signal is fed from a sensing point back to an earlier amplification stage, where it acts to reduce the gain and output.

Input and output compression amplifiers use essentially the same circuitry. The primary difference is whether the compression control signal is derived from before or after the gain control, as seen in Figure 5–10. In output compression circuits, the sensing point is after the gain control. In input compression circuits, the sensing point is before the gain control. This difference affects the output characteristics of the hearing aid, as shown in Figure 5–11.

With input compression, the output of the hearing aid varies with rotation of the gain control. As shown in Figure 5–11a, though the compression threshold stays constant, the output varies with the gain control setting. As the gain control is raised, the output increases. As the gain control is lowered, the output decreases. Therefore, it may not be a good strategy to fit a hearing aid with input compression to a user having tolerance problems for loud sounds, because the maximum output will vary with the gain control. Thus, this strategy can create the potential for presenting the user with an amplified signal that is above the uncomfortable loudness level.

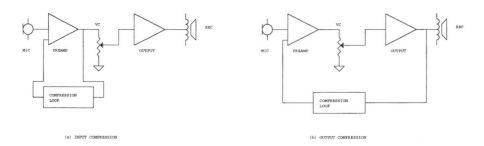

**Figure 5–10.** A comparison of input and output compression circuits showing the difference in the sensing points.

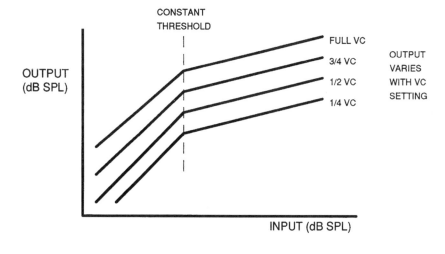

(a): INPUT COMPRESSION

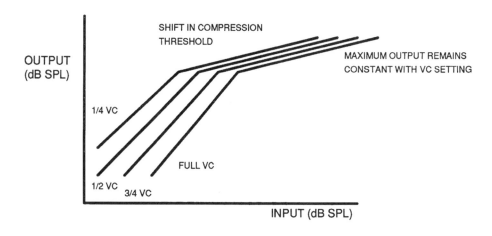

(b): OUTPUT COMPRESSION

**Figure 5–11.**   A comparison of the effects of volume control setting for input and output compression circuits.

With output compression, the SSPL of the hearing aid remains constant at the setting predetermined by the compression controls, regardless of gain control setting. However, it can be seen in Figure 5–11b that the compression threshold shifts up and down with the gain control setting. In general, it is not a good strategy to fit a hearing aid with output compression on a patient with a highly reduced dynamic range because the patient requires dynamic range reduction to compress all sounds into his or her residual dynamic range.

To accommodate patients with both a reduced dynamic range and a tolerance problem for loud sounds, a hearing aid with a combination of both input and output compression may be appropriate.

## Fitting Compression Hearing Aids

For the purpose of understanding typical settings of compression potentiometers, there are three common categories of compression (Braida et al, 1979; Walker and Dillon, 1982; Dillon and Walker, 1983): (1) syllabic compression; (2) automatic gain control (AGC); (3) compression limiting.

These categories of compression are intended for different clinical uses and, hence, the compression potentiometers are adjusted differently.

### SYLLABIC COMPRESSION

Syllabic compression uses a low compression threshold to compress the entire dynamic range of the input signal. This is also known as *whole range syllabic compression, full-range compression,* or *full dynamic range compression (FDRC).* The primary purpose for syllabic compression is to reduce the dynamic range of the input signal and, hence, to map this reduced signal into the residual dynamic range of the user. The dynamic range for normal-hearing listeners extends from 20 dB SPL (threshold) to approximately 120 dB SPL (uncomfortable loudness level). This spans a dynamic range of approximately 100 dB.

Hearing-impaired listeners lose some hearing capability both for quiet speech and for loud sounds. Their threshold of hearing is elevated due to their hearing loss. In addition, they usually experience some reduction in uncomfortable loudness level. Thus, the strategy behind syllabic compression is that the normal 100 dB dynamic range of ambient sounds should be placed in the reduced dynamic range of the hearing-impaired user.

Syllabic compression is characterized by a low compression threshold, usually below the level of soft speech sounds. Therefore, the hearing aid is in compression almost all of the time. To achieve dynamic range reduction, the compression kneepoint must be set lower than the level of the lowest sound in the range to be compressed. Practically speaking, this is usually between 40 and 50 dB SPL, so that the compression threshold is lower than soft speech.

Syllabic compression is also characterized by a relatively low compression ratio, which is usually less than 3:1. This is calculated by reducing the normal 100 dB dynamic range of the input signal into the residual dynamic range of the hearing impaired user. For example, if the residual dynamic range of the listener (UCL minus threshold) is 40 dB, then the desired compression ratio is 100 divided by 40, or 2.5:1. This is a simplistic calculation, because the dynamic range of some hearing-impaired persons may vary with frequency. Multiband compression circuits allow different compression ratios to be individually fitted to different parts of the frequency response.

Syllabic compression may be achieved with either input or output compression. Input compression is generally used if the goal is to reduce the overall dynamic range of the signal. Output compression has been recommended if the goal is to compensate for loudness recruitment (Dillon and Walker, 1983), though input compression may also be used to achieve the same result.

AUTOMATIC GAIN CONTROL (AGC) COMPRESSION

This is intended to amplify the long-term average energy of speech to a constant output level. This level is commonly set either to *most comfortable level* (MCL), or to an output level that corresponds to maximum intelligibility. Automatic gain control compression can be thought of as a linear amplifier that has slowly varying gain (Braida et al., 1979).

Automatic gain control compression is characterized by a low compression threshold, typically 40 dB SPL, because it is intended to operate on the entire dynamic range of speech. AGC compression is also characterized by a high compression ratio, typically greater than 7:1, because it is intended to maintain the output at a fixed level, regardless of the input level. Automatic gain control compression generally uses an input compression circuit.

Automatic gain control compression is also sometimes called *automatic volume control* (AVC) compression.

COMPRESSION LIMITING

Compression limiting is a compression method of limiting the SSPL90 of a hearing aid. This is also known as *compression output limiting* or *high-level limiting*. Compression output limiting reduces the maximum available hearing aid output for users who have a reduced tolerance for loud sounds, by limiting the output to a level below the user's uncomfortable loudness level. Compression limiting is a common low-distortion method for output limitation instead of peak clipping (see Fig. 5–8).

Compression limiting achieves the goal of limiting the output by means of a compression loop around the output stage, or output compression. In this way, as input signals increase, the output signal is held constant without substantially increasing distortion.

Compression limiting is characterized by a high compression threshold, because the threshold is the setting for the output limitation point. For example, it may be set at a threshold of 110 dB, to keep the output below the user's uncomfortable loudness level.

Compression limiting is also characterized by compression ratios as high as 8:1 or 10:1, or even higher. After the preset compression threshold has been exceeded, it is important that the output not rise above that level, or the user's uncomfortable loudness level will be exceeded.

Figure 5–12 is a summary of the combinations of high and low compression threshold and compression ratio reviewed in this simplified explanation of compression. The fourth combination of high compression threshold and low compression ratio, which was not discussed here, is not clinically useful.

### Potentiometers for Compression Release Time Adjustment

Another characteristic of compression that may be adjusted is *compression release time*. There are two characteristics of compression that involve the time domain.

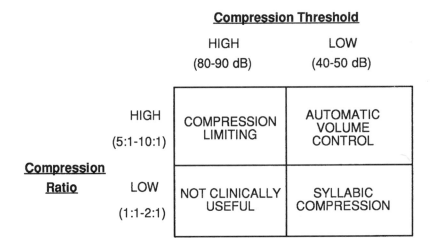

**Figure 5–12.**   Matrix of compression threshold and compression ratio for common compression settings.

One is *attack time,* which is the length of time that it takes for the compressed signal to settle to within 2 dB of its steady-state value. Attack time is usually fixed by a particular circuit design and cannot be adjusted by the audiologist. Typical attack times are less than 5 milliseconds.

The other temporal characteristic of compression is *release time,* which is the amount of time that it takes for a signal to return to within 2 dB of its steady-state value after the compression is released. Release time is often fixed for a particular hearing aid model and may commonly be set between 50 and 200 milliseconds. However, in other models, a potentiometer or rotary switch is available to vary the release time, either continuously or in discrete steps. An example of the range of adjustments might be from 25 to 400 milliseconds. The setting of such a control is open to debate; however, as a general rule, release times of 60 to 90 milliseconds are typical. Schweitzer and Causey (1977) have shown that a release time of approximately 90 milliseconds is optimum for recognizing speech. They reported that intelligibility decreased if the release time was longer or shorter than 90 milliseconds.

Further explanation of attack and release times was given in Chapter 4, or in one of the references on compression mentioned earlier in this chapter.

Though having the ability to adjust release time to a fixed setting may be questionable, there is a useful nonadjustable option that automatically selects the release time in relation to the length of time that the input signal is above the compression threshold (Teder, 1991, 1993). This may be called a *variable release option,* or by various proprietary trade names.

### Potentiometers to Change Phase Characteristics

There are two special adjustable circuits for phase manipulation that the audiologist may encounter, even though infrequently. At this point, the reader unfamiliar with the concept of phase may wish to refer back to the discussion of phase in Chapter 2.

The first circuit is an electronic circuit that simulates acoustic venting. The traditional method of reducing the occlusion effect in hearing aids is to enlarge the size of the vent (Revit, 1992). This is not always a satisfactory solution because excessive venting may lead to acoustic feedback. An alternative method is to electronically manipulate the phase of the signal for frequencies below 1000 Hz. By doing this, it is possible to electrically simulate the effect of a vent and not create a situation that could lead to acoustic feedback. This circuit option is called the *active vent circuit* (trade name AV1), and is available from several manufacturers (Schweitzer and Smith, 1992).

A second phase adjustment option is a feedback-stabilizing circuit. The circuit operates by feeding some of the output signal back to the input via a negative feedback loop. The effect of this is to produce partial cancellation of signals that could cause acoustic feedback. By adjusting the feedback potentiometer, it is possible to reduce the potential for acoustic feedback, while optimizing the high frequency response (Preves, Sigelman, and LeMay, 1986; Stearns, 1992).

## Problems with Potentiometers

Because gain controls and potentiometers are mechanical devices, they often fail because of mechanical problems. The electronic components in a hearing aid are generally very reliable and most common repair problems tend to be related to mechanical moving parts, such as battery drawers, switches, and potentiometers.

Problems with gain controls and potentiometers usually revolve around wear of the mechanical moving parts of the control due to contamination by dirt, lint, dust, and other debris over time. As the debris builds up, the hearing aid may not function at all. Foreign material entering the housing of the potentiometer promotes wear of the resistive element. This is likely to initially result in the control becoming intermittent. Wear over many rotational cycles of use of a gain control may eventually result in a dead spot, or open circuit on the element, which is audible as an intermittent sound as the gain control is rotated.

Similar to temporary switch rejuvenation, it may be possible to use a chemical switch cleaner *lightly* sprayed directly into the gain control to help to resolve the problem. However, if a gain control is intermittent, the real problem is mechanical wear of the resistive element and the problem will occur again. In addition, a lubricant is applied to the sliding contact on the resistive element during manufacture. Solvents in chemical cleaners accelerate wear of the element because they dissolve and flush away these lubricants. In the end, replacement is the most reliable and cost-effective repair.

## Adjustment of Potentiometers

One final note about adjustment of potentiometers. This may seem trite to the reader, but an audiologist must be willing and capable of adjusting potentiometers. Potentiometers are intended to be adjusted during the fitting process, and the hearing aid cannot be damaged by adjusting these potentiometers. However, it is not unusual for manufacturers to receive hearing aids back from audiologists with requests to change parameters, such as low-frequency gain or SSPL90, that could have been adjusted in the office, only to find that the potentiometers have never been moved from the original factory position!

If there is reluctance to adjust a potentiometer because of concern of losing the original adjustment position, it is easy to document the original control setting or, if there are no adjustment markings, to make a diagram of the settings. It is also possible to mark the original position of the potentiometer settings on the hearing aid case with a felt pen with water-based ink. In this way, the new setting can be returned to the original setting if the change does not result in greater user satisfaction, and then wiped clean.

To adjust potentiometers or subminiature rotary switches, it is necessary to have a set of subminiature screwdrivers. These are available from vendors of hearing supplies, from jewelers' supply houses, or from many hobby shops.

## Hearing Aids That Use Remote Controls

Some users are physically unable to manipulate the controls often found on conventional hearing aids. One method of making adjustments is the use of a remote control to communicate with the hearing aid (Wolf and Powers, 1986).

With this type of fitting, the hearing aid is combined with a small user-operated remote control (see Fig. 5–13). Remote controls typically use ultrasonic signals, radio frequency waves, or infrared light to transmit control signals to the hearing aid. The remote control either parallels or replaces the function of one or several controls on the hearing aid. These may include the gain control, on-off switch, noise suppression switch, or telephone switch. The use of a remote control sometimes allows the size of the hearing aid to be smaller, because the space for the controls on the hearing aid are not necessary.

There are several fitting situations where a remote control may be useful: (1) for very small hearing aids with controls that are not easily accessible or easily manipulated by the user, (2) for control of multiple functions of the hearing aid, and (3) for geriatric or physically handicapped users who are unable to manipulate hearing aid controls.

### INACCESSIBLE CONTROLS

As hearing aids have become smaller, they fit deeper into the ear canal, and the controls and adjustments may not be accessible to the user. An example of this is a CIC fitting. In addition, many ITC hearing aids also fall into this category. In these cases, one method for the control of overall gain may be to use a hearing aid with a remote control.

Though the gain control on the remote still varies the output SPL, the mode of operation is slightly different when compared to a mechanical gain control wheel. Instead of the continuous variation of loudness that is achieved with a conventional thumbwheel volume control, a remote volume control varies overall gain in discrete steps.

The remote control usually operates the gain function via 2 push-buttons. One button is used to raise the gain and the other button is used to decrease the gain. At each push of one of the buttons, the gain is increased or decreased in a typical

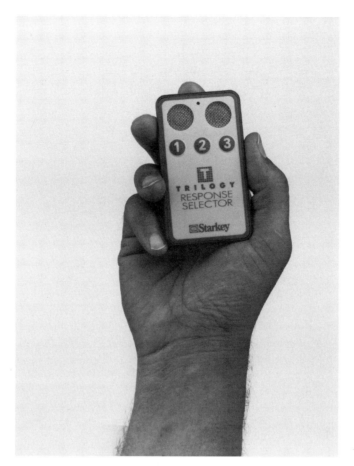

**Figure 5–13.**    An example of a hand-held remote control.

discrete step of 2 dB or 3 dB. Holding down a push-button causes the gain to increase (or decrease) continuously until the desired loudness is reached and then the push-button is released.

The remote control may also have a push-button to change the frequency response of the hearing aid. An example would be remote operation of the *N-H* switch. When the push-button is pressed once, the hearing aid may switch from the *N* position to the *H* position. When the push-button is depressed again, the frequency response is switched back to the *N* position response. Other functions, such as the telephone coil or on-off switch, may be similarly accessed.

The functioning of a remote control can usually be explained to the user in terms of common television remote controls, because a user may be already familiar with the use of these devices.

CONTROL OF MULTIPLE FUNCTIONS

This capability falls primarily into the area of programmable hearing aids, which will be discussed in the next section of this chapter.

PATIENTS WITH HANDICAPS

Another situation where a remote control may be useful is for a geriatric patient who is unable to manipulate the small gain control wheel found on many hearing aids. A similar situation would be for a patient who is physically handicapped. Other examples may be patients with Parkinson's Disease or severe arthritis. These patients may still be able to successfully operate a remote control and thus vary the desired functions of the hearing aid.

### Problems With Remote Controls

Hearing aids using a remote control are technologically more complex than hearing aids with switches or potentiometers. Problems with remote controls may seem difficult to diagnose, but there is one simple test that can be performed to help determine the cause of the problem. For troubleshooting in the office, it is often possible to determine whether the problem is in the hearing aid or in the remote control. The easiest way to determine this is to try the hearing aid with a different remote control. With most of these systems, the remote control units from a particular manufacturer are generic and may be interchanged. If a different remote control works with the hearing aid, then the trouble is with the remote control. If a new remote control does not operate the hearing aid and the problem appears to be in the hearing aid itself, the hearing aid and remote control should be returned to the manufacturer for repair.

The only simple in-office repairs to a remote control are to clean the battery contacts, check the batteries, and replace the batteries with fresh cells, if necessary. The batteries in remote controls usually last significantly longer than the batteries in the hearing aid; therefore, patients may forget about the batteries or not be in the habit of replacing them.

Some remote controls do not have user-replaceable batteries. These are designed to operate for a long time (up to 5 years), under normal operating conditions. These remotes usually have some type of indicator that inform the patient that the batteries are still functional. When the batteries on this type of remote are exhausted, some models may be returned to the factory for battery replacement, while others are intended to be discarded.

## Programmable Hearing Aids

Thus far, this chapter has covered the adjustments that may be made with potentiometers and switches. All of the adjustments discussed above can be incorporated into a hearing aid, and any hearing aid could theoretically contain all of these adjustments. However, due to size constraints, a single hearing aid usually does not contain all, or even most, of these adjustments. As hearing aids have decreased in size from BTE to CIC, the capability of providing numerous adjustments has been reduced. A typical ITC may only have space for one, or a maximum of two, potentiometers. Yet today's sophisticated consumer demands technologically advanced hearing aids that perform a variety of complex functions. The way that these conflicting requirements of small size and increased functionality have been resolved is with the recent introduction of programmable hearing aids.

As with some of the previous topics in this chapter, the focus of this section will not be specifically on programmable hearing aids, but rather will discuss some of the adjustments available on programmable hearing aids. Though it is necessary to outline the basic operation of programmable devices, these hearing aids will not be discussed extensively, and the reader is referred to comprehensive surveys available elsewhere (Sammeth, 1990; Staab, 1990; Berkey, Marion, Robinson, and Van Vliet, 1992; Sandlin, 1994).

### Basic Operation of Programmable Hearing Aids

A programmable hearing aid can broadly be defined as one in which the parameters of the hearing aid can be changed through programming. Programmability electronically performs the same functions that screwdriver potentiometers and switches perform on conventional hearing aids.

The terms *digital* and *programmable* are generic terms and need to be qualified for clearer understanding of their meaning. Programmable hearing aids are sometimes generically called *digital hearing aids, hybrid hearing aids, hybrid digital hearing aids,* or *digital/analog hybrid hearing aids.* To a hearing aid or electronics manufacturer, the term *hybrid circuit* refers to a common method of packaging subminiature electronic circuitry. This terminology may lead to confusion if used improperly.

In an effort to standardize terminology, the Hearing Industries Association (HIA) has proposed uniform terminology based on the type of signal processing and control functions present in a hearing aid. The term recommended for programmable hearing aids is *digitally controlled analog (DCA)* hearing aids (Conger, 1990). The signal path in these hearing aids is analog, as in the traditional BTE, ITE, and ITC hearing aids discussed in previous sections. However, the control functions used to alter the electroacoustic characteristics of the hearing aid are performed by digital circuitry.

This distinction forms the important difference between programmable hearing aids and true digital hearing aids. DCA hearing aids use analog amplifiers. Thus, adjustments made to these hearing aids use the adjustments possible with analog technology. However, instead of only using a limited selection of conventional screwdriver potentiometers, switches and wiring changes, a programmable hearing aid has a large number of potential adjustments built into the hearing aid at the factory. Then the audiologist determines the final adjustment of these adjustable parameters to achieve the desired fitting.

A functional block diagram of a DCA hearing aid is shown in Figure 5–14. The figure shows an analog amplification path that is very similar to Figure 5–2; the main difference is that the potentiometer adjustments shown in Figure 5–2 are replaced by electronic switching, contained in the block labeled *control function.* This switching controls the block directly below, labeled *analog filters.*

Because of the digital nature of the control circuitry, continuously variable adjustments, such as high-pass and low-pass frequency response adjustments, are replaced by stepped adjustments. The fineness of the adjustment is limited by the number of steps in the adjustment. For very fine resolution, a large number of steps can be used to approach the effect of continuous adjustment. Due to practical

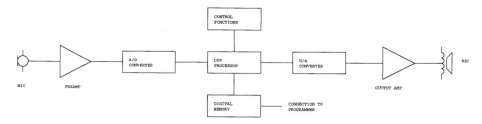

**Figure 5–14.**   Generic block diagram of a DCA hearing aid.

considerations, however, it is not cost- or user-effective to have a large number of steps in each adjustment. Adjustment steps of less than 2 dB for gain, SSPL90, and frequency response are not usually noticeable to the user. A step of 5 dB is a typical size found in programmable hearing aids.

**Programming DCA Hearing Aids**

Because the adjustments in DCA hearing aids are performed by electronic circuits, there is an electronic memory associated with the switching to remember each adjustment position to which the solid-state switches have been set.

Programming the memory in DCA hearing aids is performed by connecting the hearing aid to a computer, or to one of several proprietary programming devices. The programming device may be specific to one particular manufacturer or it may be what is often misleadingly called a *universal* programmer that can program several different models and/or brands of hearing aids from many manufacturers (Bisgaard, Christiansen, and Morison, 1993). As of this writing, there is no truly universal programmer that can program *every* programmable hearing aid, even though standardization efforts are under way. This incompatibility is primarily a result of philosophical and marketing disagreements among manufacturers, rather than the result of technological limitations.

Programmability in a DCA hearing aid implies the ability to change all the adjustable functions of a hearing aid. The comparable functions in a linear hearing aid are frequency response, overall gain, and maximum SSPL90. For a compression hearing aid, all the compression functions may be adjustable, including compression ratio, compression threshold, and compression release time. In addition, in a multiband compression hearing aid, adjustments might include crossover frequency (or frequencies) between bands, and the compression ratio and threshold in each band. Other programmable functions may include the hearing aid on-off control, a sleep circuit for reducing battery drain when the hearing aid does not have an input signal to amplify, and various options for use with the telephone. Because of this enhanced flexibility, programmers for DCA hearing aids have been nicknamed *electronic screwdrivers*.

**Programmable Adjustments**

In the context of hearing aid adjustments, the benefits of a programmable hearing aid fall into four broad categories: (1) an expanded number of switches and potentiometer adjustments, as compared to a conventional hearing aid; (2) master hearing aid; (3) multiple memories to fit different environments with a single hearing aid; and (4) remote control of hearing aid parameters.

Specific brands and models of programmable hearings aids may fall into more than one of these categories at the same time. For example, a programmable hearing aid may include remote control and have an expanded number of adjustments in the same hearing aid. Another brand or model may combine an expanded number of adjustments and multiple memories. Yet another model may combine all these categories.

## EXPANDED NUMBER OF ADJUSTMENTS

One of the primary benefits of a programmable hearing aid is that it provides the audiologist access to all the fitting parameters in the hearing aid, even if there is not enough space for potentiometer adjustments. This is a benefit for ITE and ITC hearing instruments, which are severely limited by available space on the faceplate.

An additional advantage is that, if after a trial period in the user's own environment the fitting is not optimum, it is easy to reprogram the electroacoustic characteristics of the hearing aid to fine tune the desired parameters.

Secondly, adjustments may be available on some models of DCA hearing aid that are not adjustable on conventional hearing aids. For example, the full flexibility and adjustability of multichannel amplification cannot be conveniently utilized except with programmable hearing aids.

## MASTER HEARING AID

The ability to rapidly and easily change all the potentiometer and switch settings on a DCA hearing aid offers the audiologist significant flexibility in fittings, and allows rapid evaluation of precise adjustments through comparison and forced-choice fitting strategies (Agnew, 1991). An additional advantage is that the wearer is making these choices with the exact hearing aid circuit and physical configuration that he or she will wear in their own listening situations.

## MULTIPLE MEMORIES

As mentioned at the beginning of this chapter, there is no single frequency response that is useful for all listening situations. The goal of any hearing aid fitting is to optimize communication. Though, typically, this involves speech communication, most hearing aid wearers are exposed to a variety of different listening situations. These may include listening to music and numerous ambient environmental sounds. All of these listening environments should be optimized to satisfy the user. The use of a multimemory programmable hearing aid may be one way to accomplish this goal.

Because programmable hearing aids contain electronic memory, it is easy to expand the amount of memory in the circuit to give the hearing aid the capability of storing settings for several different listening situations. The hearing aid may contain a switch or other method to choose between these memory settings.

Programmable hearing aids are commonly available that have two or three switchable memories. One has eight memories (Schnier, 1989).

Typically, the primary setting is used to store the target prescription used for normal speech communication. There are several choices for a secondary memory setting. For users who regularly listen in noisy situations, such as restaurants, it may be desirable to reduce low frequency gain and increase high frequency gain in an attempt to improve consonant recognition.

Some listeners may prefer more low-frequency gain when listening to music. Thus, an alternate secondary setting might be increase low-frequency gain by 5 or 10 dB. Other listening situations that may be optimized are communicating in a car, group meetings, church (reverberant) settings, or operating machinery. In addition to changing frequency response, the stored settings might also involve changes in SSPL90, overall gain, or changes to the compression parameters.

A common setting for the third memory is an acoustic telephone setting. For this setting, it may be useful to limit the upper end of the bandwidth to 3000 Hz to mimic the frequency response of a telephone. It may also be desirable to reduce overall gain to prevent acoustic feedback.

REMOTE CONTROL

The remote control function of programmable hearing aids can be divided into two functions that serve different purposes. One function is that the remote control may perform functions such as change the overall gain, turn the hearing aid on and off, and alter the frequency response for different environments. The other function is that the remote control may be used to switch between different memories of a multimemory DCA hearing aid, with each memory set to optimize the electroacoustic characteristics for a different listening situation. Alternatively, the remote control may also function as a combination for both of the above.

## Digital Hearing Aids

Up to this point, this chapter has described hearing aid circuits using *analog* signal paths. That is to say, circuits that process the signal through the hearing aid in a continuous fashion in the time domain. Potentiometer and switch adjustments change the circuitry to change the electroacoustic characteristics of the hearing aid. To do this, it is necessary to change a resistor value, change a potentiometer setting, open or close a switch, or make some other electronic change to these circuits to adjust their functions.

Even though digitally controlled analog circuits contain digital logic for switching functions, they process the signal in analog form. To make changes in the acoustics of the circuit, the programming in DCA hearing aid circuitry opens and closes electronic switches within the integrated circuit amplifier.

There is a limit to the amount of changes and the range of the changes that can be made in analog circuits. Even though programmable hearing aids offer the most adjustability and flexibility in current state-of-the-art hearing aids, they still use analog circuit concepts that have existed for many years. The next major change in hearing aid adjustment technology will come with the arrival of practical general-purpose *digital signal processing* circuitry in an ear-level hearing aid.

The recommended HIA terminology for hearing aids that use digital circuitry for both the signal processing and the controlling functions is a *digital signal processing (DSP)* hearing aid (Conger, 1990).

The electroacoustic characteristics of conventional analog and programmable circuits are changed by altering values of capacitors and resistors. The electroacoustic characteristics of DSP circuits are changed by altering mathematical *algorithms,* or series of computer instructions, that control the digital signal processing circuitry. Viewed simplistically, a DSP hearing aid consists of a subminiature computer inside a hearing aid case. By using the basic mathematical functions of delay, sum, and multiply, very sophisticated signal processing functions can be performed.

The description of digital hearing aids in this section, like previous sections, will be limited to a discussion of hearing aid adjustments as related to switches and potentiometers.

Digital hearing aids consist of two major components: (1) *hardware,* or the physical hearing aid itself; (2) *software,* or the instruction set stored inside the hearing aid that tells the hardware how to perform.

### Hardware

Figure 5–15 illustrates the basic block diagram of a DSP hearing aid. This diagram has no potentiometers or switch adjustments. All of the changes in frequency response shaping and other signal conditioning takes place inside the DSP block. The reader should compare Figure 5–15 with Figure 5–2 and Figure 5–14, which are block diagrams for conventional and programmable hearing aids, respectively.

To translate the analog signal received by the microphone in a usable form that the DSP can understand, it is necessary to convert the analog signal from the microphone into a string of binary codes, consisting of 1s and 0s. This is the function of the *analog-to-digital (A/D)* converter. When the DSP has performed its

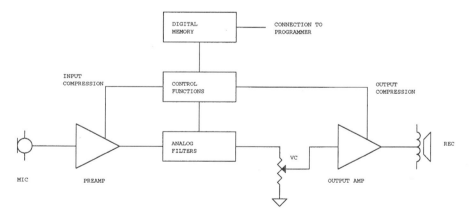

**Figure 5–15.**   Generic block diagram of a DSP hearing aid.

mathematical tasks, the signal is reconverted to the analog domain by an inverse process called *digital-to-analog (D/A)* conversion.

Further detailed information on digital hearing aid circuitry may be found in Staab (1985), Levitt (1987), Hecox and Punch (1988), and Agnew (1991).

## Software

The major hardware component of a DSP hearing aid is the *digital processor*. Software is the set of instructions stored inside the hearing aid that tell the digital processor how to process the signal. In some hearing aids, these instructions are loaded into the hearing aid memory from an external *programmer*, often based on a personal computer (PC). Multiple instruction sets, each one containing processing for a particular environment, may be stored and may be selected by the user (often via a switch or push-button), depending on the listening situation.

DSP hearing aids can perform precisely the same functions as analog filters or compression circuits. Thus, a DSP hearing aid could be built that is indistinguishable to the user from today's analog hearing aids. In this way, hardware could be built as one universal circuit and then individually programmed to account for all the fitting variations that are required for different patients. However, the real power of digital signal processing is that by manipulating the calculations inside the DSP processor, variations in the circuit can be made that are not possible in conventional analog hearing aids. These adjustments may include formant enhancement, improved spectral contrast, alteration of consonant–vowel ratios, and manipulation of the time domain. Sophisticated signal processing schemes can be customized for individuals to perform any conceivable processing of the signal in either the time, amplitude, or frequency domain. Further information on signal processing algorithms for hearing aids may be found in Lim (1982), Williamson (1986), Preves (1990), Williamson and Punch (1990), and Murray and Hanson (1992).

## Problems With Digital Technology

The potential future power of DSP hearing aids is very great. However, in reality, severe technical limitations have so far prevented practical implementation of generalized DSP functions in ear-level hearing aids.

The limitations of technology are primarily related to power and size (Nielsen, 1986; Agnew, 1991). General-purpose DSP circuits are currently available; however, even so-called "low-power" off-the-shelf circuits operate at a minimum of 3 volts and may require a supply current of up to 150 milliamps. This is several orders of magnitude above the 1.2 volt supply and 1.0 milliamp current drain available from a #13 zinc-air battery.

The problem of size is strictly one of placing all the necessary processing power and support circuitry into the small space available inside BTE or ITE hearing aids. Off-the-shelf DSP circuits are not available that will fit the subminiature requirements of current advanced hearing aid packaging.

Though these are currently real and practical problems in successfully achieving DSP technology in hearing aids, these problems will diminish as end users of technology push progress towards lower voltages and lower power dissipation.

As a step towards this future, 3 digital hearing aid circuits have already made their appearance. The first wearable DSP hearing aid was announced in 1983, but was not pursued into production (Nunley, Staub, Steadman, Wechsler, and Spencer, 1983). The second was the Phoenix, which used a body-style case containing the DSP processing attached via wires to a BTE hearing aid case that contained ear-level transducers (Vekovius and Mendoza, 1989; Sandlin, 1994). This unit is no longer available. The third example is the Genius, a BTE unit containing limited signal processing intended primarily to reduce acoustic feedback (Smriga, 1993).

Although conventional hearing aids, with switches and potentiometers, and programmable hearing aids, with computer-controlled adjustability, will continue to dominate hearing aid hardware for some years to come, the future of adjustability in hearing aids is digital signal processing. As a better fundamental understanding of the functioning of the impaired hearing mechanism is gained and, as advanced hearing aid fitting algorithms are developed, the flexibility of DSP will allow truly customized and optimized fittings for the user. Instead of a mechanical screwdriver for conventional hearing aids, or an electronic screwdriver for programmable hearing aids, the hearing aids of the future will use a computer to determine the optimum fitting parameters and processing type, and then program the hearing aid. One such early fitting system has been described by Popelka and Engebretson (1983). The emerging flexibility of such systems and hearing aids heralds the truly adjustable fittings of the future.

## *References*

Agnew J. (1991). Advanced digital signal processing schemes for ITEs. *Hear Instrum* 42(9):13–14, 16–17.

Agnew J. (1992). Advances in programmable canal hearing instrument technology. *Hear Instrum* 43(1):18–20.

Agnew J. (1993). Application of a notch filter to reduce acoustic feedback. *Hear J* 46(3):37–40, 42–43.

American National Standards Institute (ANSI). (1987). Specification of Hearing Aid Characteristics. ANSI S3.22-1987. New York: Acoustical Society of America.

ASHA Forum. (1993). Telecoils: Past, present & future. *Hear Instrum* 44(2):22–23, 26–27, 40.

Berkey DA, Marion MW, Robinson ME, Van Vliet DD (eds). (1992). New Technology: Programmable hearing aids. *Semin Hear* 13(2):105–192.

Bisgaard N, Christiansen C, Morrison P. (1993). A universal interface for programmable hearing instruments. *Hear Instrum* 44(1):14, 16–17.

Braida LD, Durlach NI, Lippmann RP, Hicks BL, Rabinowitz WM, Reed CM. (1979). *Hearing Aids—A Review of Past Research on Linear Amplification, Amplitude Compression, and Frequency Lowering. ASHA Monographs Number 19.* Rockville, MD: American Speech-Language-Hearing Association.

Brander R, Briskey R. (1988). The design of an adjustable behind-the-ear hearing instrument. *Hear Instrum* 39(4):27–28.

Bunker EJ. (1982). The loop: A boon to the hearing impaired. *Hear Instrum* 33(1):10–11.

Byrne D, Dillon H. (1986). The National Acoustics Laboratories' (NAL) new procedure for selecting the gain and frequency response of a hearing aid. *Ear Hear* 7:257–265.

Compton CL. (1994). Providing effective telecoil performance with in-the-ear hearing instruments. *Hear J* 47(4):23–26, 28–29, 32–33.

Conger C. (1990). Understanding digital technology in hearing instruments. *Hear Instrum* 41(3):21–22.

Cranmer-Briskey KS. (1992). The ADA spells urgency for telecoil use. *Hear Instrum* 43(8):8, 12.

Dillon H, Walker G. (1983). Compression—Input or output control? *Hear Instrum* 34(9):20, 22, 42.

Gilmore RA, Lederman N. (1989). Induction loop assistive listening systems. Back to the future? *Hear Instrum* 40(3):14, 16, 18, 20.

Gladstone VS. (1985). Variables affecting hearing aid telephone induction coil performance. *Hear Instrum* 36(9):18–19.

Gold S, Phipps-Davis A. (1990). Volume control taper characteristics of BTE hearing instruments. *Hear Instrum* 41(9):23–24, 26–27.

Hahn SB, Thorpe L, Fitch A. (1993). Digital cordless telephones and hearing aids: compatibility issues. *Vibrations* Spring:14–18.

Hawkins DB, Naidoo SV. (1993). Comparison of sound quality and clarity with asymmetrical peak clipping and output limiting compression. *J Am Acad Audiol* 4:221–228.

Hecox KE, Punch JL. (1988). The impact of digital technology on the selection and fitting of hearing aids. *Am J Otolaryngol (Suppl)* 9:77–85.

Herbst G. (1983). Hearing aid control systems—How do they work? *Hear Instrum* 34(9):9–10, 12, 14.

Hogg DC. (1976). Putting compression into perspective. *Hear Aid J* 29(5):11, 36–39.

Joyner KH, Wood M, Burwood E, Allison D, Le Strange. (1993). *Interference to Hearing Aids by the New Digital Mobile Telephone System, Global System for Mobile (GSM) Communication Standard.* Sydney: National Acoustic Laboratories.

Kates JM. (1986). Signal processing for hearing aids. *Hear Instrum* 37(2):19–20, 22.

Krutt JM. (1986). Direct audio input: An opportunity for hearing aid wearers in adverse-listening situations. *Hear J* 39(7):12–14.

Leavitt RJ, Hodgson WR. (1984). An effective home FM induction loop system. *Hear Instrum* 35(7):14–15, 47.

Leidy GA. (1984). Client volume-control adjustment: When, where, how often? *Hear J* 37(2):26–27, 30–32.

Levitt H. (1987). Digital hearing aids: A tutorial review. *J Rehab Res Dev* 24(4):7–20.

Libby ER, Sweetow R. (1987). Fitting the environment—Some evolutionary approaches. *Hear Instrum* 38(8):8–16.

Licklider JCR. (1946). Effects of amplitude distortion upon the intelligibility of speech. *J Acous Soc Am* 18(2):429–434.

Lim JS. (1982). Signal processing for speech enhancement. In: Studebaker GA, Bess FH, eds. *The Vanderbilt Hearing Aid Report.* Upper Darby, PA: Monographs in Contemporary Audiology, pp. 124–129.

Marutake Y, Fukutome T, Inaba Y. (1983). Flat loop system group hearing aid. *Hear Instrum* 34(3):28, 30.

McCandless GA, Lyregaard PE. (1983). Prescription of gain/output (POGO) for hearing aids. *Hear Instrum* 34(1):16–17, 19–21.

Murray DJ, Hanson JV. (1992). Application of digital signal processing to hearing aids: A critical survey. *J Am Acad Audiol* 3:145–152.

Nielsen B. (1986). Digital hearing aids: Where are they? *Hear Instrum* 37(2):6, 45.

Nunley J, Staab W, Steadman J, Wechsler P, Spencer B. (1983). A wearable digital hearing aid. *Hear J* 36(10):29–31, 34–35.

Pascoe DP. (1975). Frequency responses of hearing aids and their effects on the speech perception of hearing-impaired subjects. *Ann Otol Rhinol Laryngol (Suppl)* 23:84.

Pimental, RG. (1980). Alternative hearing systems for the mainstreamed classroom. *Hear Instrum* 31(6):8–9, 37.

Pimental RG. (1984). Direct audio input: A new communications system for the hearing impaired. *Hear Instrum* 35(7):20, 22, 24.

Popelka GR, Engebretson AM. (1983). A computer-based system for hearing assessment. *Hear Instrum* 34(7):6–7, 9, 44.

Powers TA, Sacca D. (1983). Circuit modification for feedback reduction in ITE instruments. *Hear Instrum* 34(4):40.

Premanand V, McLinn J. (1984). Automation: resistive element processing for use in hearing aid potentiometers and trimmers. *Hear Instrum* 35(2):23–24.

Preves, DA. (1990). Approaches to noise reduction in analog, digital and hybrid hearing aids. *Semin Hear* 11(1):39–67.

Preves DA. (1993). Flexibility in frequency response shaping and signal processing with analog hearing aids. *Am J Audiol* July:29–40.

Preves DA, Sigelman JA, LeMay PR. (1986). A feedback stabilizing circuit for hearing aids. *Hear Instrum* 37(4):34, 36–41, 51.

Revit LJ. (1992). Two techniques for dealing with the occlusion effect. *Hear Instrum* 43(12):16–18.

Rodriguez GP, Holmes AE, Gerhardt, KJ. (1985). Microphone versus telecoil performance characteristics. *Hear Instrum* 36(9):22–24.

Ross M. (1982). Communication access for the hearing impaired. *Hear Instrum* 33(1):7, 9.

Sammeth CA. (1990). Current availability of digital and hybrid hearing aids. *Semin Hear* 11(1):91–99.

Sandlin RE (Ed). (1994). *Understanding Digitally Programmable Hearing Aids.* Boston: Allyn and Bacon.

Schnier WR. (1989). Practical experience with a digital/analog hybrid instrument. *Hear Instrum* 40(10):31–32.

Schweitzer HC. (1979). Tutorial paper: Principles and characteristics of automatic gain control hearing aids. *J Am Audiol Soc* 5(2):84–94.

Schweitzer HC, Causey GD. (1977). The relative importance of recovery time in compression hearing aids. *Audiology* 16:61–72.

Schweitzer C, Smith DA. (1992). Solving the "occlusion effect" electronically. *Hear Instrum* 43(6):30, 32–33.

Smith CF. (1985). Induction loop systems. *Hear Instrum* 36(2):26, 31, 36.

Smriga D. (1985a). Modern compression technology, developments and applications. Part I. *Hear J* 38(6):28–32.

Smriga D. (1985b). Modern compression technology, developments and applications. Part II. *Hear J* 38(7):13–16.

Smriga D. (1993). Digital signal processing to suppress feedback: Technology and test results. *Hear J* 46(5):28–33.

Staab WJ. (1985). Digital hearing aids. *Hear Instrum* 36(11):14, 16-20, 22–24.

Staab WJ. (1990). Digital/programmable hearing aids—An eye towards the future. *Br J Audiol* 24:243–256.

Stearns WP. (1980). Enhancing speech understanding in high noise environments with adjustable aids. *Hear Instrum* 31(10):36, 38–40.

Stearns WP. (1992). Tri-frequency tuning for half-shell/canal instruments. *Hear Instrum* 43(3):30–31.

Sweetow, RW. (1990). Set screw volume controls, continued. *Hear Instrum* 41(1):27.

Teder H. (1991). Hearing instruments in noise and the syllabic speech-to-noise ratio. *Hear Instrum* 42(2):15–18.

Teder H. (1992). Reduction of high-frequency gain can help solve feedback problems. *Hear J* 45(3):28–30.

Teder H. (1993). Compression in the time domain. *Am J Audiol* July:41–46.

Vekovius GT, Mendoza L. (1989). Digital amplification: Clinical perspectives. *Hear Instrum* 40(10):23–24, 58.

Walker G, Dillon H. (1982). Compression in hearing aids: An analysis, a review and some recommendations. *National Acoustic Laboratories Report Number 90.* Australian Government Publishing Service, Canberra.

Williamson MJ. (1986). Review of noise reduction schemes. *Fourth Annual Digital Processing Symposium.* Madison, WI.

Williamson MJ, Punch JL. (1990). Speech enhancement in digital hearing aids. *Semin Hear* 11(11):68–78.

Wolf HP, Powers TA. (1986). Remote control: The invisible touch. *Hear J* 39(10):18–20.

# 6

## *Options: Earhooks, Tubing, and Earmolds*

### MICHAEL VALENTE
### MAUREEN VALENTE
### LISA G. POTTS
### EDWARD H. LYBARGER

## Introduction

The electroacoustic characteristics of a hearing aid, measured according to ANSI S3.22-1987 specifications (ANSI, 1987a) (see Chapter 1) in either HA-1 or HA-2 couplers, can be significantly altered by the manner in which the hearing aid is coupled to the ear (deJonge, 1983). As reported in Chapter 2, some alterations of the electroacoustic characteristics (i.e., from head diffraction, concha and ear canal resonances, head shadow and body baffle, residual ear canal volume, and the impedance of the eardrum and middle ear) may be unpredictable and are beyond the control of the audiologist. However, the audiologist can alter, in a fairly predictable way, the electroacoustic characteristics of the hearing aid via changes in the transmission line (i.e., earhook, tubing, and earmold), relative to the electroacoustic characteristics originally measured in the coupler.

This chapter will attempt to provide a comprehensive overview of how altering the earhook, tubing, and earmold may affect the electroacoustic characteristics of the delivered signal to the eardrum. The goal of this chapter, combined with the information presented in the other chapters, is to provide the audiologist the tools necessary to provide a hearing aid fitting which: (1) allows aided performance, in "quiet," to be significantly better than unaided performance in the same listening situation, (2) allows aided performance, in many "noisy situations," to be significantly better than unaided performance in the same listening situation. However, it is important for the patient to understand that aided performance in "noise" will not be as satisfactory as aided performance in "quiet."

In addition, users should be counseled that some listening situations may be so adverse that they probably would perform better (or at least find it less annoying) without using the hearing aids, (3) allows soft speech to be soft, but audible, average speech to be comfortable, and loud speech to be loud, but not uncomfortably loud, (4) provides excellent sound quality and good intelligibility of speech, (5) is relatively distortion free (10% or less) at high input levels, (6) is free of feedback throughout the useable range of the volume control wheel, (7) preserves the balance between the low and high and frequency regions of the average speech spectrum, (8) when appropriate, extends the high frequency range of the hearing aid, (9) when appropriate, minimizes excessive gain at around 1500 Hz, (10) when appropriate, maintains a gently rising frequency response, (11) creates a comfortably fitting earmold or shell, and (12) eliminates the sensation that the patient's head is "at the bottom of the barrel."

As mentioned earlier, the primary goal of this chapter is to provide a comprehensive overview of the transmission line from the earhook to the earmold. Because little has changed over the years regarding the acoustics of the transmission line, the authors do not feel it necessary to "rewrite" this information. If the reader is interested in this area, he should consult the excellent works of Cox (1979), Egolf (1979a, 1979b, 1980), Lybarger (1979, 1980), Mynders (1985), Leavitt (1986), and Staab and Lybarger (1994).

## *Dimensions of the Typical Transmission Line*

The tubing from the receiver encased in the behind-the-ear (BTE), in-the-ear (ITE), or in-the-canal (ITC) hearing aid is typically 8 to 15 mm long and has an internal diameter (ID) of 0.5 to 1.5 mm wide (Cox, 1979; Killion, 1982). The sound bore of the earhook is typically 20 to 30 mm long and 1.2 to 1.8 mm wide (Cox, 1979; Killion, 1982). The tubing from the earhook to the tip of earmold is usually 40 to 45 mm long and 1.93 mm wide (Cox, 1979; Killion, 1982). This latter dimension should be compared to the ANSI S3.22-1989 standard that requires 25 mm of 1.93 mm tubing connected to an HA-2 coupler, which is designed to simulate the average earmold with a bore length of 18 mm and ID of 3 mm. Thus, the transmission line of a typical BTE is approximately 75 mm long. In an eyeglass fitting, the transmission line is about 20 to 30 mm shorter, due to the absence of an earhook (Staab and Lybarger, 1994). Finally, the dimensions of the typical ear canal from the earmold tip to the eardrum is 13 to 15 mm long and 7.5 mm wide (Cox, 1979; Killion, 1982). Figure 6–1 (Valente, 1984c) provides a schematic drawing of the typical dimensions of the transmission line from the tubing to the eardrum.

## *Earhook*

### Introduction

The earhook is a semirigid acoustic connector used to retain the hearing aid over the ear and to conduct sound to tubing that is connected to the earhook. Earhooks are available in a variety of shapes (1/4 and 1/2 moon) and materials.

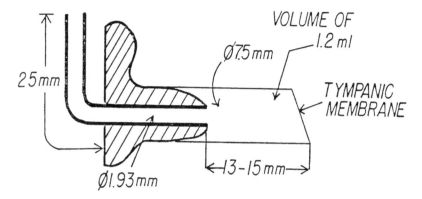

**Figure 6–1.**  Schematic drawing of an earmold coupled to the ear canal.

The bore diameter of the earhook usually tapers at the tubing end, although some earhooks have minimal tapering (i.e., 2.25 mm at the start and 1.83 mm at the end). Cox (1979) compared the output of a hearing aid-earmold system with a variety of earhooks ranging in length from 20 to 30 mm and with constant diameters of 1.2 to 1.5 mm. She reported 1 to 2 dB greater high frequency output when using the shorter and wider earhooks.

Some earhooks are delivered with dampers, and others allow the audiologist to add or change the damper. Some earhooks are threaded, and others are of the snap-on type. ANSI S3.37-1987 (ANSI, 1987b) specifies a preferred earhook nozzle thread (5-40 UNC-2A; modified and unmodified) to reduce the number of different earhook styles currently stocked by audiologists in their clinics for replacing damaged earhooks.

### Tubing Resonances

As stated earlier, one of the goals for providing a successful fitting is delivering a smooth and gently rising frequency response to the eardrum of the listener. Unfortunately, many hearing aids provide a frequency response that is characterized by numerous sharp resonant peaks that can hamper a successful hearing aid fitting.

As mentioned earlier, the typical length of the transmission line from the receiver to the tip of the earmold is approximately 75 mm, with an ID ranging from 1.0 to 1.93 mm. In a tube open at both ends, a length of 75 mm and diameter of 1.93 mm will produce 1/2 wave resonances at approximately 2300, 4600, and 6900 Hz (Cox, 1979). Half wave resonances will occur at frequencies that are two times the effective length of the tubing. In a hearing aid fitting, the tube is closed at the receiver end with relatively low acoustic impedance in the ear canal and eardrum. The presence of the closed tube and the impedance mismatch will create a 1/4 wave resonance where the wavelength of the incoming signal is four times the effective length of the tube. Additional resonances will occur at odd-number intervals of this fundamental frequency. Thus, for a 75-mm effective length tube closed at both ends, a 1/4 wave resonance will produce resonances between 1000 to 10,000 Hz at approximately 1100, 3300, and 5500 Hz (Walker, 1979). Figure 6–2 (Valente, 1984c) illustrates the presence of these resonances for a BTE hearing aid when damping was not placed in the earhook (solid line).

### Damping

FUSED MESH DAMPERS

To reduce the sharp resonant peaks in the frequency response to achieve a smooth and gently rising frequency response, several types of damping materials have been introduced in the past. The use of damping allows the user to increase the volume control setting with less probability of feedback and, thus, achieve greater useable gain and output. In addition, the reduction of gain at 1000 Hz will reportedly reduce the upward spread of masking and improve word recognition in noise.

These peaks are undesirable because they reportedly degrade sound quality, introduce transients, and allow the output to exceed the listener's loudness discomfort level. Knowles Electronics introduced fused mesh dampers to reduce the gain and output to acceptable levels and smooth the frequency response (Gastmeirer, 1981; Killion, 1982, 1988a). The fused mesh damper is a finely woven plastic screen held in place by a stainless steel screen and encased in a

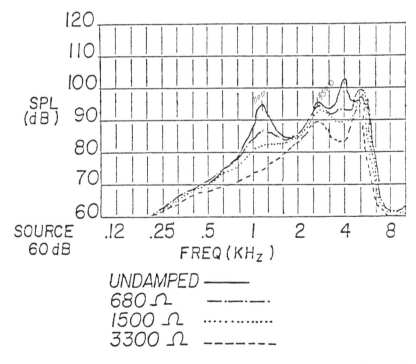

**Figure 6–2.** Frequency responses of a hearing aid with an undamped and damped earhook. For the damped conditions, a 680, 1500, and 3300 ohm fused mesh damper was placed at the earhook.

2.5 mm long and 2.0 mm wide metal ferrule. The fused mesh damper provides a pure acoustic resistance and negligible reactance and, therefore, does not attenuate the high-frequency region of the frequency response; this was one of the problems with previous materials used for damping. They were originally designed to fit snugly inside #13 tubing which has an ID of 1.93 mm. These dampers are available in five discrete resistances of 680, 1500, 2200, 3300, and 4700 ohms, which are color coded as white, green, red, orange, and yellow, respectively. These dampers allow greater high frequency output and a smoother frequency response. Figure 6–2 (Valente, 1984c) illustrates the smoothing of the frequency response and increased low frequency attenuation by adding 680, 1500, or 3300 ohm dampers to the earhook. From Figure 6–2 it can also be seen that the 3300 ohm damper decreased output at 4000 Hz, which may be considered undesirable.

Currently, inserting the damper at the tip of the earhook is the most common position. Inserting the damper further along the transmission line will increase its ability to dampen the peaks, but will increase the probability of the damper becoming clogged with moisture and/or debris.

The effectiveness of dampers is determined by the density (i.e., resistance in acoustic ohms) of the material and the number and location of the damper(s). Killion (1988a) reported using two fused mesh dampers (one at the tip of the earhook and another at the threaded end) to reduce the gain and output by approximately 15 dB and provide a smoother frequency response. As a cautionary note, if resonances do not appear when electroacoustically analyzing a BTE hearing aid, the manufacturer has probably provided damping; inserting additional dampers will further reduce the gain and output of the hearing aid.

Briskey (1982) reported that a 680-ohm damper reduces average full-on gain and SSPL90 by 3 dB, while the remaining four dampers reduce the gain and output by 4, 5, 6, and 9 dB, respectively.

Libby (1979) and Teder (1979) reported that by reducing the peak in the frequency response, the audiologist can increase the "headroom" (i.e., output) of the aid and expand the range of linear amplification. Further, Teder (1979) reported that a peak in the SSPL curve can cause a "volume expansion effect" when high intensity sounds occur at the peak frequency (i.e., dishes clattering, automobile horns, and typewriters). These sounds are then limited by the output, but are higher in intensity than the remainder of the output curve, which is relatively flat.

One of the disadvantages of using dampers, as reported by Chasin (1983a), is that dampers can easily become plugged with moisture and/or debris. Thus, dampers usually need to be changed often and the patient must be counseled regarding this problem and informed of the steps necessary to follow when the aid does not appear to be functioning properly.

OTHER DAMPING MATERIALS

1. LAMB'S WOOL: This is the earliest damping material. It is usually placed in the earhook or tubing and is typically used on a trial-and-error basis. It is an effective and inexpensive method of damping, but the effect can be very unpredictable.

2. SINTERED STEEL PELLETS: These are small cylinders of stainless steel, welded together in such a manner that their specified resistance in acoustic ohms offers specific amounts of attenuation (Goldstein, 1980; Mynders, 1985). In our clinic, we use sintered filters, which are available in different colors and provide progressively greater degrees of attenuation at 1000 Hz (orange = 3 dB; green = 6 dB; brown = 9 dB; yellow = 12 dB; grey = 15 dB; and red = 18 dB). The greatest attenuation occurs at 500 to 1000 Hz and, as the sintered filter is placed further down the transmission line, it provides greater attenuation.

3. STAR DAMPER: This is a flexible silicone material that is usually placed in the earhook and does not permit moisture buildup because its design allows drainage of moisture. This damper provides some gain at 2700 Hz to compensate for the loss of the ear canal resonance. The star damper must be cut to different lengths and electroacoustic measures made to assure that the desired effect has been achieved.

4. DAMPERS IN CUSTOM HEARING AIDS: A variety of dampers are now available in custom hearing aids, which reduce the peak around 2000 Hz. These include, from one manufacturer, a white damper that reduces the output by 3 to 5 dB; a green damper, which reduces the output by 7 to 8 dB, and a red damper, which reduces the output by 10 dB.

### Dampers: Effect Upon Speech Intelligibility and Clarity

As mentioned earlier, research has suggested that improved speech intelligibility, greater clarity of speech, and increased user satisfaction will result when using dampers. However, Decker (1975) reported no significant differences in word recognition scores (W-22) for 10 subjects who listened to the monosyllabic words using broadband and high-frequency emphasis hearing aids with and without the insertion of sintered filters.

Cox and Gilmore (1986) reported that damping could improve speech intelligibility and/or sound quality by reducing the effects of the upward spread of masking. Suppression of the peaks by damping should reduce these effects and improve the overall fidelity of amplification. They utilized 10 subjects with sensorineural hearing loss, who evaluated 1-1/2 minutes of male-connected discourse embedded in multitalker babble presented at 55 and 70 dB Leq using a paired comparison paradigm. In general, they reported that damping the frequency response did not provide improved clarity of speech or a more advantageous preferred listening level. However, they reported that reducing resonant peaks by damping could be useful in reducing feedback.

### Special Purpose Earhooks

Killion, Berlin, and Hood (1984), Killion and Wilson (1985), and Killion (1988c) introduced four special oversized earhooks using open canal fittings or closed earmolds to provide solutions for four hard-to-fit hearing losses (see Fig. 6-3). However, for these earhooks to be useful, they must be coupled to hearing aids using threaded earhooks. Each earhook costs approximately $25, or five may be purchased for $110. These special earhooks include the:

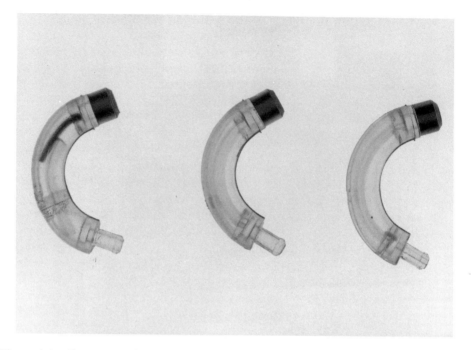

**Figure 6–3.**    Etymotic earhooks. Left: ER12-1; middle: ER12-2; right: ER12-3.

1.  ER12-1 (Low-Pass or K-Bass): was designed for patients with normal hearing at 2000 to 3000 Hz and hearing loss up to 40 to 65 dB at 250 to 1000 Hz. In the high-frequency region, the patient should have hearing thresholds of 0 to 25 dB at 4000 Hz and 0 to 60 dB at 8000 Hz (Killion et al., 1984; Killion and Wilson, 1985). This earhook can be coupled to the ear canal using Lybarger's 1.5 LP open canal reverse horn tube fitting (Lybarger, 1980), which is comprised of #15 tubing coupled to 12 mm of #20 tubing having an ID of 0.86 mm and extending into the ear canal by at least 16 mm. An alternative tube fitting (Janssen free field) is #13 tubing and an 18 mm insert of #18 tubing. These tube fittings reduce the gain in the midfrequency region by 10 to 15 dB and shift the first resonant peak at 1000 Hz downward to 500 Hz. The ER12-1 is identified with a silver band with one red stripe at one end that screws onto the hearing aid and has a clear disk in the middle of the earhook (left earhook in Fig. 6–3). The ER12-1 should be used with power aids having adequate low frequency gain and a maximum SSPL90 of 130 dB. Killion and Wilson (1985) reported a 76% acceptance rate in 68 fittings.

2.  ER12-2 (2 kHz Notch Filter): this is identified by a silver band with two red stripes and has no clear center disk (middle earhook in Fig. 6–3) (Killion and Wilson, 1985). This earhook is used with a conventional earmold and is used for patients with normal or near normal hearing at 2000 Hz (10 to 40 dB HL) with hearing loss up to 40 to 60 dB at 500 to 1000 Hz and 3000 to 4000 Hz. The ER12-2 reduces the gain by 20 dB at 2000 Hz. It produces an acoustic signal that is very similar to the Macrae 2 k notch-filter earmold (Macrae, 1981, 1983) which will be discussed in a later section.

3. ER12-3 (High Pass): can be identified with gold band having three red stripes and a small barb at the end (right earhook in Fig. 6–3) (Killion and Wilson, 1985). This earhook is designed to be used with Lybarger's nonoccluding dual diameter earmold (see Fig. 6–4), which uses tubing with an ID of 0.8 mm coupled to 15 mm of #13 tubing that should be inserted minimally to obtain maximum high frequency gain before feedback (i.e., insertion of only 4 to 8 mm). This configuration changes a wideband aid hearing aid into a high-pass aid with reduced output below 3000 Hz, to eliminate excessive gain in the frequency region where the patient may have normal hearing. This combination also provides 12 dB of additional gain at 4000 to 7000 Hz. The ER12-3 is designed for patients who have hearing thresholds of 25 to 35 dB at 500 to 2000 Hz and 50 to 90 dB HL at 4000 to 8000 Hz.

4. ER12-4 (Cookie Bite): is the opposite of the ER12-2 and is designed to be used with patients with reduced hearing at 2000 Hz and better hearing in the frequency regions above and below 2000 Hz. This earhook is used with an open earmold with 1/32 inch tubing coupled to a Lybarger high-pass eartube. It has a silver band on one end that screws onto the hearing aid and has no disk in the center of the earhook.

Finally, Bergenstoff (1983) introduced the "E-Hook" in which a wedge-shaped filter is placed in the earhook. Also, an acoustic resistance element is permanently mounted inside the tubing end of the earhook. Using #13 tubing from the end of the earhook to the tip of the earmold, a very smooth real ear insertion response (REIR) can be obtained when coupled to a hearing aid having a wideband receiver.

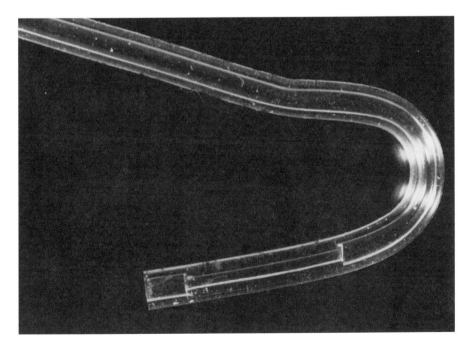

**Figure 6–4.**   Example of a Lybarger high-pass eartube.

## Tubing

### NAEL SIZES

Table 6–1 reports the numerical system used by the National Association of Earmold Laboratories (NAEL) to identify the various tubing sizes. As can be seen, as the number increases, the ID decreases. For example, #9 tubing has an ID of 2.4 mm, while #13 tubing has an ID of 1.93 mm. The outside diameter (OD) can be thin, standard, medium, thick, or double walled. The thick and double-walled tubing are often used for power BTEs to reduce the probability of feedback and vibration.

### TUBING STYLE

Tubing can be ordered as bulk, preformed, quilled, single bend, double bend, or triple bend. Tubing can also be ordered as clear or tinted or with a cut-tapered end for easier insertion into the earmold sound bore. Tubing is also available as a "dri-tube." This type of tubing is made from a more dense and more rubbery material that is reported to eliminate or reduce condensation and is available in the 3 or 4-mm horn, #13 medium, and thick walled.

### TUBING ADAPTORS

Several variations of adaptors are available to connect to tubing. For example, male and female adaptors (large and miniature sizes) are available to be used with receiver-type earmolds. These fit onto the tubing to allow direct snap-in connectors to the receiver earmold. In addition, elbows made of hard vinyl with gradual or sharp right angle bends can be ordered that are threaded or cemented into a hole in a lucite earmold for easier changing of tubing. Another possibility of a tubing adaptor is the Bakke horn, which is a hard plastic, stepped-bore permanent elbow that creates an acoustic effect similar to the Libby 4-mm horn, which will be discussed in a later section.

**Table 6-1.** Inside Diameter (ID) and Outside Diameter (OD) of Tubing Sizes as Standardized by the National Association of Earmold Labs (NAEL)

| Tubing No. | ID | | | OD | |
| --- | --- | --- | --- | --- | --- |
| | *Inches* | *mm* | | *Inches* | *mm* |
| 9 | 0.094 | 2.4 | | 0.160 | 4.1 |
| 12 | 0.085 | 2.2 | | 0.125 | 3.2 |
| 13 standard | 0.076 | 1.9 | | 0.116 | 2.9 |
| 13 medium | 0.076 | 1.9 | | 0.122 | 3.2 |
| 13 thick wall | 0.076 | 1.9 | | 0.130 | 3.3 |
| 13 double wall | 0.076 | 1.9 | | 0.142 | 3.6 |
| 14 | 0.066 | 1.7 | | 0.116 | 2.9 |
| 15 | 0.059 | 1.5 | | 0.166 | 2.9 |
| 16 standard | 0.053 | 1.3 | | 0.166 | 2.9 |
| 16 thin | 0.053 | 1.3 | | 0.085 | 2.2 |

TUBING CEMENT

Generally, cementing tubing into the bore of an earmold is a relatively simple task when using hard lucite earmolds. However, for polyvinyl and other soft ear-molds, the dispenser should use "sheer" tubing cement. Another solution is to use "tube-lock," "tube-lock plus," and "tubing retention systems," that have recently been introduced. These use a small 14-carat gold-coated brass ring containing a small flange. It is assembled and permanently affixed by the earmold laboratory. Using this system, the tubing can never be loosened or pulled out. It is available in two sizes (regular and double walled), and requires a special tool for insertion and removal of tube-lock. The tube-lock can be used with any size tubing and is highly recommended for materials where glue will not easily adhere. More recently, several earmold manufactures introduced a special tube lock ("EZ Tube") for the JB1000 and other soft earmolds designed for patients with severe to profound hearing loss. This is a permanently installed nozzle in the sound bore of the earmold and the audiologist can remove the old tubing from the nozzle and replace it with new tubing. Another possibility is ordering Continuous Flow Adaptor (CFA) earmolds, which will be explained in greater detail in a later section.

TUBING LENGTH

Recall that ANSI S3.22-1987 (ANSI, 1987a) requires BTE hearing aids to be elec-troacoustically analyzed using 25 mm of #13 tubing coupled to an HA-2 coupler. In reality, changing tubing length is limited because tubing length is related to anatomical dimensions of the head. However, as Figure 6–5 (Valente, 1984c)

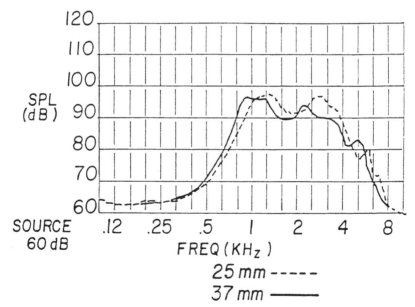

**Figure 6–5.** Frequency response of a hearing aid coupled to an HA-2 coupler with 25 mm and 37 mm of #13 tubing.

illustrates, if the length is increased (re: 25 mm), the primary resonant peak will shift downward and the output will increase in the lower frequencies and decrease in the mid and high frequencies. Also, the amplitude of the second and third peaks will be reduced (Egolf, 1980; Lybarger, 1985; Valente, 1984c). If the tubing is shortened (re: 25 mm), the primary and secondary peaks will shift upward in frequency. Also, the output will decrease in the low frequencies and increase in the mid and high frequencies. Table 6–2, Section I, summarizes the effect changing tubing length may have upon four regions of the frequency response curve.

TUBING DIAMETER

ANSI S3.22-1987 (ANSI, 1987a) also requires BTE hearing aids to be electro-acoustically analyzed using 25 mm of #13 tubing, which has an ID of 1.93 mm. Using tubing with a wider ID (#9, #11, or #12 tubing) will increase the gain between 1000 to 2000 Hz and decrease the gain in the lower frequencies. Using tubing with a narrower ID (#14 to #16 tubing) will increase the gain in the lower frequencies and decrease the gain in the higher frequencies (Lybarger, 1979, 1980, 1985; Austin, Kasten, Wilson, 1990c). Table 6–2, Section II, summarizes the effect changing tubing diameter may have upon 4 regions of the frequency response curve.

TUBING LENGTH AND DIAMETER

Changes in length and diameter are consistent with when either length or diameter is varied independently. That is, a long tube with a narrow ID will shift the frequency peaks downward. Using a short tube with a wider ID will shift the frequency peaks upward.

## Minimal Insertion of Tubing

Up to this point, the discussion has assumed that the audiologist has inserted the tubing to the tip of the earmold. Another strategy is to insert the tubing minimally into the sound bore and create a "dual tube" fitting (Lybarger, 1979, 1985; Valente, 1984b, 1984c). This strategy takes advantage of the fact that when there is a significant step-up in diameter toward the ear canal, there is a quarter wave open-end resonance in the larger bore section that exits into the ear canal. This can result in considerable high-frequency amplification above 2000 Hz.

An example of such a strategy would be inserting #13 tubing only 3 mm into the sound bore. Figure 6–6 (Valente, 1984b, 1984c) illustrates 2-cc coupler measures of a BTE hearing aid when #13 tubing was inserted 3 mm, 9 mm, and 16mm (tip) into the sound bore. Notice the improved high-frequency output when the tubing was inserted only 3 mm (solid line) into the sound bore in comparison to when the tubing was inserted to the tip (dashed line). In this case, there is 10 to 12 dB greater output at 5000 to 6000 Hz than when the tubing was cemented to the tip. Table 6–2, Section V, summarizes the effects insertion of tubing in the sound bore has upon four regions of the frequency–response curve. As a cautionary note, when using the strategy of minimal insertion of tubing into the

**Table 6-2.**    Effect of Various Modifications Upon Four Regions
of the Frequency Response

| Change | *Frequency Region (Hz)* | | | |
| | *<750* | *750–1500* | *1500–3000* | *>3000* |
| --- | --- | --- | --- | --- |
| I. Tubing length | | | | |
| Short | Slight decrease | Moves peak to higher Hz | Moves peak to higher Hz | Minimal |
| Long | Slight increase | Moves peak to lower Hz | Moves peak to lower Hz | Decrease |
| II. Tubing diameter | | | | |
| Wider | Minimal | Moves peak to higher Hz | Moves peak to higher Hz | Increase |
| Narrower | May decrease | Moves peak to lower Hz | Reduces height of Peak and moves to lower Hz | Decrease |
| III. Bore length | | | | |
| Short | Slight decrease | Moves peak to higher Hz | Moves peak to higher Hz | Increase |
| Long | Slight increase | Moves peak to lower Hz | Moves peak to lower Hz | Decrease |
| IV. Bore diameter | | | | |
| Wider | Minimal | Moves peak to higher Hz | Moves peak to higher Hz | Increase |
| Narrower | Minimal | Moves peak to lower Hz | Moves peak to lower Hz | Decrease |
| Belling | Minimal | Minimal | Minimal | Increase |
| V. Tubing insertion | | | | |
| Medial | Minimal | Minimal | Shift peak to lower Hz | Decrease |
| Lateral | Minimal | Minimal | Shift peak to higher Hz | Increase |
| VI. Venting | | | | |
| Small[1] | Minimal | Minimal | Minimal | Minimal |
| Medium[2] | Decrease | Increase peak height | Minimal | Minimal |
| Large[3] | Decrease | Increase peak height | Minimal | Minimal |
| Parallel | Less attenuation of low-frequency SPL than diagonal ventng, but no attenuation of high-frequency SPL | | | |
| Diagonal | Greater attenuation of low-frequency SPL than parallel venting, but greater attenuation of high-frequency SPL | | | |

[1] 0.8 mm.
[2] 1.6 mm.
[3] 2.4 mm.
Adapted from Microsonic, 1994

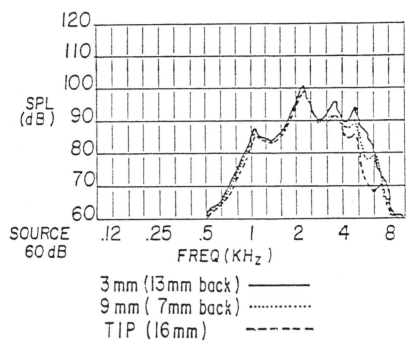

**Figure 6–6.**   Change in output when inserting #13 tubing 3 mm, 9 mm, and to the tip of an earmold when the bore length is 16 mm.

sound bore, it is very important that a high quality cement be used to anchor the tubing into the sound bore.

Figure 6–7 (Valente, 1984b, 1984c) reveals that the effect of minimal insertion of the tubing is directly related to the length of the sound bore. That is, as the bore length increases, the effect of minimal insertion becomes greater. As bore length is reduced, the advantage of this strategy is diminished. Finally, the magnitude of the effect is dependent upon the length and diameter of the second segment. The longer and wider the second segment, the greater the high-frequency boost (Valente, 1984b, 1984c).

### Open Canal Fittings

TUBE FITTING

One method of tube fitting is to use a free-field mold that is adjusted in varying lengths to create the desired change in the frequency response and then cemented in place to a nonoccluding earmold (see Fig. 6–8 middle and Fig. 6–9d). When used with a conventional BTE, this would be classified as an IROS (ipsilateral routing of the signal) fitting. Another method is using a tube fitting (Fig. 6–8 left)

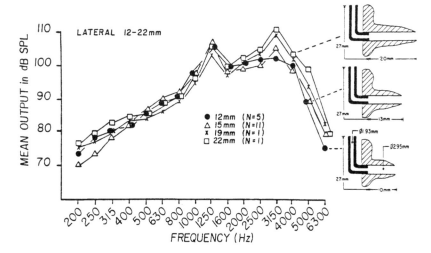

**Figure 6–7.**   Change in output when inserting #13 tubing 2 mm into the sound bore for four earmolds in which bore length is 12 mm, 15 mm, 19 mm, and 22 mm long.

in which the tubing is not cemented (Staab and Nunley, 1982). The rationale is to achieve maximum high-frequency gain without feedback, obtain maximum low-frequency attenuation (up to 30 dB at 500 Hz), and provide maximum comfort. This type of tube fitting will not occlude the ear canal, which can reduce the transmission of low-frequency sounds by as much as 15 to 30 dB, depending upon the magnitude of occlusion by the earmold. This type of tube fitting also takes advantage of the natural resonance of the ear canal, which is around 17 dB at 2800 Hz. For some patients, greater retention of a nonoccluding earmold may be necessary. A design offering the benefits of a nonoccluding earmold, but with greater retention, is illustrated in Figure 6–9c.

Tube fittings should be considered when the patient has a ski-slope audiometric configuration with hearing loss up to 50 dB above 2000 Hz. If the hearing loss

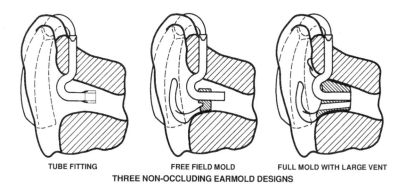

**Figure 6–8.**   Three nonoccluding earmold designs. Left: tube fitting; middle: free field; right: full mold with a large vent. (Printed with permission from Microsonic, Inc.)

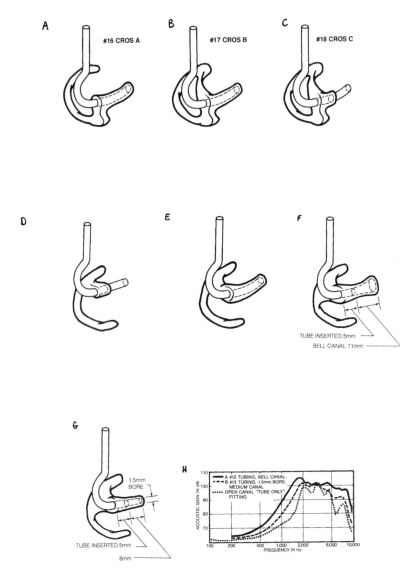

**Figure 6–9.** Examples of seven nonoccluding earmolds: (a) CROS A; (b) CROS B; (c) CROS C; (d) free field; (e) Janssen; (f) extended range earmold; (g) another extended range earmold; (h) frequency response of three nonoccluding earmolds. (Printed with permission from Microsonic, Inc.)

is greater than 50 dB, then the audiologist should not consider using a tube fitting but, instead, use a conventional earmold with some degree of venting because of acoustic feedback. Also, tube fittings can theoretically eliminate the upward spread of masking by reducing low-frequency amplification and, thus, improve word recognition. Other advantages of this type of fitting may include reduction of harmonic distortion due to minimal gain below 1000 Hz and providing improved sound quality.

A tube fitting may be considered when an earmold is contraindicated due to middle ear drainage, irritations in the ear canal, allergic reactions to earmold materials, psoriasis, eczema, and scars. It should not be used with a high-frequency emphasis hearing aid but, instead, should be used with a broadband hearing aid. Further, for tube fittings to provide adequate high-frequency gain, insertion of the tubing must be greater than 15 mm beyond the orifice of the ear canal. As the tubing is moved closer to the eardrum, the frequency response below 1500 Hz is shifted downward, producing a broader response. As the tubing is placed further away from the eardrum, there is greater low-frequency attenuation. Also, its use in smaller ear canals will produce greater high-frequency gain than in longer canals, with tubing length held constant.

To properly fit tube fittings, it is suggested that the audiologist first use #15 tubing (ID = 1.5 mm) and then try tubing with a wider ID (#9) to achieve even greater high-frequency emphasis. To achieve maximum comfort, it is necessary to properly bend the tubing to comfortably fit in the ear canal. In order to do this, it is suggested to wipe isopropyl alcohol over solid core solder wire whose outside diameter is sufficiently wide enough to fit snugly inside the tubing. The audiologist should then bend the tubing to the desired configuration and add heat via an air blower with a heat directing shield. Cool the tubing in alcohol or water to preserve the configuration and then remove the solder. At this point the tubing will maintain its shape.

TRADITIONAL CROS OPEN MOLD

Harford and Barry (1965), Harford and Dodds (1966), Green and Ross (1968), and Green (1969) introduced the CROS (see Fig. 6–9a–c) earmold for unilateral and high-frequency hearing loss. They reported that the CROS mold can improve aided word recognition scores in noise due to significant low-frequency reduction. Courtois, Johansen, Larsen, Christensen, and Beilin (1988) advocated use of CROS molds for patients with mild to moderate hearing loss to attenuate low frequencies, thereby reducing both the amplification of ambient noise and the occlusion effect. They measured the sound pressure level (SPL) in closed and open molds and found differences of 30 to 40 dB below 125 Hz, and these differences disappeared at around 2000 Hz. They also reported that a 2 mm vent reduces the occlusion effect at 250 to 500 Hz and a 3 mm vent reduces the occlusion effect to 750 Hz.

The CROS mold is similar to a parallel-vented earmold which has a vent so large that only a small piece of earmold is left to hold the tubing in place (Cox, 1979). Cox (1979) and Lybarger (1979) reported that the acoustic difference between a CROS mold and a tube fit is minimal providing the ear canal is not so small as to be occluded by the small retention portion of the open mold fitting. If retention does occlude the ear canal, a tube fitting is preferred to obtain the desired acoustic effect. The tube fitting will significantly reduce low-frequency amplification and provide some high-frequency emphasis above the vent-associated resonance. This effect is dependent upon the depth of insertion, the ID of the tubing, and the size of the ear canal. As insertion depth is closer to the eardrum, less low-frequency energy will escape but, more importantly, greater high-frequency amplification will occur. As tubing diameter is reduced, there will be an overall reduction in output and a shift of the first peak to a lower frequency. If no gain is required below 2000 Hz, the audiologist should use tubing with a narrower ID for greater user satisfaction. However, this strategy will reduce the overall SPL and provide less high-frequency gain. Low-frequency attenuation will be less for a tube fit when fitted to a small ear canal than if the ear canal is of average length.

### Libby 3 mm and 4 mm Horns

Libby designed injection-molding techniques to obtain a one-piece 3 mm and 4 mm tapered horn (see Fig. 6–10). The 4-mm design is comprised of 21 mm of #13 tubing, enlarged to 22 mm of tubing 4-mm wide. The 3-mm horn has 21 mm of #13 tubing followed by 22 mm of tubing 3 mm wide. The 3-mm horn will provide 5 to 6 dB less gain at 2500 to 3000 Hz in comparison to the 4-mm horn. Both styles are designed to work best with a 1500 ohm fused mesh damper at the tip of the earhook. Libby advocated that the stepped diameter earmold should be used with a hearing aid having a wideband receiver to obtain high fidelity sound

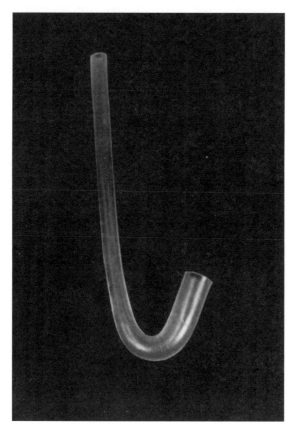

**Figure 6–10.** Example of a Libby 4-mm horn.

quality, an extended frequency response, and reduced battery drain. The first 2 rows in sections A and B in Table 6–3 report the relative changes in the output of a hearing aid produced by the Libby 3-mm and 4-mm designs relative to the output measured in an HA-1 (section A) or HA-2 coupler (section B).

Valente (1983) reported 0.9 to 8.4 dB greater mean functional gain (Fig. 6–11) using an earmold design similar to the Libby 3 mm horn in comparison to when #13 tubing was inserted to the earmold tip. For the same subjects with sensorineural hearing loss, the mean word recognition scores (NU-6) were 8.3% better in quiet and 12.1% better in noise (multitalker babble at a +6dB signal-to-noise ratio) using the Libby 3-mm horn (Fig. 6–12).

Usually, the Libby 3-mm or 4-mm horn is ordered without a vent. However, Pedersen (1984) reported that a 2-mm diagonal vent intersecting near the end of the earmold did not affect the high frequency gain provided by the 3-mm or 4-mm horn. The mean difference was less than 1 dB at 6 discrete frequencies between 250 to 4000 Hz. To reduce the likelihood of inducing the occlusion effect, the authors suggest that 3-mm and 4-mm horns be ordered with some degree of venting. The authors of this chapter routinely order Select-A-Vent (SAV) or Positive-Venting-Valve (PVV) vent "trees" for all horn fittings. The advantage of this strategy will be presented in a later section.

**Table 6–3.** Changes in Gain/Output (dB) for Several Acoustically Tuned Earmolds Relative to the Response Obtained Using an HA-2 Coupler or #13 Tubing to the Tip of the Earmold Measured in an HA-1 Coupler

| Design | 250 | 500 | 1000 | 2000 | 3000 | 4000 | 6000 |
|---|---|---|---|---|---|---|---|
| Earmold Design | | | | | | | |
| A. Re: #13 Tubing to the Tip (HA-1 Coupler) | | | | | | | |
| Libby 4 mm | –1 | –2 | –3 | –2 | –6 | 10 | 6 |
| Libby 3 mm | –1 | –2 | –2 | 0 | 6 | 8 | 2 |
| 8CR[1] | –2 | –2 | –3 | 0 | 7 | 7 | 2 |
| 6R12 | –1 | –2 | –1 | –2 | 1 | 5 | 7 |
| 6B10 | –2 | –2 | –2 | –2 | 1 | 7 | 0 |
| 6B5 | 0 | 0 | 2 | 1 | 2 | 4 | 3 |
| 6B0 | 0 | 0 | 0 | 0 | 0 | 0 | 0 |
| 6C5 | 0 | 1 | 0 | 0 | –4 | –6 | –11 |
| 6C10 | 0 | 2 | –2 | –5 | –10 | –12 | –17 |
| B. Re: 3 mm x 18 mm (HA-2 Coupler) | | | | | | | |
| Libby 4 mm | –1 | –1 | –2 | 0 | 2 | 3 | 0 |
| Libby 3 mm | 0 | 0 | 0 | 1 | 3 | 2 | –4 |
| 8CR[1] | –1 | –1 | –2 | 0 | 4 | 0 | –6 |
| 6R12 | 0 | 0 | 0 | 0 | 0 | 0 | 1 |
| 6B10 | 0 | 0 | 0 | 0 | 0 | 1 | –5 |
| 6B5 | 1 | 2 | 3 | 2 | 0 | –1 | –2 |
| 6B0 | 0 | 1 | 1 | 0 | –2 | –5 | –7 |
| 6C5 | 1 | 2 | 1 | 2 | –5 | –10 | –16 |
| 6C10 | 1 | 3 | 0 | –3 | –11 | –17 | –22 |

[1] 680 ohm damper at earhook tip; dimensions of Libby 4 mm

Dillon, 1985, 1991.

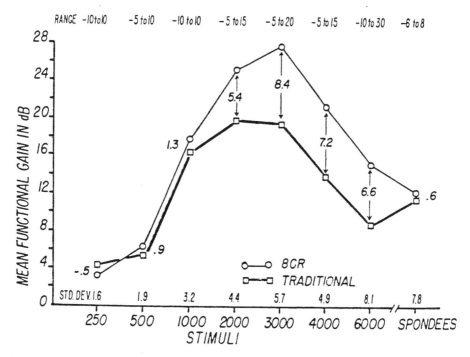

**Figure 6–11.** Mean functional gain for warble tones and spondee words utilizing conventional and 8CR earmolds. Also provided is the mean difference in warble tone thresholds between the two earmold designs, standard deviation, and range.

Burgess and Brooks (1991) reported that the sound quality from a hearing aid using the Libby horn was rated clearer, more natural, undistorted, and more acoustically comfortable when compared with an earmold where the tubing was cemented to the tip of the earmold. Objectively, real ear and functional gain measures reported greater gain (mean of 8 dB) in the higher frequencies (1,500 to 6000 Hz). They also reported improved recognition of phonemes, especially the fricatives and affricates.

Mueller, Schwartz, and Surr (1981) compared the Libby 3-mm horn to a free-field mold for 24 subjects with high-frequency sensorineural hearing loss. Functional gain measures revealed 5 to 10 dB greater functional gain at 3000 Hz with the Libby horn in comparison to the free-field earmold. However, there were no significant differences in word recognition scores or subjective ratings between the 2 earmold designs.

Robinson, Cane, and Lutman (1989) compared the performance of 21 inexperienced users with the Libby 4-mm horn and an earmold where #13 tubing was cemented to the tip of the earmold. Aided scores for speech in noise (+5 dB SNR) using CVC words were, on average, only 2.4% better with the Libby 4-mm horn. However, two thirds of the subjects preferred the sound quality of the 4-mm horn. After a 4-week trial period, the 4-mm horn was preferred by those subjects who had poorer hearing above 2000 Hz. They concluded that improved word

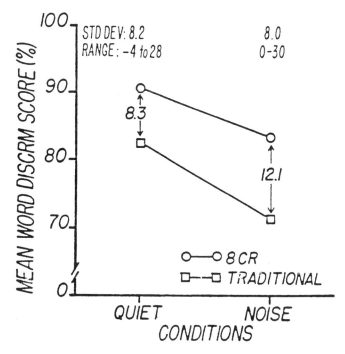

**Figure 6–12.** Mean word recognition score in quiet and noise utilizing conventional and 8CR earmolds. Also provided is the mean difference in word recognition scores between the two earmold designs, standard deviation, and range.

recognition could be achieved with a hearing aid providing a smooth rising frequency response in which the response extended the higher frequencies.

Bergenstoff (1983) reported that the real ear gain above 2000 Hz for a hearing aid coupled to an earmold in which #13 tubing is inserted to the tip was as much as 20 dB lower than the gain reported in a 2-cc coupler whose dimensions are 18 mm long and 3-mm wide. When using a 4-mm horn coupled to a hearing aid having a narrow frequency range, the frequency response was extended by almost an octave, the gain was increased by 10 to 15 dB and the midfrequency resonant peak was reduced by 4 dB. When the same earmold was coupled to a hearing aid providing a wideband response, the 4-mm horn extended the frequency response by almost 2 octaves, increased high-frequency gain by 20 dB, and reduced the midfrequency resonant peak by 8 dB.

Sung and Sung (1982) compared the performance of the Libby 3-mm and 4-mm horns to a conventional earmold with #13 tubing to the tip on 28 subjects with sensorineural hearing loss. Word recognition scores (NU-6 and high-frequency word lists) presented in quiet at 70 dB SPL and noise (SNR of +6 dB) were improved only 0.9–4.9%. Functional gain increased by 0.5 dB at 1,500 Hz to 6.4 dB at 4000 Hz. For some subjects, the improvement was as large as 15 dB. In addition, 54% of the subjects expressed a preference for the Libby designs.

Fernandes and Cooper (1983) reported on the successful use of an undamped Libby 4-mm horn in nine subjects with severe hearing loss in comparison to their performance with the same hearing aid coupled to #13 tubing to the earmold tip. They reported minimal differences in functional gain below 2000 Hz, but 15 dB greater functional gain at 3150 Hz when using the 4-mm horn. There were no significant differences in speech reception threshold (SRT), most comfortable level (MCL), or loudness discomfort level (LDL). However, there was an overwhelming preference for the 4-mm horn because it reportedly provided better sound quality and clarity.

Lyregaard (1982) reported that the effectiveness of the horn is not diminished significantly if small variations are present in the dimensions of the horn or if different hearing aids with different receivers are used. He reported that the horn effect can improve the high-frequency response by 10 dB. Finally, some audiologists might question the feasibility of the average ear canal being wide enough to accommodate an earmold requiring a 4-mm bore and venting. He concluded that an earmold requiring an ID of 4 mm is feasible for a majority of adult subjects. Clearly, this may be a viable concern when providing services to a pediatric population.

### Bakke Horn

Another method of achieving the acoustic benefits of a 4-mm horn in the transmission line is using a Bakke horn. This is a rigid plastic tube, or horn, which is glued directly into lucite or soft (Bakke horn-S) earmolds. This horn is designed so that the ID is 2-mm at the tubing end and 3-mm at the earmold end. The Bakke horn is then followed by 4-mm wide and 11-mm long sound bore. These are the same dimensions as the Libby 4-mm horn. However, there is a major difference between the Libby and Bakke horns. With the Bakke horn, it is very efficient and inexpensive to change the tubing from the earhook to the Bakke horn. However, with the Libby horn it is necessary to replace the entire 4-mm tubing. This can be more expensive because the cost for a 3-mm or 4-mm horn is significantly greater than the cost of #13 tubing. Finally, when used with a conventional hearing aid, the Bakke horn extends the frequency response by almost one octave and provides 10 to 15 dB greater high frequency gain. When used with a wideband hearing aid, it extends the frequency response by almost two octaves and increases the high frequency gain by 20 dB.

### Reversed Horn

Libby (1990) designed injection molding techniques to obtain a one-piece reverse tapered horn (i.e., the diameter of the tube at the tip is narrower than the diameter of the tube at the earhook) for patients with severe to profound hearing loss, to reduce the likelihood of feedback for BTE fittings caused by the peaks in the high-frequency region of the frequency response. The reverse horn reduces the gain above 2000 Hz and shifts the energy toward the lower frequencies (8 dB to 10 dB shift in low-frequency gain). This is appropriate for patients who cannot achieve sufficient gain prior to feedback and must reduce the volume control to eliminate feedback. When feedback is reduced via a reversed horn, the subject can achieve sufficient low-frequency gain where their hearing is typically better.

## *Earmolds*

### Introduction

Early earmold selection in this country was rather simple. The hearing aid fitter poured plaster of Paris to cast the impression and the completed earmold was fabricated from a black hard rubber material. The only style available was a "regular" earmold and a large button receiver, painted in a bright pink and optimistically called "flesh," which was attached to the earmold. An alternative fitting used a flat 2-inch diameter earphone, which covered most of the pinna and was held in place by a 19-mm wide spring steel headband. By World War II, plastics technology grew to include thermosetting acrylic impression materials and methyl methacrylate (lucite) earmolds.

Today, audiologists have a wide range of material and style options available to them. However, this technology is used in only a quarter of the hearing aid fittings because approximately 75% of hearing aid fittings in the United States incorporate custom hearing aids. This may be unfortunate, because when an audiologist sends an impression to a manufacturer, the audiologist has little say in the final configuration of the custom shell. The decision is made by the manufacturer based upon accommodation of the circuitry, power supply, and venting. If space is available, then the manufacturer can consider patient needs or preferences. In addition, in comparison to earmolds, shell options are small in number. Finally, in a large hearing aid manufacturer, a particular shellmaker may never consistently interact with an individual audiologist to get to know the audiologist's needs and impressions.

Earmolds are designed to seal the ear canal, correctly couple the hearing aid to the ear from an acoustical viewpoint, retain the hearing aid on the pinna, be comfortable for an extended period of time, modify the acoustic signal produced by the hearing aid, be able to be easily handled by the patient, and be cosmetically appealing.

Recall that ANSI S3.22-1987 (ANSI-1987) specifies the use of a HA-2 2-cc coupler in which the final segment is 18 mm long and 3 mm wide. These dimensions reportedly represent the average length and diameter of an earmold. However, Cox (1979) reported an average length of 14.3 mm for 52 ears. Dalsgaard (1975) reported an average length of 21.9 mm on 100 ears and Valente (1984c) reported an average length of 15.3 mm for 55 ears. Lybarger (1979) and Killion (1981) reported that if earmolds with dimensions of 18 mm by 3 mm were used instead of #13 tubing to the tip, they would provide 5 to 7 dB greater high-frequency gain. Table 6–3 reveals a 2 to 7 dB decrease in output at 3000 to 6000 Hz for the 6B0 earmold design (same as #13 tubing to the tip of the earmold) in comparison to an earmold with dimensions of 18 mm by 3 mm. Figure 6–13 (Valente, 1984c) reports the dimensions of a "2-cc earmold," which was manufactured in the clinic by using the appropriate lengths of #13 (ID = 1.93 mm) and #9 (ID = 3.0 mm) tubing. Figure 6–14 (Valente, 1984c) shows the frequency response of the same BTE hearing aid measured in HA-1 (without the earmold) and HA-2 (with "2-cc earmold") couplers. It can be seen that the 2 responses are quite similar.

# 2 CC EARMOLD

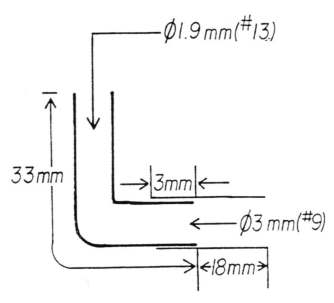

**Figure 6–13.**   Schematic diagram of a "2-cc earmold" simulating the dimensions of a HA-2 coupler.

## Changing Bore Length

Lybarger (1979, 1985) reported that changing the bore length from minimum to maximum will increase or decrease the overall gain by no more than 2 dB in either direction. However, increasing bore length will increase low-frequency gain and decreasing bore length will increase high-frequency gain. Table 6–2, Section III, summarizes how changing the bore length may affect four regions of the frequency response curve.

## Changing Bore Diameter

Lybarger (1979, 1985) reported that the wider the diameter of the bore, the greater the high-frequency emphasis. The narrower the diameter of the bore, the greater the low-frequency emphasis. Table 6–2, Section IV, summarizes how changing the bore diameter may affect four regions of the frequency response curve.

## Changing Length and Diameter

Changes in length and diameter are consistent when either length or diameter is varied independently. That is, a long bore with a narrow ID will shift the frequency response downward. Using a short bore with a wider ID will shift the frequency response upward.

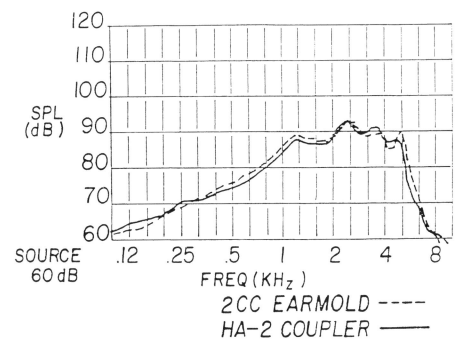

**Figure 6–14.** Frequency response of a hearing aid measured in a HA-2 coupler and the "2-cc earmold" described in Figure 6–13.

### Belled Bore

Another method of increasing high-frequency amplification is to drill, or "bell," the last segment of the earmold with a burr to create a wider diameter than at the entrance of the earmold. Lybarger (1980) and Cox (1979) reported that belling the end of the earmold effectively produces a limited horn effect that can increase high-frequency amplification, but its effectiveness depends upon the length of the bore. Killion (1980) suggested that a bore length of 17 mm is required for the belling effect to be beneficial. Lybarger (1980) stated a length of 16–19 mm is required to obtain maximum benefit when using this strategy. Figure 6–15 (Valente, 1984a) illustrates a belled bore with minimal insertion of tubing and a parallel vent. Figure 6–16 illustrates such an earmold that was prepared for a patient with a gently sloping audiogram. Figure 6–17 (Valente, 1984a) illustrates the performance of a BTE hearing aid measured in a HA-1 2-cc coupler under two conditions. First (dotted line), the hearing aid was measured using #13 tubing and a 1000 ohm damper at the tip of the earmold. Second, the same hearing aid was measured using a configuration illustrated described in Figures 6–15 and 6–16, but with the vent closed with putty. Notice how the belled bore increased high-frequency output and extended the high-frequency response (dashed line).

### Earmold Impressions

To develop the skills required in taking an acceptable impression of the ear, it is necessary for the audiologist to become familiar with the anatomy of the external

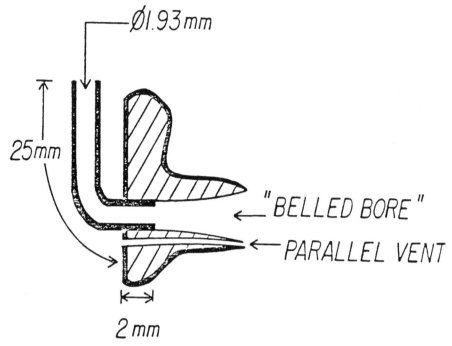

**Figure 6–15.** Schematic diagram of an earmold with a belled bore, parallel vent, and inserting the tubing 2-mm into the sound bore.

ear and have a good knowledge of the vocabulary used to identify key anatomical sites (Fig. 6–18). This is necessary to communicate with the earmold laboratory how the earmold needs to be modified because the earmold/shell is preventing a comfortable and/or appropriate fit. Therefore, it is necessary for the audiologist to become familiar with the terminology used by earmold manufacturers to describe important segments of the earmold in relation to the anatomy of the ear (Fig. 6–19).

EXAMINATION OF THE EAR CANAL

Thoroughly perform an otoscopic observation. For an adult, pull the pinna upward to straighten the ear canal. For a child, pull the pinna downward to straighten the ear canal. Be sure the ear canal of free of cerumen or other foreign objects. Inspect the ear canal to determine if deformities (i.e., atresia), pathologies (warts, moles, tumors), infections (drainage, irritations, redness of the canal wall or eardrum), or abnormalities of the ear canal (stenosis, prolapsed canal, surgically altered canal) are present. If any of the conditions are present, the audiologist should not proceed with the impression and, instead, refer the patient to an otolaryngologist for consultation.

SELECTION AND PLACEMENT OF AN OTOBLOCK

One of the first decisions made when preparing an earmold impression, is to select the appropriate otoblock, which is placed in the ear canal to prevent the

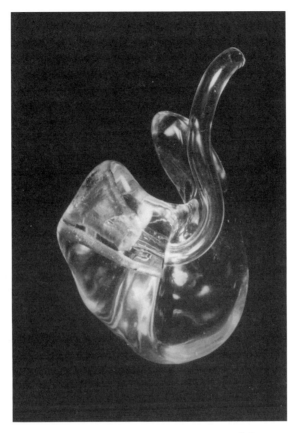

**Figure 6–16.**   Example of an earmold with a belled bore, parallel vent, and minimal insertion of tubing ordered for a patient with a gently sloping audiogram.

impression material from coming into contact with the eardrum. Attached to the otoblock is thread or dental floss, which helps in the removal of the impression from the ear canal. This thread should be placed along the floor of the ear canal and draped over the intratragal notch of the pinna.

Morgan (1994) reminded us of the importance of selecting the correct otoblock. An undersized otoblock will allow impression material past the otoblock or push the otoblock too deep into the ear canal, resulting in an uncomfortable situation for both the patient and audiologist. An oversized otoblock will abnormally expand in the ear canal or prevent the otoblock from being placed sufficiently deep. He suggests that the otoblock be correctly placed using an earlite, to beyond the first bend of the ear canal and optimally to at least the second bend.

IMPRESSION MATERIALS

The audiologist has a choice of using either powder (polymer) and liquid (monomer) or silicone impression materials. In recent years, the advantages and disadvantages of these two impression materials has become a controversial issue for which uniform agreement is not about to occur in the near future. However,

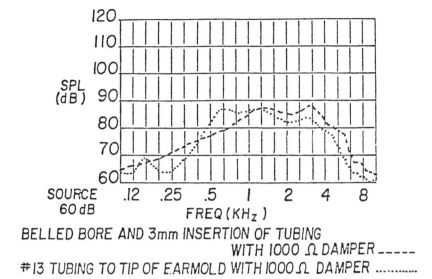

**Figure 6–17.** Frequency response using an earmold with a belled bore, 3 mm insertion of tubing and a 1000 ohm damper at the tip of the earhook. Also illustrated is the frequency response generated when using an earmold with #13 tubing to the tip of the earmold and a 1000 ohm damper at the tip of the earhook.

there is agreement in that for whichever material the audiologist chooses to use, it is imperative that he or she carefully follows the instructions provided by the earmold laboratory.

Figure 6–20 illustrates the step-by-step procedure for using the syringe techniques for taking an earmold impression. Using this technique, the impression material is carefully mixed and placed in the syringe and the nozzle of the syringe is placed in the ear canal. Gently press the plunger and gradually withdraw the nozzle as the material fills the ear canal and begins to flow out into the concha. Finally, fill the entire outer ear, especially the helix area. Keep the nozzle submerged in the impression material at all times for better filling of the ear. Do not press the outer surface of the impression because any pressing may lead to distortion of the impression. Allow at least 10 minutes for the impression to set. Gently break the seal by asking the patient to yawn or use exaggerated facial expressions. Remove the impression by grasping the pinna firmly with one hand and the impression with the other. Rotate the impression slowly with an upward and outward motion. The otoblock should remain on the tip of the impression. Figure 6–21 provides several illustrations of correct and incorrect earmold impressions. Finally, inspect the ear canal with an otoscope to be sure no impression material remains in the ear canal.

Morgan (1994) reported that silicone impression material retains a highly accurate and dimensionally stable impression of the ear canal from the clinic to the earmold laboratory. Many audiologists are hesitant to use silicone impression material because it is relatively messy in that it requires the proper mixing of two "pastes." One paste is a base material (silano-terminated gum) that is measured in

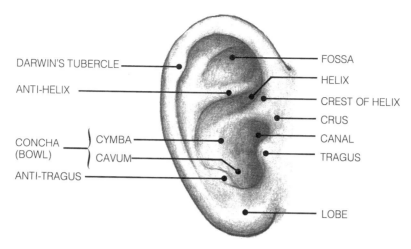

**Figure 6–18.** Illustration of the anatomical sites of the outer ear. (Printed with permission from Microsonic, Inc.)

a scoop, and the second paste is an activator agent that is spread over the base material. The two pastes are mixed together by hand for 20 to 30 seconds until an even, consistent color is reached (Figure 6–22) and then it is inserted into a syringe that is specially designed for silicone impressions. Trade names for silicone impression material across earmold laboratories include XL-80, X-SIL, Otoform A/K, XL-100, XL-200, Micro-SIL, Blue Velvet, Gold Velvet II, and Silicast™. Prepackaged silicone is available. This material is delivered in prepacked, self-mixing cartridges and is injected into the ear canal using an injection gun illustrated in Figure 6–23.

Although there is a growing consensus on the advantages of silicone impression material, it is the opinion of the authors that powder (polymer) and liquid (monomer) impression material can provide an excellent impression if the audiologist uses the proper mix of powder and liquid and the resulting mixture is correctly syringed into the ear canal in a timely fashion. If the mixture of powder

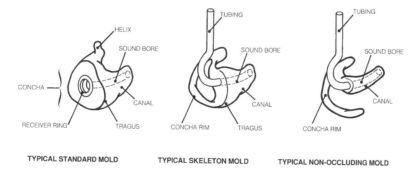

**Figure 6–19.** Terminology commonly used by earmold laboratories to relate the anatomical sites of the ear with various sections of three common earmolds. (Printed with permission from Microsonic, Inc.)

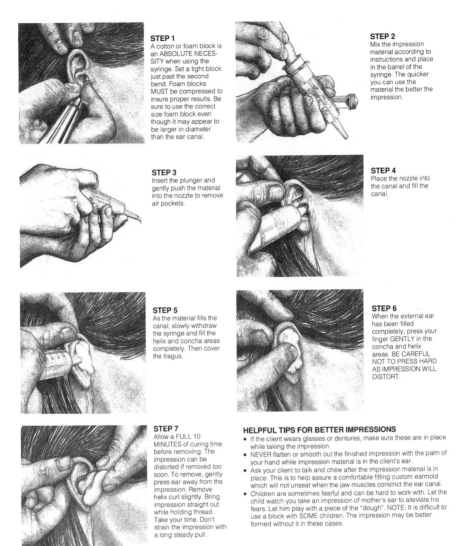

**STEP 1**
A cotton or foam block is an ABSOLUTE NECESSITY when using the syringe. Set a tight block just past the second bend. Foam blocks MUST be compressed to insure proper results. Be sure to use the correct size foam block even though it may appear to be larger in diameter than the ear canal.

**STEP 2**
Mix the impression material according to instructions and place in the barrel of the syringe. The quicker you can use the material the better the impression.

**STEP 3**
Insert the plunger and gently push the material into the nozzle to remove air pockets.

**STEP 4**
Place the nozzle into the canal and fill the canal.

**STEP 5**
As the material fills the canal, slowly withdraw the syringe and fill the helix and concha areas completely. Then cover the tragus.

**STEP 6**
When the external ear has been filled completely, press your finger GENTLY in the concha and helix areas. BE CAREFUL NOT TO PRESS HARD AS IMPRESSION WILL DISTORT.

**STEP 7**
Allow a FULL 10 MINUTES of curing time before removing. The impression can be distorted if removed too soon. To remove, gently press ear away from the impression. Remove helix curl slightly. Bring impression straight out while holding thread. Take your time. Don't strain the impression with a long steady pull.

**HELPFUL TIPS FOR BETTER IMPRESSIONS**
- If the client wears glasses or dentures, make sure these are in place while taking the impression.
- NEVER flatten or smooth out the finished impression with the palm of your hand while impression material is in the client's ear.
- Ask your client to talk and chew after the impression material is in place. This is to help assure a comfortable fitting custom earmold which will not unseat when the jaw muscles constrict the ear canal.
- Children are sometimes fearful and can be hard to work with. Let the child watch you take an impression of mother's ear to alleviate his fears. Let him play with a piece of the "dough". NOTE: It is difficult to use a block with SOME children. The impression may be better formed without it in these cases.

**Figure 6–20.** Illustrating the syringe techniques for making an earmold impression. (Printed with permission from Microsonic, Inc.)

and liquid is incorrect and not properly cured (at least 10 minutes), the impression can stretch during removal. If the mixture is too dry (too much powder or too little liquid), it will be difficult to push through the syringe and, thus, cause voids. On the other hand, too much liquid makes the impression susceptible to melting.

To reinforce these points, Agnew (1986) reminded us that ethyl methacrylate will shrink if the proportion of the powder and liquid are poorly mixed. The magnitude of shrinkage can be 2 to 3% in 24 hours and 4 to 5% in 48 hours. One key factor for increased shrinkage is increased use of liquid in proportion to the

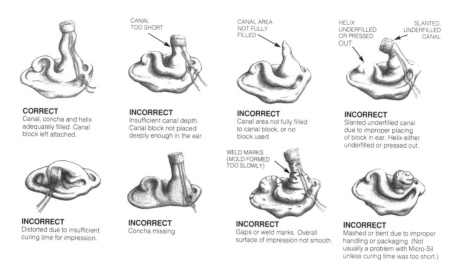

CORRECT
Canal, concha and helix adequately filled. Canal block left attached.

INCORRECT
Insufficient canal depth. Canal block not placed deeply enough in the ear.

INCORRECT
Canal area not fully filled to canal block, or no block used.

INCORRECT
Slanted underfilled canal due to improper placing of block in ear. Helix either underfilled or pressed out.

INCORRECT
Distorted due to insufficient curing time for impression.

INCORRECT
Concha missing

INCORRECT
Gaps or weld marks. Overall surface of impression not smooth.

INCORRECT
Mashed or bent due to improper handling or packaging. (Not usually a problem with Micro-Sil unless curing time was too short.)

**Figure 6–21.** Several examples of correct and incorrect earmold impressions. (Printed with permission from Microsonic, Inc.)

amount of powder. Other reasons may include not shaking the liquid and/or powder before using or loss of liquid via evaporation due to a poorly sealed container.

Another key factor in providing a good impression of the ear canal is "gel time" or "set-up time." This is the time it takes for the mixing of the powder and liquid to become solidified or "cured" in the ear canal. As a general rule, gel time is at least 10 minutes. Gel time decreases with increased temperature and humidity. Thus, on a hot and humid summer day, the impression will gel faster than in winter. To retard gel time, some audiologists increase the amount of liquid. To evaluate this strategy, Agnew increased the liquid amounts by 10% and 20% and found that shrinkage increased by 12 and 22%, respectively in comparison to when the correct mixture ratio was used.

Excessive heat (i.e., impression placed in a mailbox outside) will increase warpage and distortion of the impression. Excessive heat may cause the tip of the impression to distort toward the body via warpage and drooping (1.0 mm) after 5 days. For this reason, it is important to keep the impression in a cool place. Also, it is important not to use excessive force during the impression. This will "balloon" the ear canal and the resulting earmold will cause the ear canal to become sore.

Morgan (1994) also reminded us to encourage the patient to talk, turn his head in all directions, smile, and chew while the impression material is setting in the ear canal. This will result in a more accurate impression of the dynamics of the ear canal and reduce the probability of feedback when the patient moves his jaw when wearing the hearing aids.

When shipping, it is necessary to glue the powder and liquid impression, but a silicone impression can be shipped loose in the box. Finally, it is important not to allow the order form to come into contact with the impression while in the shipping box because this may result in the order form pressing against the impression and cause distortion.

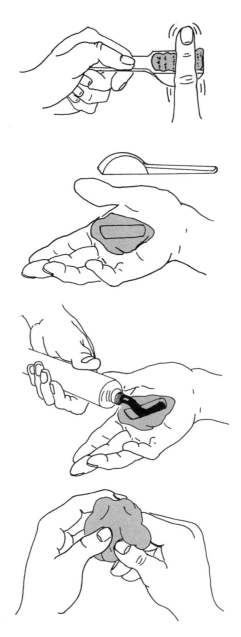

**Figure 6–22.** Mixing the "base" material and "activator" agent when making an impression using silicone material. (Printed with permission from Microsonic, Inc.)

EARMOLD MATERIALS

Earmolds are available in both hard and soft materials, and it is not a simple task to select the appropriate earmold material for a patient. For example, if the pinna is hard, then a soft earmold material may be more appropriate. Conversely, if the pinna is soft, then a hard earmold material may be more appropriate. If the

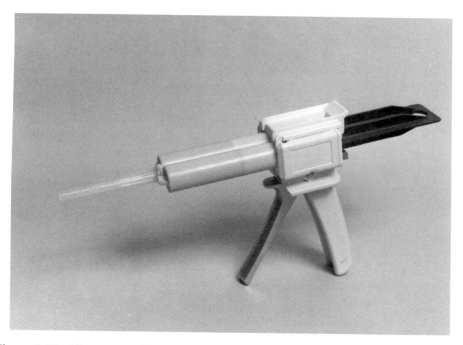

**Figure 6–23.**  Illustration of an impression gun used when making earmold impressions with premixed silicone material.

gain/output requirements of the hearing aids are "high" (usually 70 dB of gain and 125 dB SPL of output), then the audiologist might consider ordering a hard lucite body with a soft canal or a material that softens to the heat of the ear canal, which provides a better seal to prevent feedback. For mild to moderate gain aids, a lucite earmold might be considered. If there is any indication of an allergic reaction to the earmold material, then the audiologist might consider polyethylene (hard) or silicone (soft) material. If the patient indicates difficulty with inserting an earmold, then a lucite material may be considered because it is easier to insert earmolds made of hard material. If the audiologist prefers the flexibility of having the ability to make modifications (venting, changing bore length or diameter, and belling) then ordering a lucite material may be better because of its greater ease in allowing for such modifications. Finally, the audiologist needs to be familiar with the terminology used by his or her earmold laboratory because there is quite a variance in terminology across earmold laboratories. Provided in the next section is a description of the various earmold materials provided by one manufacturer.

1.  LUCITE: This is a polymethyl methacrylate dental acrylic. It is a hard material that is easily modified, easy to insert and remove, and it is very durable. It is available in clear, various tints, and opaque. It is also available as a nontoxic material in clear or opaque. The canal portion is rigid and may lead to sound leakage during chewing or other facial movement if applied to a high-gain hearing aid.

2. LUCITE BODY WITH VINYLFLEX CANAL: This earmold combines the body of the earmold made with poly methyl methacrylate (lucite) material and the canal made with poly ethyl methacrylate (vinylflex) material. This combination of materials is designed for patients who want the comfort and increased sealing capacity of the vinylflex material when fit with hearing aids having greater gain and output.

3. VINYLFLEX: This is a poly ethyl methacrylate material that is a heat-cured semisoft plastic that will soften with body temperature. It is available in clear, beige, and tint. Finally, it is not easy to modify.

4. SEMI-SOFT: This is a fairly rigid vinyl material which softens at body temperature. This is typically used for additional comfort, while maintaining ease of insertion. Finally, it is fairly easy to modify.

5. SOFT VINYL: This is the most common soft material where allergies are not a concern. This material will shrink with body contact and age, and can become discolored over time. Cementing tubing can cause some problems and, therefore, a tube locking system is recommended.

6. SILICONE: This is a flexible, inert rubber material. It is available in clear, opaque, pink, beige, and brown. It has very little shrinkage and is good for high-power aids and it is not easy to modify. Silicone material will solve most allergy problems. Finally, a tubing lock method is required because cement does not adhere to this material.

7. SOFT SILICONE: This material is recommended for the highest gain requirements. It is most effective when used in a canal or canal-shell earmold design, but is not easy to modify. This material also requires an accurate impression to at least the second bend of the ear canal.

8. POLYETHYLENE: This is a hard material that is appropriate for severe cases of allergy and it is easy to modify. It is only available in opaque white or pink.

Recently, E-Compound material was introduced by Emtech Laboratories (Letowski and Burchfield, 1991; Letowski, Richards, and Burchfield, 1992) (see address in Table 6–4). E-Compound is produced by filling a polymeric matrix (lucite or silicone) with hollow glass microspheres. This new material is reported by the manufacturer to provide better sound quality than conventional materials. Letowski, Burchfield, and Hume (1991) reported the results of 10 normal listeners who provided sound-quality judgments of eight stimuli, recorded through KEMAR fitted with lucite and silicone earmolds made with and without E-Compound. Results indicated that only a few of the listeners could detect differences in sound quality between the earmold materials when signals comprised of "noise" were presented. However, they could not detect differences when "non-noise" signals were presented. The authors reported that E-Compound seems to provide better results with silicone material than with lucite material.

Ridenhour (1988) reported that 76% of 25 subjects wearing ITE hearing aids revealed improved NU-6 word recognition scores, embedded in cafeteria noise at a SNR of +10 dB when wearing E-Compound lucite shells in comparison to conventional lucite shells. He reported that the average improvement was 12% and that 68% of the users preferred the shell made with E-Compound.

**Table 6–4.**  List of Several Earmold Manufacturers

| | |
|---|---|
| All American Mold Labs<br>226 S.W. Sixth Street<br>P.O. Box 25751<br>Oklahoma City, OK 73125<br>405-232-8144 | Mid-States Labs, Inc.<br>P.O. Box 1140<br>Wichita, KS 67201<br>800-247-3669 |
| Earmold Designs, Inc.<br>3424 East Lake Street<br>Minneapolis, MN 55406<br>800-721-5711 | Pacific Coast Labs, Inc.<br>P.O. Box 7981<br>San Francisco, CA 94120<br>510-351-2770 |
| Earmold and Research Labs, Inc.<br>P.O. Box 12368<br>Wichita, KS 67277<br>316-682-9587 | Precision Mold Labs<br>830 Sunshine Lane<br>Altamonte Springs, FL 32714<br>800-327-4792 |
| Emtech<br>P.O. Box 12900<br>Roanoke, VA 24022<br>800-336-5719 | Starkey Labs<br>6700 Washington Ave, South<br>Eden Prairie, MN 55344<br>800-328-8602 |
| Microsonic<br>P.O. Box 184<br>1421 Merchant Street<br>Ambridge, PA 15003<br>800-523-7672 | Westone Labs, Inc.<br>P.O. Box 15100<br>Colorado Springs, CO 80935<br>800-525-5071 |

Williams and Gutnick (1990) reported the results of 10 listeners who were fitted with conventional lucite and E-Compound lucite earmolds. Seventy percent of the patients preferred the E-Compound earmolds, although none of the objective data (functional gain, *in situ* gain, word recognition scores at 50 dB HL in quiet and noise at +5 and +8 SNR) could reveal statistically different performance between the two materials.

**Two-Stage Versus One-Stage Impressions**

Custom earmolds require two stages. First, there is the impression of the ear by the audiologist. The impression is then mailed to an earmold laboratory where it is wax dipped and invested in a matrix medium that is either silicone or plaster. A polymeric material is cured in plaster or silicone and then it is drilled, tubed, and polished. Many problems may arise that will not allow the finished product to "duplicate the ear." These include poor impression-taking techniques; shrinkage of the impression and/or earmold; incorrect trimming of the impression; and changes in the dimensions of the ear canal between the time of the impression and the fitting.

Single-stage earmolds (i.e., the impression is the earmold) include such commercially available products as Instamold™, Silisoft™, and Otozen™. These earmolds have been used in our clinic as temporary earmolds to allow patients to continue using their hearing aids while waiting for a custom mold to be delivered. We have also used single-stage earmolds instead of stock earmolds for evaluating benefit from amplification during a hearing aid evaluation (HAE).

Some single-stage earmolds have reportedly presented problems such as producing a high degree of heat related to setting reaction that may cause burns to the ear; a high degree of shrinkage; too great a degree of hardness; and poor resistance to tearing, which may lead to difficulties in removal of the earmold (Okpojo, 1992).

Okpojo (1992) reported on a new material for one-stage earmolds that is used in the United Kingdom. This material is reportedly nontoxic, nonirritant, and the setting reaction has a low exothermal release. It is a "polymer power and monomer liquid" mixture that sets in 4 to 7 minutes. Shrinkage is reportedly less than 1 to 2% and it has suitable mechanical and rheologic properties (elastic, resilient, adequate strength to resist tearing, and comfortable). All of these properties led to the development of the soft Otana™ material.

**Custom Versus Stock Earmolds**

Stock earmolds are available in skeleton, shell, or regular designs and typically are available in a set of five earmolds for each ear. The purpose of these earmolds is to conveniently assess benefit with a BTE hearing aid during an HAE, when the patient does not have a custom earmold. Konkle and Bess (1974) reported better performance with custom earmolds in comparison to stock earmolds. They reported that using stock earmolds instead of custom earmolds presented several problems, which include differences in (a) the dimensions between the stock versus custom earmold; (b) vent length and diameter; (c) tubing length and diameter; (d) the size of the residual volume between the tip of the earmold and the eardrum; and (e) sealing capacity. All of these differences led the authors to conclude that custom and stock earmolds will deliver different acoustic signals than were evaluated at the time of the HAE with the stock earmold and, therefore, the results from the HAE may not be valid. They highly recommended using the custom earmold during the HAE. To punctuate this point, they evaluated 17 patients with sensorineural hearing loss. They compared the performance of six soft and hard acrylic stock earmolds against custom earmolds. They reported no significant differences in functional gain, although mean aided warble tone and speech reception thresholds were lower for the custom earmolds. They also reported that the mean word recognition score was significantly better for the custom earmold.

**Disposable Foam Earmolds**

Another method of providing a temporary and, in some cases, a permanent earmold is using disposable foam earmolds. Smolak, Iserman, and Hawkinson (1987) reported on seven subjects that used the 3M Comply™ disposable foam earmold. This earmold incorporates retarded recovery foam technology to provide a comfortable fit and eliminate the need for an earmold impression. Venting (four vents) is provided by the use of trench vents in the foam to control the low frequency response. They reported that differences between a custom earmold and foam earmold was, at its greatest, less than 2 dB. The four vents provided by the disposable foam earmold yielded an average reduction of 3.1 to 6 dB at 250 to 1000 Hz. However, 25% of the ears did not achieve as satisfactory a fit with the disposable foam earmold as they did with their custom earmold. These differences were attributed to the inability of the disposable foam earmold to adequately address ear canals that were unusually narrow or tortuous. These types of ear canals reduced retention and provided inadequate venting. Finally, it was found that the disposable foam earmold was more effective in reducing feedback due to the adaptive sealing capabilities of the disposable foam and the excellent sealing capability that prevents acoustic signals from reentering the ear canal via a vent or slit leak.

Oliveira, Hawkinson, and Stockton (1992) reported on results with the Comply™ disposable foam earmold versus custom earmolds at 15 test sites. They reported significantly better performance of the disposable foam earmold in providing greater comfort and in reducing feedback. However, the disposable foam earmold did present some problems with retention and proper insertion for patients over 75 years of age.

Another option for a disposable earmold is the ER-13 Generic BTE earmold kit, which is delivered with small, medium, and large disposable foam eartips and #13 or 3 mm Continuous Flow Adaptor (CFA) elbows.

## Earmold Styles

### Introduction

Sullivan (1985a, 1985b, 1985c) suggested that all hearing aid fittings can be categorized into four classes according to the type of coupling employed:

Class I includes earmolds where there is no loss in transmission of the acoustic signal; pinna, concha, and ear canal effects are retained; maximum venting is used; an hermetic seal is not necessary; the volume between the tip of the earmold and the eardrum (V3) is maximum due to the need for a short bore length; maximum *in situ* gain is 10 to 25 dB, and usable *in situ* output is 75 to 90 dB. Class I fittings are appropriate for hearing loss between 15 to 40 dB HL. Examples of Class I fittings would be tube fittings, free field, Janssen, and other nonoccluding designs.

Class II fittings include earmolds where there is a slight reduction in high-frequency transmission; minimal venting is required; the pinna effect is retained, but the concha and ear canal effects are modified; hermetic sealing is not required; there is some reduction in V3 due to the need for a longer bore; maximum *in situ* gain is 20 to 35 dB; and useable *in situ* output is 80 to 100 dB. Class II fittings are appropriate for hearing loss between 30 to 55 dB HL and include the use of acoustic modifiers, Select-A-Vent (SAV), Variable-Venting-Valve (VVV), Positive-Venting-Valve (PVV), and fixed venting.

Class III fittings include earmolds where there is significant loss of high-frequency and midfrequency transmission; the pinna, concha, and ear canal effects are not useable; a limited hermetic seal is required; there is further reduction of V3 due to the need for a longer bore; maximum *in situ* gain is 30 to 55 dB; and useable *in situ* output of 95 to 115 dB. Class III fittings are appropriate for hearing loss between 45 to 85 dB HL and include closed molds and use of pressure equalization venting (0.05 mm).

Class IV fittings include earmolds where there is complete loss of the transmission loss of the frequency response; the pinna, concha, and ear canal effects are not useable; a tight hermetic seal is required; V3 is reduced further due to the need for further increases in bore length; maximum *in situ* gain is 50 to 65 dB; and useable *in situ* output of 110 to 135+ dB. Class IV fittings are appropriate for hearing loss between 70 to 95+ dB HL and include earmolds requiring a closed mold with no venting, tight hermetic seal, and a deep canal fit.

### NAEL Earmold Designs

Coogle (1976) reported the nomenclature for earmold designs as agreed to by the National Association of Earmold Laboratories (NAEL). These include:

1. Regular, Receiver, or Standard Earmold (Fig. 6–24a): This earmold design is typically used for fitting body aids and BTEs. It is usually ordered with a vinyl or metal snap ring that is either 1/4 or 3/16 inch wide. In a body aid fitting, the external receiver from a body aid snaps into the snap ring. For BTE fittings, a plastic nub attached to tubing from the earhook snaps into the snap ring or it can be ordered with glued tubing. The plastic nub over which the tubing from the earhook slips onto can be ordered in several sizes (standard, D90, 8080, etc.). An alternative may be a regular earmold with a wire hook for cases where the pinna has little cartilage (i.e., a young child), and this style will hold the weight of the receiver and earmold in place.

   For a regular earmold, bore dimensions of 18 mm by 3 mm will produce a relatively flat frequency response to 3400 Hz. When the bore length is longer and the diameter narrower (23.4 x 2.4 mm), a loss in the high-frequency response occurs. Actually, the use of a long bore may be in the best interest of a patient with a severe hearing loss. This is because attenuating the high-frequency response would reduce the possibility of feedback. In addition, the benefits from high-frequency amplification are questionable in patients with profound hearing loss.

   Lybarger (1979) reported that regular earmolds containing a snap ring can reduce the high-frequency gain by 8 to 10 dB above 2800 Hz and increase gain around 1000 Hz by about 4 dB relative to when #13 tubing is inserted to the earmold tip. The magnitude of the high-frequency reduction is related to the volume of the cavity in front of the receiver, which has been denoted as V2 by Lybarger (1979). The smaller the V2, the less the reduction of high-frequency gain. Again, as noted earlier, the reduction in high-frequency gain for patients with severe to profound hearing loss may be desirable.

2. Skeleton (Fig. 6–24b): This is similar to the shell, but the center of the concha section is removed to provide less bulk and greater comfort.

3. Semi-Skeleton (Fig. 6–24c): This earmold is the same as the skeleton, but the upper portion of the concha ring is removed. It is appropriate for patients who have reduced manual dexterity or hardened ear texture.

4. Canal (Fig. 6–24d): This is designed for mild to moderate gain hearing aids. It is easy to insert, but retention may be poor and is prone to problems with feedback. This is also available in Canal-Lock (Fig. 6–24e).

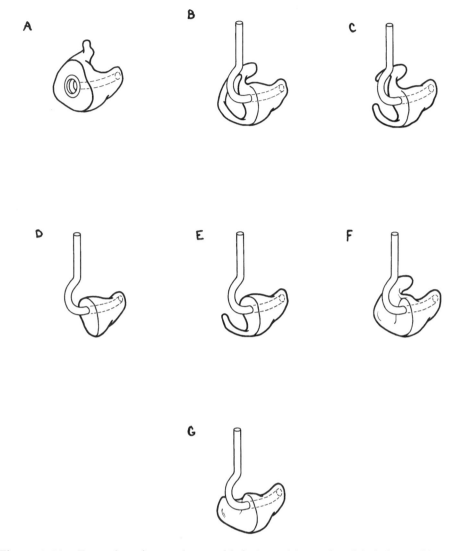

**Figure 6–24.** Examples of several earmold designs: (a) regular; (b) skeleton; (c) semi-skeleton; (d) canal: (e) canal-lok; (f) shell; (g) canal-shell. (Printed with permission from Microsonic, Inc.)

5. Shell (Fig. 6–24f): This earmold fills the concha completely. It can be ordered with or without the helix segment. Adding the helix improves retention of the earmold to reduce the possibility of feedback. However, the addition of the helix increases the probability of discomfort in the helix region. It usually selected for high gain hearing aids.

6. Half-Shell or Canal Shell (Fig. 6–24g): The entire helix area is removed and the earmold covers the bottom half of the concha bowl. It is recommended for patients with reduced manual dexterity.

7. Nonoccluding Earmolds: as presented earlier in the sections discussing tubing and earhooks, there are a variety of nonoccluding earmolds. These include tube fitting, free field, CROS, Janssen, Lybarger dual-diameter, Lybarger 1.5LP, and extended range earmolds (see Figs. 6–8 and 6–9).

### Non-NAEL Earmold Designs

ACOUSTICALLY TUNED EARMOLDS

In the typical BTE fitting, the output from the receiver is transmitted to the earhook by tubing having a length of 10 mm and diameter of 1.0 mm. The earhook typically has a length of 23 mm and diameter of 1.3 mm. The tubing from the earhook to the tip of the earmold is approximately 40 to 45 mm long and 1.93 mm wide. Finally, the signal is delivered to the ear canal, which is typically 13 mm long and 7.5 mm wide (see Fig. 6–1). Thus, the typical hearing aid fitting already has a stepped diameter design. Killion (1980, 1981, 1982, 1984, 1988a, 1988b), Killion and Monser (1980), Killion and Revit (1993), and Libby (1980, 1981) advocated that the stepped diameter design should be extended to the earmold when used with a hearing aid having the newer wideband receiver to obtain maximum high-fidelity sound quality, extended frequency response, and reduced battery drain. Up to that time, receivers had a high-frequency cutoff at 4000 to 4500 Hz. Killion presented 12 new earmold designs that varied in the dimensions of sections of tubing and the placement of damping in either the earhook or tubing. These designs include the 6R12, 6R10, 6K14, 16KLT, 8.5R8, 8CR, 6AM, 6B10, 6B5, 6B0, 6C5, and 6C10; their dimensions have been outlined by Valente and DeJonge (1981). The last seven rows of sections A and B of Table 6–3 report the relative change in output for the 8CR, 6R12, 6R10, 6B5, 6B0, 6C5, and 6C10 earmold designs relative to measures made in HA-1 and HA-2 couplers.

The 6R10, 6R12, and 6K14 earmold designs provide a smooth rising frequency response resulting in 10, 12, or 14 dB greater gain at 6000 Hz than at 1000 Hz. The 16KLT provides gain to 16,000 Hz and can only be used if coupled to a receiver whose frequency response extends to 20,000 Hz. The 8.5R8 is a shorter bore design providing a smooth rising frequency response where the gain is 8 dB greater at 8500 Hz than at 1000 Hz. The 8CR is designed to provide a smooth frequency response, with the greatest gain at 2,00 to compensate for the loss of the ear canal resonance, which is eliminated with the introduction of the earmold. It also extends the frequency response to 8000 Hz (see Fig. 6–25; Valente, 1983). The 6AM is an acoustic modifier earmold that extends the frequency response to 6000 Hz. Five additional designs (6B10, 6B5, 6B0, 6C5, and 6C10) either boost (B) or cut (C) the gain at 6000 Hz relative to the gain at 1000 Hz by using either a horn (Boost) or reversed horn (Cut) design. As mentioned earlier, the 6B0 is a conventional earmold with #13 tubing cemented to the tip of the earmold.

Preves (1980) reported that the advantages of the stepped diameter design could be extended to ITE fittings. He reported that using a stepped bore increased gain by 10 dB at 6000 Hz. In addition, placement of a 2200 ohm damper in the receiver reduced the amplitude of the resonant peak at around 2000 Hz by 4 to 8 dB.

Rezen (1980) evaluated the performance of the 6R12 on 11 subjects with sensorineural hearing loss. She reported functional gain increased from 3.5 dB at

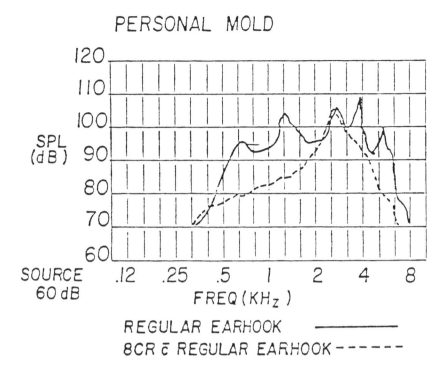

**Figure 6–25.** Frequency response of a hearing aid coupled to an 8CR earmold and an earmold using #13 tubing cemented to the tip.

2500 to 4000 Hz to 19.5 dB at 6300 to 10,000 Hz relative to an earmold with #13 tubing cemented to the tip. She also reported improved word recognition scores (NU-6; Nonsense Syllable Test; and SPIN) of 8.1 to 15.5% relative to the earmold using #13 tubing to the tip of the earmold.

To illustrate the advantages of providing greater high-frequency gain, Schwartz, Surr, Montgomery, Prosek, and Walden (1979) evaluated 12 subjects using conventional high-frequency emphasis amplification versus an experimental high-pass hearing aid that extended the frequency response to 6000 Hz. They reported similar performance between the two hearing aids for word recognition scores in quiet, but the experimental aid provided an average of 9% better word recognition scores in noise. In addition, the experimental aid provided greater functional gain above 4000 Hz and 15 to 20 dB greater high-frequency coupler gain. Finally, eight subjects preferred the sound quality of the experimental aid.

Harford and Fox (1978) fitted nine subjects having a flat moderate to severe sensorineural hearing loss with a conventional hearing aid and an experimental high-frequency hearing aid that extended the frequency response to 6500 Hz. They reported increased functional gain of 1 to 23 dB at 2000 to 8000 Hz and a mean improvement of 13.5% in word recognition scores (NU-6) embedded in competition. Also, they reported that seven subjects revealed word recognition scores that were 18% or greater than their performance with the conventional aid. Finally, they pointed out that most subjects preferred the performance of the experimental aid in noise, but did not prefer the experimental aid in quiet because it was perceived as "too tinny."

Killion and Tillman (1982) compared the performance of an experimental high-frequency emphasis BTE coupled to an 8CR earmold and ITE hearing aids to high-quality loudspeakers, a pocket radio, a discount stereo, a simulated audiometer, popular headphones, and a monitor loudspeaker. Comparisons were based upon six speech samples (nonsense sentences, speech spectrum noise, and four musical passages) recorded through the various listening devices. Subjective fidelity ratings were obtained from three groups of listeners (24 untrained listeners; five "golden ears," and six trained listeners). Results revealed that ratings for the hearing aids and high-fidelity loudspeaker were equal. Mean fidelity ratings were 82% for the BTE and 91% for ITE. The scores were 63 to 93% for the "low-end" loudspeaker and 89% for high-fidelity loudspeaker. For the 24 untrained listeners, the ITE had a mean subjective fidelity rating of 76%, followed by the BTE, which had a mean rating of 75%. The monitor speakers had a mean rating of 73%, and the popular earphones had a mean rating of 60%. Similar findings were revealed for the "golden ear" and trained listener groups. The results of this study revealed that "high-fidelity" performance was possible with well designed BTEs and ITEs.

EXTENDED RANGE EARMOLD (ERE)

This is a specially designed earmold that provides a smooth frequency response between 2000 to 5000 Hz and extends the effective frequency response to 9000 Hz. It is available in 2 versions from several earmold laboratories. In the first version, #13 tubing is inserted to within 5 mm from the lateral end of the earmold and it is followed by a wide diameter belled canal that is 11 mm long (Fig. 6–9f). The second version contains a narrower and shorter sound bore that has #13 tubing inserted 5 mm into the sound bore followed by a bore length of 8 mm, which is reduced in diameter to 1.5 mm (Fig. 6–9g). This version provides slightly less high frequency amplification than the first version. Because it is a nonoccluding design, it provides a fair degree of low-frequency attenuation. It is very similar in performance to the Janssen earmold (Fig. 6–9e), which is very similar to a CROS mold except that the canal portion of the mold runs along the top of the ear canal. Figure 6–9h illustrates the improved high-frequency gain with either extended range earmold designs in comparison to a tube-fitting (dotted line).

WIDE RANGE MOLD (WRM)

This is a special resonator earmold that is designed to provide maximum gain at 5000 Hz. It uses #13 double-walled tubing inserted 3.2 mm into the sound bore and followed by a short bore 3.4 mm wide. If the audiologist wants a smoother response, the WRM can be ordered with two dampers in the sound bore that are placed between the end of the #13 tubing and the beginning of the 3.4 mm sound bore. The WRM also contains a vent, which is 1.35 mm in diameter.

## LYBARGER DUAL DIAMETER SYSTEM

This is an open canal earmold that is appropriate for patients having normal hearing from 250 to 2000 Hz followed by a precipitous decrease in hearing above 2000 Hz. This earmold contains a section of tubing with an ID of 0.8 mm, which is cut to the required length and cemented between two sections of #13 tubing (see Fig. 6–4). The upper section of #13 tubing is connected to the earhook (containing a 1500 ohm damper), and the lower section of #13 tubing is cemented into the nonoccluding earmold and extends between 6.3 to 9.5 mm into the ear canal. The 0.8 mm section of tubing moves the first resonant peak downward and the open mold design provides 20 to 25 dB of attenuation at 500 Hz. The 1500 ohm damper provides a broad and smooth frequency response. Finally, this design provides 12 dB of gain between 4000 to 7000 Hz when used with a wideband receiver (Mynders, 1985).

## FREQUENCY GAIN MODIFIER (FGM)

This earmold is available in numerous occluding and nonoccluding designs. Its construction is highlighted by using a stepped bore, belled canal, and a plastic elbow for efficient changing of tubing. Some designs use venting and others do not. This earmold is designed to damp the low-frequency region and amplify the high-frequency region.

## VOGEL MOLD

This is designed for severe to profound hearing loss and for patients who illustrate "excessive" mandibular jaw movement. It is comprised of a lucite base for rigid retention in the outer ear and a soft, flexible silicone section in the ear canal portion that reportedly moves with the ear canal to maintain a constant acoustic seal.

## CONTINUOUS FLOW ADAPTORS™ (CFA)

These earmolds are ordered in various numbers (i.e., CFA #1, CFA #2, etc.) and contain a single snap-in/snap-out elbow that has a constant internal diameter to incorporate the earmold designs of Killion, Libby, and Janssen discussed earlier. The advantages of CFA are the ease of changing tubing and the elimination of damping in the earhook or tubing to smooth the frequency response. Another advantage is the inability of the tubing to become crimped or pinched, which is a common problem when inserting Libby 3-mm or 4-mm tubing inside the sound bore.

It is important for the audiologist to consult his earmold laboratory manual to determine the dimensions and purpose of the various CFA designs because the nomenclature can vary from manufacturer to manufacturer. However, for one manufacturer, CFA #1 has a small bore of 1.93 mm that provides high-frequency emphasis at 2000 to 5000 Hz and a smooth frequency response. CFA #2 has a belled bore of approximately 4.0 mm, which also provides high-frequency emphasis at 2000 to 5000 Hz and a smooth frequency response. CFA #3 has a sound bore between 1.93 to 4.75 mm to provide greater high-frequency emphasis.

CFA #4 also contains a large open bore of 4.75 mm to provide even greater high-frequency emphasis. CFA #5 is designed for rising configurations and uses venting and a short-wide bore that removes 8 dB to 10 dB of gain at 2000 to 5000 Hz. For all CFA designs it is not necessary to remove the damaged tubing. The audiologist simply needs to pull out the old CFA (with the attached tubing) and snap the new CFA (with the attached tubing) into the seating ring above the sound bore.

BAKKE HORN

As previously discussed, this is a hard plastic elbow having a stepped bore design (2 mm at the tubing end and 3 mm at the earmold end), which snaps into the final segment of the earmold having a 4.0-mm sound bore. It provides an acoustic signal that is very similar to the Libby 4-mm horn.

MACRAE 2K NOTCH FILTER

Macrae (1983) reported an earmold designed for hearing losses having an inverted trough configuration (best hearing at 2000 Hz). To accomplish this, the earmold has a Helmholtz resonator that band-rejects the frequency response around 2000 Hz (1400 to 2600 Hz) by 18 dB. His design places a coiled tubing, connected to the sound bore by a T-connector, and recessed into the cavity of the earmold. Then a faceplate was glued over the recess to hide the coiled tube. The reader should be reminded that the Macrae earmold provides the same frequency response as the ER12-2 earhook that was discussed in an earlier section.

EARMOLDS USED WITH STETHOSCOPES

In our clinic, based in a large medical center, it is common for physicians, nurses, or anesthetisologists to request an earmold that can be used concurrently with their hearing aids or stethoscope because they report difficulties due to their hearing loss or the presence of excessive ambient noise. Mullin, Gorlin, and Lassiter (1986) described an earmold designed for simultaneous use with a stethoscope and BTE. The earmold (lucite or soft) accepts the plastic tips (i.e., lug) of stethoscopes. For this earmold design, the rubber tips of the stethoscope are removed and the ends of the stethoscope are inserted into 6.4 mm holes drilled in the earmolds. Peck (1986) described a similar earmold ("stethomold") that does not require the stethoscope's plastic tip to be removed. These earmold designs are available from a number of the earmold laboratories listed in Table 6–4.

PATRIOT™ MOLD

This was introduced by Emtech Laboratories as a means to control feedback and is available from several earmold laboratories. The Patriot™ uses E-Compound™ material and is unique in that the earmold is hollow in the canal area that reportedly enables it to move with face and jaw movement. The fitting range is reportedly up to 110 dB HL at 250 to 4000 Hz. The manufacturer requests the audiologist to use a cotton otoblock, silicone material, and to have the patient chew while the ear impression is made.

## Other Issues Related to Earmolds

ATTENUATION OR SEALING CAPACITY OF EARMOLDS

As stated earlier, earmolds are designed to provide (1) an adequate seal, (2) comfort, (3) appropriate gain throughout the entire frequency range, (4) prevention of feedback, and (5) prevention of the sensation that the earmold is "blocking" the ear (i.e., occlusion effect). Macrae (1990, 1991), in a series of studies, reminded us that the seal provided by earmolds and shells has become increasingly important as the microphone has gotten closer to the receiver, and for patients with severe to profound losses who require greater gain and output.

Sound can propagate through the earmold, vibrate the earmold as a whole, radiate through tissues, cartilage, or bone surrounding the ear canal, and pass through the air pathway between the earmold and the walls of the ear canal via unintentional slit leaks. Some of these paths of propagation can cause feedback. The presence of feedback results in the need for the patient to reduce the volume control setting, which results in inadequate amplification. Another outcome of these problems may be unintentional attenuation of low-frequency amplification, which is necessary for patients with severe to profound hearing loss who need as much low-frequency amplification as possible. For these patients, there is a need for earmolds with minimal pathway for leaks between the sides of the earmold and walls of the ear canal. The ability to achieve this goal depends upon the impression material and technique, as well as the earmold material and style.

To evaluate static pressure seal, Macrae (1990) used an immittance meter attached to the tubing and earmold. With the air pump and manometer connected to the tubing of the earmold, pressure was increased to 200 daPa and maintained for 5 seconds. During this time, the subject was encouraged to talk to determine if jaw movements broke the seal. If there was no loss of pressure in five seconds, it was concluded that the earmold created an adequate static pressure seal. He evaluated two impression materials (silicone and dental impression) and four earmold materials (hard acrylic, silicone rubber, polyvinyl chloride, and Microlite). For 16 subjects, he found that 12 of the 128 earmold combinations provided an adequate seal and, for those earmolds that did provide an adequate seal, the average length and width of the ear canal was larger. Thus, he felt that the dimensions of the ear canal may be a better predictor of maintaining an adequate seal than the impression or earmold materials. He concluded that, because only 12 earmolds provided an adequate seal, the chance of sealing the ear with a two-stage earmold process with only a general buildup of the earmold was small. Also, using different impression material or earmold materials did not significantly improve the chances.

In another experiment, Macrae (1991) ordered two earmolds for one impression. He concluded that this method did not improve the chances of maintaining a static seal. In a final experiment, he "patted down" the surface of the impression material after it was syringed into the ear, but before the impression set. He then asked the earmold laboratory to apply a wax buildup to the impression with a hot wax knife. The results of this experiment revealed that "patting down" the impression did not increase the probability of a seal, but the special buildup did increase the probability of maintaining an adequate seal. In fact, in

55% of the cases, a buildup applied to the impression at the earmold laboratory resulted in an adequate seal. He also found that earmolds with round tips are more likely to seal than those with more elliptical tips.

As mentioned earlier, unintentional leaks can occur around the periphery of the earmold. Some estimate that the average leak is equivalent to the presence of a 1.4 mm vent. Lybarger (1979) reported that a vent this wide will have minimal effect on the output of a hearing aid coupled to an unvented earmold. However, when a unintentional leak is presented around an already vented earmold, low-frequency transmission is increased and the effectiveness of the vent is diminished (Cox, 1979).

Frank (1980) compared the performance of lucite and vinylflex earmolds (shell and skeleton) with and without the presence of a tragus lock against the performance of an E-A-R disposable foam earmold. In 20 subjects, he found that the custom earmolds provided approximately 17 dB less attenuation than the E-A-R disposable foam earmold. In addition, he warned against the commonly held belief that an earmold provides adequate hearing protection. The custom earmolds revealed a mean noise reduction rating of 3.3 dB, while the E-A-R disposable foam earmold had a mean noise reduction rating of 18.2 dB.

Letowski, Burchfield, and Hume (1991) evaluated the attenuation of silicone and lucite earmolds on real ears and KEMAR. They reported that silicone earmolds provided greater attenuation than lucite earmolds with differences ranging from 13 dB at 500 Hz to 3 to 4 dB at 4000 Hz.

Trychel and Haas (1989) used Bekesy tracking procedures at 250 to 8000 Hz on four subjects in which a hearing aid was coupled to silicone and lucite earmolds manufactured in several styles (regular, shell, nonoccluding, and skeleton). In 85% of the comparisons, silicone provided greater attenuation. Also, the regular earmold design provided the greatest attenuation in 63% of comparisons, followed by the shell, skeleton, and nonoccluding earmolds. They cautioned that the audiologist should not overfit a regular or shell earmold because these styles provide greater high frequency attenuation and theoretically could have a deleterious effect on word recognition in noise.

Parker, Okpojo, Nolan, Combe, and Bamford (1992) compared two forms of commercially available silicone impression materials (Amsil™ and Otoform™) to determine differences in accuracy and stability. They used several earmold materials (hard acrylic, soft acrylic, Otofozm™, Amsil™, and Molloplast™) on 27 subjects with severe to profound hearing loss. They found that Otoform™ provided about 4 dB greater attenuation than Amsil™. They also suggested that using silicone impression material may improve hearing aid fittings by reducing the likelihood of feedback due to improved attenuation and acoustic seal.

MAXIMUM REAL-EAR GAIN

For patients with severe to profound hearing loss, the audiologist wants to select an earmold that will provide the greatest useable gain prior to feedback. Madell and Gendel (1984) reminded us that hearing aids, at that time, were available that provided maximum gain in excess of 60 dB and SSPL90, which was greater than 130 dB. For these patients, these authors believe that a soft (vinyl or silicone) earmold used with double-walled tubing, is the most suitable because it provides the tightest fit and offers the greatest retention and, therefore, the greatest useable gain.

Kuk (1994) reported on the maximum usable real ear gain for 10 occluding earmolds (regular with helix lock and #13 tubing; shell with helix lock; canal, skeleton without helix lock; skeleton with helix lock; CROS with extended canal; CROS with partial IROS vent; tube mold; and the Oticon E43 earmold designed for patients with hearing loss above 2000 Hz). Kuk reported there is a tendency among audiologists to believe that a bulkier earmold (regular or shell) will result in greater user gain than those with less bulk (canal or skeleton). His findings revealed that the greatest real-ear gain was achieved by the skeleton and shell earmolds followed by the canal and regular earmold. Further, he reported that the average high-frequency gain was 44 dB for the skeleton and canal earmold, 46 dB for the shell earmold, and 40 dB for the regular earmold. In addition, he reported little advantage of using the helix lock because this addition resulted in increased difficulty in correctly inserting the earmold into the ear canal, increased user discomfort, and increased the possibility of feedback.

EARMOLD DESIGN AND WORD RECOGNITION

As mentioned earlier, past research has implied that earmold designs may have an effect on improved word recognition scores. Northern and Hatler (1970) and Hodgson and Murdock (1972) could not demonstrate significant differences in word recognition scores between unvented and vented earmolds in 18 subjects with high-frequency hearing loss. Similar findings were reported by Revoile (1968) using W-22 and CNC word lists at a –6 dB SNR to evaluate 4 earmold designs (regular with a narrow bore; hollow cavity with a 5.6 mm diameter bore; regular with a diagonal vent of 1.9 mm near the base; and regular with a diagonal vent of 2.2 mm near the base). However, many of the subjects thought the vented earmold provided greater comfort.

If greater gain is desired by the audiologist, then the following suggestions may be beneficial. First, if the pinna is hard, use a softer earmold material. Second, useable gain can be increased by using a lucite body with a soft canal. Third, consider using one of the "newer" earmold materials where the material expands in response to the heat of the ear canal. Examples include the JB1000, MSL90, Audtex, M2000, or Patriot™ earmolds, which are available from a number of earmold manufacturers (see Table 6–4). Fourth, order an earmold with a long bore that will reduce the likelihood of the occlusion effect and feedback, while at the same time, allow the patient the opportunity to achieve greater useable gain. Finally, the earmold design should allow the tip of the earmold to be round and face the eardrum and not the ear canal wall. If the tip of the earmold faces the ear canal wall, it will reflect sound back and cause feedback.

## Problems With Earmolds

IMPRESSIONS AND THE PRESENCE OF PERFORATIONS

Occasionally, audiologists will observe an eardrum perforation during otoscopic observation while in the process of taking an earmold impression. This should present some concerns for at least two reasons. First, the audiologist clearly needs to select the appropriate block so that the impression material does not pass through the perforation into the middle ear space or expand the width of the perforation. Either event would cause discomfort and increase the possibility of middle ear infection. The second concern is related to the possibility that the presence of the earmold in the ear canal will enhance the probability of creating middle ear infections. Alvord, Doxey, and Smith (1989) reported that placement of earmolds in the ear canal will increase the risk of infection because the earmold reduces normal ventilation by creating a warm and moist environment for infectious growth. They also stated that bacteria may be introduced by the earmold or the earmold can induce allergic, irritating, or foreign body reactions. They evaluated six subjects with perforations. Four of the six subjects had a regular earmold with no vent, and two subjects had a regular earmold with a 2-mm vent. Their greatest success was with subjects with smaller perforations and vented earmolds. Also, the authors reported that pressure vents of 1 mm or less did not solve the problem and often became plugged. They suggested counseling patients on not using earmolds full time to provide ventilation during times when communication needs are less stressful.

ALLERGIES TO IMPRESSION AND EARMOLD MATERIALS

Occasionally, patients will report that use of the earmold or shell will cause discomfort to the ear or ear canal. Cockerill (1987) reported on patient allergic reactions to earmold materials. He wanted to determine if patient complaints of allergic reactions to earmolds were related to "true" allergic reactions or were due to irritation caused by a tight fit, surface roughness, lack of hygiene, or simple inflammation due to constant tissue coverage.

Often, the acrylic resins used in the manufacture of earmolds are in the form of a powder (polymer) and liquid (monomer). Polymerization is the process whereby the monomer is converted into a polymer or the solid end-product. The main component of both the polymer and monomer is methyl methacrylate, with other ingredients being hydroquinine, dibutylphthalate, and benzoyl-peroxide acting as inhibitors, activators, and catalysts. Nonallergic materials may be vulcanite, silicone rubber, gold, and polyvinyl chloride (PVC), which is usually in the form of a thin coat brushed over the earmold or shell.

Cockerill (1987) evaluated 25 subjects who were divided into three subgroups. Group 1 were subjects who reported other skin problems, but did not report problems relating to the earmold. Group 2 contained subjects who had or had a history of external otitis or seborrheic dermatitis. Subjects in Group 3 had or encountered otorrhea and had persistent reactions to earmolds. He performed skin patch tests and found reactions to eight substances specifically related to the ingredients used in earmolds. Reactions ranged from dry itchy skin with a slight inflammation of the concha to painful edema of the pinna, cheek, or neck area, which prevented the use of the earmold. Fourteen subjects (55%) showed a reaction to methyl methacrylate. One subject (4%) had a reaction to vulcanite, and two subjects (8%) had a reaction to polyvinyl chloride.

Meding and Ringdahl (1992) reported 22 subjects who had long-standing and severe dermatitis in the ear canal. Patch testing indicated that nine subjects had

15 positive reactions in the standard series. Six patients (27%) had contact allergy to the earmold materials. Four of these six patients had a reaction to methyl methacrylate (sensitizer), and two also had a reaction to ethyleneglycol dimethacrylate and triethyleneglycol dimethacrylate. The diagnosis was allergic contact dermatitis in seven cases and seborrheic dermatitis in six other cases. For the remaining nine subjects, the diagnosis was not obvious, although irritation from occlusion was probable. These authors recommended making another impression using less monomer (liquid) or silicone material. They also recommended consideration for a bone conduction hearing aid and patch testing in cooperation with dermatologists.

When a patient reports an allergic reaction to earmold or shell materials from previous experiences or due to current soreness of the ear, a polyethylene earmold should be ordered in either white or pink opaque colors.

## THE ELDERLY

Fitting the elderly can create some special concerns. One of these concerns is manual dexterity and its effect upon ease of insertion of the earmold. Meredith and colleagues (1989) evaluated three groups of elderly patients with 20 subjects per group. For each group, they compared ease of handling, comfort, and the general effectiveness of the half shell, skeleton, and skeleton without the tragus notch. Results indicated that the skeleton with the tragus notch removed provided the greatest benefit in all three areas. However, the removal of the tragus notch did increase the possibility of feedback, and it was suggested that this mold would only be appropriate for low-gain hearing aids. Other generic problems associated with correctly inserting earmolds by the elderly population in this study included: (1) placing the tragus notch outside the crus of the tragus rather than underneath; (2) the presence of the concha rim, heel, and helix lock prevented easy insertion into the antitragus and antihelix areas; (3) inserting earmolds back to front or upside down; and (4) incorrect placement of the BTE hearing aid over the ear.

## FEEDBACK

In the beginning of the chapter, the authors stated that a "successful" hearing aid fitting would be one where there was no feedback present in the useable range of the volume control wheel.

There are a number of solutions available to combat the problem of feedback. Some have been discussed earlier, which may include the sealing ability of the earmold, special earmold designs and materials, dampers, and the depth of insertion of the sound bore. To combat feedback the audiologist might also consider:

1.  Using antifeedback kits where sleeves (available in four sizes) are snugly fit over the earmold or shell and cemented in place. This strategy has disadvantages because the sleeves are often uncomfortable, develop "ripples," fall off, or cause allergic reactions.

2.  Applying a "soft seal" liquid around the surface of the shell or earmold to reduce or eliminate the spaces between the earmold or shell and the canal wall. Other types of "sealing" compounds include (a) soft or hard Addco Addon for a minor buildup of soft or hard earmolds; (b) Adcobuild for a

major buildup; (c) Addco Sheen, which is applied over Adcobuild products as a sealer to prevent discoloration.

3.  Applying ER-13R E-A-R Ring Seal Kit or "seal rings" around the shell or earmold with tetrahydrofuron (C4H8O) in small quantities. They are available in sizes of 8 mm, 10 mm, 12 mm, 14 mm, 16 mm, 20 mm, and 22 mm.

4.  Using a ER-13MF microphone filter kit, which reportedly reduces gain by 10 to 15 dB at 5000 to 10,000 Hz.

5.  Remaking the impression for a new earmold or shell because the original earmold or shell was too loose.

6.  Narrowing the diameter of the vent if using any of variable venting schemes, which will be discussed later.

7.  Decreasing the overall gain and/or output.

8.  Placing a damper along the transmission line or in the vent.

9.  Electronically reducing high-frequency gain via a high-cut potentiometer, feedback reduction circuit, or feedback notch filter, which are available from a number of ITE and ITC manufacturers. One additional possibility is using digital feedback suppression, which was recently introduced by Danavox, Inc.

10. Making sure the opening from the receiver of the ITE or ITC is not facing the canal wall. This will result in reflection of the amplified sound off the canal wall and induce feedback. The same can be suggested as a cause for feedback with an earmold in a BTE fitting.

11. Ordering all ITE and ITC hearing aids with receiver extension tube (see Fig. 6–26). This places the output closer to the eardrum and typically results in a lower volume control setting. The lower setting typically results in the patient using less overall gain and, thus, reduces the chances for feedback. In our clinic, receiver extension tubes are ordered for all ITE and ITC fittings. An additional benefit of using receiver extension tubing is reducing the possibility that the receiver will be clogged with cerumen because the opening of the tubing is further away from the receiver.

OCCLUSION EFFECT

Again, as stated earlier in this chapter, one of the goals for a "successful" fitting is eliminating the sensation that the patient's head is "at the bottom of a barrel," which is commonly referred to as the occlusion effect (OE). Killion (1988d) and Revit (1992) reported that placing an earmold or shell in the ear canal can amplify the patient's own voice by 20 to 30 dB in the lower frequencies. Further, Revit (1992) reminded us that only a 10 dB increase results in a doubling of the perceived loudness of a signal. In this case, inserting the earmold or shell in the ear canal can cause the perceived loudness to be four times as great in comparison to when the hearing aid is not in the ear canal. This perceived increased in loudness is especially true for the closed vowels /i/ (ee) and /u/ (oo).

Westermann (1987) measured the OE and reported it was 4 to 10 dB at 200 Hz, 2 to 24 dB at 300 Hz, 11 to 17 dB at 400 Hz, and –1 to 20 dB at 500 Hz. When a 2-mm vent was introduced to the earmold, the trapped sound in the ear canal was

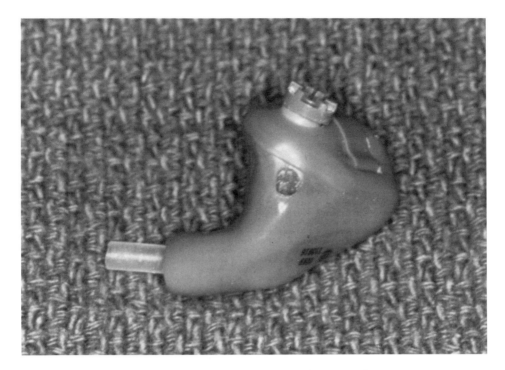

**Figure 6–26.**   Use of extended receiver tube on an ITC hearing aid.

"short-circuited" and the subject reported that his voice sounded more natural. Wimmer (1986) reported an overall OE of about 20 dB at 250 to 500 Hz for an occluded earmold on four ears. The mean OE was 22 dB at 250 Hz, 15 dB at 500 Hz, and 6 dB at 1000 Hz. When a 3-mm vent was added, it decreased the OE by 19 dB at 250 Hz, 6 dB at 500 Hz, and 0 dB at 1000 Hz. Staab and Finlay (1991) report that the OE can be 13 to 21 dB for an ITE and 20 dB for a deeply inserted ITC.

In the past, the only tool the audiologist had in dealing with the OE had been subjective reports by the patient because objectively measuring the OE was a challenge. However, Revit (1992) reported on how a real-ear analyzer could perform spectrum analysis of externally generated signals, with and without the hearing aid in place, to objectively measure the OE. First, the patient is asked to vocalize a sustained vowel ("eee" or "ou"), which is self-monitored at 70 dB (A) on a sound level meter held 1 meter from the lips (see the thicker line in the upper graph of Fig. 6–27). With the hearing aid in place, but turned off, the procedure is repeated (see the thin line in the upper graph of Fig. 6–27). The difference between the two measures, or the OE, is displayed as "insertion gain" in the lower graph of Fig. 6–27. For this patient, approximately 15 dB of OE is seen at 800 to 900 Hz. At this point, the audiologist can attempt several steps described below and repeat the measures to determine if the lower graph can be reduced to as close to 0 dB as possible.

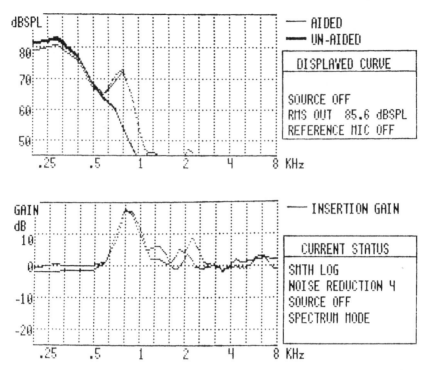

**Figure 6–27.** Measurement of the occlusion effect using a real-ear analyzer. The upper graph displays the spectrum of an /ou/ sound measured in the ear canal without the hearing aid in place (dark line). The light line displays the spectrum of the same sound, but with the hearing aid in place and the volume control turned off. The lower graph displays the resulting occlusion effect.

REDUCING THE OCCLUSION EFFECT

One way to reduce or eliminate the OE is to apply venting of the earmold or shell to reduce low-frequency amplification. For example, a 2-mm vent can decrease the measured SPL at 200 Hz by 8.5 dB. Dempsey (1990) reported that venting options to reduce the OE in ITCs are limited due to space restrictions and the close proximity of the microphone and receiver and the resulting problems of feedback. Usually, vent diameter in ITCs is limited to 2 to 3 mm and, therefore, reducing the OE via venting is limited. In this study, shells for ITEs and ITCs were manufactured for 10 subjects, and 1.5 to 3 mm vents were introduced. The mean OE was 5.4 dB for the ITEs and 8.6 dB for the ITCs with the vents in place.

Another method for reducing the OE is making a silicone impression and placing a cotton otoblock beyond the second bend of the ear canal in the osseous segment of the ear canal to provide the patient with a deep canal fitting (Killion, Wiber, and Gudmunsen, 1988). In addition, it is important to allow jaw movement during the impression and ask the patient to yawn when removing the impression in order to reduce the effect of the vacuum created by the deep impression technique. Also, the audiologist should request a parallel pressure vent of 0.05 to 1.5 mm. Revit (1992) reported a 15 dB reduction in the OE at 200 Hz when the patient was fit with a deeply inserted foam tip in comparison to a medium-length bore that was seated in the cartilaginous portion of the ear canal. Staab and Finlay (1991) reported that a properly seated deep canal fitting where the tip is sealing the ear canal can reduce the OE by 19 to 22 dB at 200 Hz in comparison to a medium-length fit.

COMPLETELY-IN-THE-CANAL (CIC) HEARING AIDS

A recent development to partly address the issue of reducing the OE has been the completely-in-the-canal (CIC) hearing aid (Northern, Kepler, and Gabbard, 1991; Roesel, 1994). In these hearing aids, the visible end of the hearing aid is 1 to 2 mm inside the opening of the ear canal. On the other hand, as described earlier, a deep canal hearing aid or earmold is simply one in which the tip of the shell or earmold is very close to the eardrum (i.e., past the second bend into the osseous portion of the ear canal). The reported advantages of the CIC include (a) cosmetic appeal, (b) reduction of the OE, (c) lower requirements for coupler gain and output to achieve the same real ear gain, and (d) increased gain of 5 dB at the lower frequencies and increased gain of 13 dB at 4000 Hz. Because of the reduced volume of air, the CIC will produce 9 dB greater output than an ITE and 20 dB greater output at the eardrum than is measured in a 2-cc coupler at 4000 Hz. The increased gain occurs because of the deep placement of the shell, whereas the increased output occurs from the increase in gain plus the increased SPL at the higher frequencies resulting from the deep concha placement of the microphone. Thus, a CIC fitting requires less coupler gain and output to achieve the same level of real-ear performance for an ITE or ITC (Gudmundsen, 1994).

Agnew (1994) also reported that the CIC provides less distortion and better sound quality due to its higher amplifier headroom capabilities. He also reported the elimination of wind noise due to the deep placement of the microphone and better use of the telephone without feedback. In agreement with past research, Agnew reported that the volume between the shell and the eardrum can be as small as 0.25 cc, which may result in a 12 dB increase in SPL at the eardrum, relative to an ITE fit where the same volume might be 1.0 cc. This may represent as much as a four-fold decrease in volume from an ITE to CIC fitting. Agnew reported that peak gain, as measured in KEMAR, increased from 20 dB to 45 dB as the volume was reduced from 2.0 to 0.12 cc.

Preves (1994) reported that a long bore length (mean of 22.4 mm) provided an average of 6.4 dB greater overall real-ear root mean square (RMS) output when compared to the RMS output measured for five bore lengths that were significantly shorter (mean = 15.2 mm). He reported a 6 dB difference in the higher frequencies and a 3 to 4 dB difference in the lower frequencies. In addition, he found that there is a 4.4 dB mean overall RMS advantage for the CIC microphone inlet position compared to the typical ITE microphone inlet position. Finally, he reported that the overall RMS output SPL for coupler to real-ear differences (RECD) for the CIC is 25.3 dB, whereas for the ITC it is 17.0 dB and for the ITE it is 11 dB. On average, the CIC provided 8 dB and 14 dB more output SPL than the ITC and ITE, respectively. Thus, a CIC fitting would require 14.3 dB less overall gain than an ITE and 8.3 dB less overall gain than an ITC, as measured in a 2-cc coupler.

MINIMAL CONTACT TECHNOLOGY (MCT)

Another method for reducing the OE has been the recent introduction of Minimal Contact Technology (MCT) by Emtech Laboratories for earmolds and shells. This earmold design reportedly reduces contact between most of the earmold body and the cartilaginous portion of the ear canal. The only point of contact between the body of the earmold and the ear canal wall is the bony portion of the ear canal. The fitting range is reportedly up to 60 dB HL at 250 to 1000 Hz and 90 dB HL at 2000 to 4000 Hz. This earmold is made with E-Compound, which has been described earlier, and the bore length must be between 15 to 20 mm long.

Bryant, Mueller, and Northern (1991) evaluated eight subjects fit with ITEs manufactured with a conventional shell and a MCT shell. The subjects were asked to wear the aids for four weeks and provide their judgments. Real ear insertion responses were equivalent for both sets of aids with the exception of 4000 Hz, where an average of 12 dB greater gain was reported with the shell made with MCT material. All eight subjects reported that the MCT earmold was initially more difficult to insert and remove. Also, most subjects reported that their voices sounded more natural with the MCT shells. The authors measured OE using real-ear measures while asking the subjects to sustain the /ee/, /um/, /oo/, and /ah/ sounds at a level of 90 dB SPL. They reported that the OE was smaller for the MCT shells for the closed vowels (ee, um, oo), but there was little difference between the shells for the open vowel (ah). The differences in OE varied from 10 dB for the /um/ and 4 dB for the /ee/.

## Venting

### Introduction

It is the belief of the authors that virtually every hearing aid fit should have some degree of venting. Dillon (1991) reminded us of the many roles of venting. First, the vent allows some of the low-frequency amplified sound to dissipate outside the ear canal instead of contributing to the sound pressure level buildup at the eardrum. The vent will reduce low-frequency gain and output relative to a closed earmold fitting. Second, the vent allows unamplified signals to enter the ear canal through the vent. This results in less attenuation of the low frequencies and greater attenuation for the higher frequencies. Third, the volume of the vent tube combines with the cavity of the ear canal to produce a Helmholtz resonator to create a vent associated resonant frequency at 250 to 1000 Hz. At the vent-associated resonant frequency, the vented mold provides greater gain than would have been present if the vent were blocked. Fourth, the vent can reduce or eliminate the occlusion effect. Other advantages of venting include providing pressure release to prevent a sensation of pressure buildup near the eardrum and ventilation to minimize the buildup of moisture in the ear canal.

On a negative note, the presence of a vent can allow the amplified sound in the ear canal to pass back to the hearing aid microphone and lead to suboscillatory (heard by the patient as a "ringing," but not heard by the audiologist) or oscillatory (heard by the audiologist, family members, and, perhaps, the patient) feedback. As vent size increases, the amount of acoustic leakage increases and the probability of feedback heightens. Oscillatory feedback will occur at any frequency when the attenuation along the feedback path is less than the gain of the hearing aid in the ear canal. In BTE fittings, the gain has to be greater or the attenuation along the path less, because the length of the path from the ear canal to the microphone of the hearing aid is greater than it is for an ITE or ITC fitting. Even for vents slightly smaller than this critical size, feedback will produce an additional peak in the frequency response and add a "ringing" or transient tone to the sound quality. For many low- to medium-gain hearing aids, it is necessary to specify a vent large enough to minimize the OE, but small enough to avoid feedback.

## Effect of Vent Diameter

PRESSURE EQUALIZATION

As a general guideline, a pressure vent is approximately 0.06 to 0.8 mm and it will have no measurable effect upon the frequency response. Kuk (1994) reported that the pressure vent changed the low-frequency real-ear response by 1 to 6 dB. For a medium length bore (16.6 mm), Lybarger (1977, 1979, 1980) suggested a pressure equalization vent diameter of 0.64 mm (#72 drill). Use of a 1.0-mm vent will be too wide because it will change the low-frequency response for earmolds with a short bore length (see Table 6 to 5). Even "tight" earmolds will provide some degree of "slit leak," which will attenuate the frequency response around 100 Hz by 6 dB and be reduced to 0 dB of attenuation at 250 Hz (Lybarger, 1979).

LOW-FREQUENCY ENHANCEMENT

Lybarger (1977, 1979) reported that measurements of venting on 2-cc couplers have shown an increase of low-frequency gain as vent diameter increases. However, when the measurements were performed on a Zwislocki coupler, the increase in low-frequency gain was not as apparent (Studebaker, Cox, and Wark, 1978; Lybarger, 1979). As seen in Table 6 to 5, With the same 16.6 mm bore length described above, a 1.0-mm vent will increase gain at 250 to 300 Hz with little effect on the frequency response above 500 Hz. A 2.0 mm vent will result in greater low-frequency attenuation below 500 Hz and increased gain between 500 to 700 Hz. A 3.0 mm will not provide amplification above the vent-associated resonance, but will provide greater attenuation below 550 Hz. Similar low-frequency enhancement is seen for long (22.0 mm) and short (12.2 mm) bore lengths.

MODERATE LOW-FREQUENCY REDUCTION

A 2.0-mm vent will provide considerable low-frequency reduction below 500 Hz, depending upon the length of the sound bore (see Table 6–5). Also, as the vent size increases, there will be an increase in the height of the vent- associated resonance. To reduce or eliminate the undesired peak, Lybarger (1977, 1979, 1980) recommended placing light cloth damping over the lateral end of the vent.

**Table 6–5.**  Vent Minus Unvented Response (dB) for Simulated Earmolds Using Parallel and Diagonal Vents (1–3 mm) with Bore Lengths (L) of 6.0 mm, 12.2 mm, 16.6 mm, and 22 mm and Bore Diameters (D) of 1.0 mm, 2.0 mm, and 3.0 mm as Measured in a DB 100 Coupler

| | | | | | | | Parallel Vents | | | | | |
|---|---|---|---|---|---|---|---|---|---|---|---|---|
| Bore L | 6.0 | | | 12.2 | | | 16.6 | | | 22.0 | | |
| Vent D | 1 | 2 | 3 | 1 | 2 | 3 | 1 | 2 | 3 | 1 | 2 | 3 |
| Freq (Hz) | | | | | | | | | | | | |
| 200 | −8 | −22 | −29 | −2 | −17 | −25 | 0 | −15 | −23 | 2 | −14 | −22 |
| 250 | – | – | – | 4 | −13 | −20 | 6 | −11 | −19 | 6 | −10 | −18 |
| 315 | – | – | – | 7 | −8 | −16 | 6 | −6 | −14 | 5 | −4 | −13 |
| 400 | 8 | −9 | −16 | 5 | −2 | −12 | 4 | 0 | −10 | 3 | 3 | −8 |
| 500 | 6 | −2 | −11 | 3 | 6 | −6 | 2 | 9 | −4 | 2 | 9 | −2 |
| 630 | – | – | – | 2 | 9 | 1 | 1 | 5 | 5 | 1 | 5 | 6 |
| 800 | 1 | 5 | 1 | −1 | 3 | 4 | 1 | 2 | 3 | 0 | 1 | 1 |
| 1000 | 1 | 4 | 1 | 1 | 3 | 3 | 1 | 3 | 3 | 0 | 2 | 2 |
| 1250 | 1 | 3 | 4 | 0 | 2 | 4 | 0 | 2 | 4 | 0 | 1 | 3 |
| 1600 | 0 | 2 | 3 | 0 | 1 | 3 | 0 | 1 | 2 | 0 | 1 | 2 |

| | Diagonal Vents | | | | | |
|---|---|---|---|---|---|---|
| Bore L | | 16.6 | | | 22.0 | |
| Vent D | 1 | 2 | 3 | 1 | 2 | 3 |
| Freq (Hz) | | | | | | |
| 200 | −6 | −15 | −21 | −8 | −17 | −23 |
| 250 | 0 | −11 | −17 | −2 | −13 | −20 |
| 315 | 6 | −4 | −11 | 4 | −6 | −13 |
| 400 | 6 | 3 | −5 | 5 | 1 | −7 |
| 500 | 3 | 6 | 2 | 2 | 4 | 2 |
| 630 | 1 | 2 | 3 | 0 | 0 | −1 |
| 800 | 0 | 0 | −1 | −1 | −2 | −3 |
| 1000 | −1 | −1 | −2 | −1 | 0 | −4 |
| 1250 | −1 | −2 | −4 | −2 | −4 | −6 |
| 1600 | −1 | −2 | −5 | −3 | −5 | −8 |

For the two diagonal configurations, vent length was 11.9 mm, while the bore length medial to the intersection was 6.3 mm and 11.7 mm, respectively, for the 16.6 mm and 22 mm conditions.

(+) measured SPL is greater.

(–) measured coupler SPL is less.

Lybarger, 1985; Mueller et al., 1992.

STRONG LOW-FREQUENCY REDUCTION

As a general rule, a medium size vent is 1.6 to 2.4 mm wide. A vent this wide will reduce amplification below 500 Hz and result in a vent-associated resonance that will increase amplification at 500 to 1000 Hz. As a general rule, a large size vent is 3.2 to 4.0 mm, which will reduce amplification below 500 Hz, and its vent-associated resonance will increase amplification at 500 to 1000 Hz (see Table 6–5). A wide-short vent will provide strong low-frequency reduction. Extreme low-frequency reduction will occur with an open or nonoccluding earmold. The magnitude of low-frequency reduction will be 25 dB at 250 Hz with a cutoff at 500 Hz. For a long bore (22 mm), there will be an 18 dB reduction at 250 Hz, and the cutoff frequency begins at 800 Hz (Lybarger, 1977, 1979, 1980; Staab and Nunley, 1982).

EXTREME LOW-FREQUENCY REDUCTION

For patients with normal hearing up to 1500 Hz, the use of a tube fitting would be very appropriate because it provides the greatest low-frequency reduction and greatest high-frequency enhancement. For maximum benefit of this strategy, the diameter of the tubing be should wide and the depth of insertion minimal.

LENGTH AND DIAMETER OF VENTS

The length of the vent is related to the length of the bore and is not really the critical factor in decisions concerning vents. However, as a general rule, as bore length increases, there is less low-frequency attenuation when vent diameter is held constant (see Table 6–5). The crucial decision is usually the diameter of the vent. Chasin (1983b) reported that venting can create a high-frequency antiresonance (notch) that may fall within the frequency range of the hearing aid. All vents have a characteristic vent-associated antiresonance frequency that produces a decrease in gain and whose frequency depends upon the length and volume of the vent. The frequency of this vent-associated antiresonance is inversely related to the effective length of the vent. Shortening the effective length of the vent may increase the frequency of the antiresonance until it is above the frequency response of most hearing aids. As a general rule, for each 1.0 mm decrease in vent length, the frequency of the vent-associated antiresonance is increased by 400 Hz. One effective way to eliminate the vent-associated antiresonance is to bell the vent at the medial side of the earmold.

Another issue related to vent diameter is how much gain is available as the diameter is increased before feedback is present. Lybarger (1977) measured the sound pressure level at a point 2.5 cm from the tip of the earmold in which the length of the sound bore was described as "short." He reported that maximum gain before feedback using a 0.8 mm vent was 43 dB, with a reserve gain of 10 dB. For a 3.2-mm vent, maximum gain before feedback was reduced to 36 dB, with a reserve gain of 10 dB.

Finally, as vent length is decreased, there will be a segment of the frequency response at which there is no further reduction in gain caused by the presence of the vent. This is referred to by some as the high-frequency cutoff. For example, in Table 6–5, when the vent length is 22 mm, the high-frequency cutoff for a 2-mm vent is approximately 315 Hz. However, when the vent is shortened to 6 mm, the high frequency cutoff is increased to approximately 500 Hz. Also, as vent length is decreased, there is increased attenuation of the low-frequency response (Egolf, 1980; Lybarger, 1985; Mynders, 1985). This latter effect also occurs when the vent is widened.

## Types of Venting

DIAGONAL VERSUS PARALLEL VENTING

Aside from deciding the length and/or diameter of the vent, the audiologist needs to inform the earmold laboratory if the vent should run parallel (lower example of Fig. 6–28) to the sound bore or if the vent needs to intersect (i.e., diagonal; see upper example in Fig. 6–28) the sound bore at some point between the

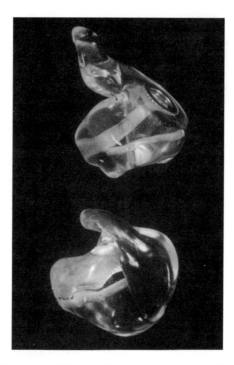

**Figure 6–28.**    Example of diagonal (upper) and parallel (lower) venting.

lateral and medial end. Most research indicates that the primary choice should be a parallel vent because a diagonal vent, relative to a parallel vent, will decrease high-frequency gain by as much as 10 dB and the effect increases as vent diameter increases (see Table 6–5). Most researchers recommend diagonal venting only if space limitations (i.e., narrow ear canal) prevent the use of a parallel vent. If a diagonal vent is the only choice, minimizing high-frequency reduction can be achieved by ordering a shorter bore length or having the vent intersect the sound bore as close to the medial end possible and then belling the final section of the sound bore (Studebaker and Cox, 1977; Cox, 1979; Egolf, 1980; Valente, 1984a; 1984c).

Studebaker and Cox (1977) and Cox (1979) reported the results of measuring the effects of parallel versus diagonal venting on three earmolds measured in a Zwislocki coupler and the real ear. One earmold had a parallel vent of 16.8 mm. The second earmold had a diagonal vent that was 13.2 mm long and intersected the sound bore 7.6 mm from tip of the earmold. The third earmold had a diagonal vent 8.5 mm long and intersected the sound bore 9.5 mm from the tip of the earmold. Results for the parallel vent showed the expected reduction in low-frequency output below 400 Hz, and a vent-associated resonance was seen between 300 to 700 Hz with little high-frequency attenuation. For the first diagonal condition, there was the same low-frequency reduction below 400 Hz, and a vent-associated resonance as was measured with the parallel vent. However, above the vent-associated resonance there was a 3 to 5 dB attenuation of 3000 Hz. For the second diagonal condition, there was greater low-frequency reduction and a similar vent-associated resonance. However, there was a 10 to 11 dB attenuation in output between 2000 Hz to 3000 Hz. Thus, the three venting conditions yielded similar low-frequency reduction and vent-associated resonances, but the diagonal vent revealed high-frequency attenuation that increased as the point of intersection moved more laterally in the sound bore. Above the vent-associated resonant frequency, the parallel vent did not reduce high-frequency gain, whereas the diagonal vent did yield greater reduction in high-frequency transmission as the point of intersection was moved more laterally. The magnitude of the high-frequency loss in diagonal vents is related to the diameter of the vent in relation to the diameter of the sound bore. As seen in Table 6–5, reduction in high-frequency gain increases as the vent diameter increases when vent length is held constant. Further, the loss of high-frequency transmission can be as great as 15 to 20 dB if the diagonal vent intersects the main sound bore at a very lateral position and the diameter of the vent is large (3 mm or greater).

Studebaker and Zachman (1970) reported that as the diameter of the diagonal vent increased (0.75 mm, 1.5 mm, and 3.0 mm) there was (1) greater low-frequency attenuation, (2) a shift in the vent-associated resonance to a higher frequency, (3) amplitude of the vent-associated resonance became greater, and (4) greater reduction in high-frequency transmission. During real ear measures, there was the same low-frequency reduction as was measured in the 2-cc coupler, but the height of the vent-associated resonances was smaller or was not present.

EXTERNAL VENTING

Occasionally, the dimensions of the ear canal will be so small that neither parallel nor diagonal venting can be used. In these cases, a "V-shaped groove" can be cut into the bottom surface of the earmold from the outside to the tip. This method of venting is also suggested in cases where the ear may be draining.

CUSTOM VENTING

For audiologists who prefer to specify the exact length and diameter of venting, Table 6–6 can be used for ordering vent sizes to specify the vent cutoff frequency at either 250, 500, 750, or 1000 Hz. For example, if the audiologist wants the low frequency attenuation to extend to 1000 Hz (i.e., greater low-frequency reduction because the patient has normal or near normal hearing at 1000 Hz and below), he could specify that the bore length should be 8.9 mm and the vent diameter should be 3.0 mm. To achieve the same degree of low-frequency attenuation in an earmold with a shorter bore (i.e., 4.4 mm), the vent diameter would be reduced to 2.1 mm. For example, let us assume the patient has some hearing loss in the lower frequencies and the audiologist wants less low-frequency attenuation. In the case of the patient with the longer bore (8.9 mm), the audiologist would order a vent diameter of 0.8 mm. In the case of the patient with the shorter bore length (4.4 mm), the audiologist would order a vent diameter of 0.5 mm.

## Adjustable Venting

As mentioned earlier, it is the strong belief of the authors that virtually all earmolds/shells should be delivered to the patient with some degree of venting. An

**Table 6-6.** Custom Venting

| Frequency (Hz) | Vent Diameter (mm) | Vent Length (mm) |
|---|---|---|
| 250 | 1.1 | 17.8 |
| | 0.8 | 8.9 |
| | 0.5 | 4.4 |
| 500 | 2.2 | 17.8 |
| | 1.5 | 8.9 |
| | 1.1 | 4.4 |
| 750 | 3.0 | 17.8 |
| | 2.3 | 8.9 |
| | 1.6 | 4.4 |
| 1000 | 4.3 | 17.8 |
| | 3.0 | 8.9 |
| | 2.1 | 4.4 |
| | 1.5 | 2.2 |

Adapted from Microsonic, 1994.

issue to consider is "should the diameter of the vent be fixed or should the audiologist order a method of adjustable venting to better meet the needs of the patient as well as the audiologist?" The next section will discuss several methods to vary the vent diameter at the time of the hearing aid fitting.

VARIABLE VENTING VALVE

Although not commonly used today, Griffing (1971) and Griffing and Shields (1972) introduced the Variable Venting Valve (VVV), which is a gold-plated, brass-tooled threaded valve that is recessed in the earmold in a cavity 4.0 mm deep and 6.4 mm wide. The valve is manipulated by the user to adjust the low-frequency response yielding the most pleasing sound quality for that listening situation. The valve can be rotated 540° from fully open to fully closed. By rotating the valve, the piston is simply moved from a point where it completely seals the 1.5 mm vent to a point where the vent is fully open.

Cooper, Franks, McFall, and Goldstein (1975) reported that the VVV was ineffective in reducing low-frequency gain at 400 to 900 Hz in 12 patients, regardless of whether the earmolds had parallel or diagonal vents. These results are not unexpected in view of the fact that the range of adjusting the diameter of the vent is only 1.5 mm from fully open to fully closed.

SELECT A VENT (SAV)

In the past, audiologists often drilled their own vents on a trial and error basis. Table 6–7 provides guidelines for readers who may wish to drill their own vents and the drill size required to accomplish the task. Figure 6–29 illustrates examples of drill sets used in our facility to vent and modify earmolds and shells. Today, however, most audiologists order earmolds or shells with either PVV, SAV, select-a-tube (Fig. 6–30), or Mini-SAV changeable venting systems, which

**Table 6–7.** Common Drill Sizes and the Resulting Vent Diameter

| Drill Size | Vent Diameter (mm) |
|---|---|
| 31 | 3.17 |
| 33 | 2.93 |
| 47 | 2.00 |
| 53 | 1.57 |
| 61 | 1.00 |
| 65 | 0.89 |
| 68 | 0.79 |
| 70 | 0.72 |
| 75 | 0.54 |
| 76 | 0.51 |
| 80 | 0.35 |

eliminate the trial-and-error methods associated with drilling vent holes. For one manufacturer of ITE hearing aids, the ID of the select-a-tubes are 1.9 mm, 1.6 mm, 1.3 mm, 0.77 mm, and a plug. Variable venting techniques provide the audiologist with greater flexibility to experiment with different vent diameters and their effect upon (a) reducing low-frequency gain, (b) reducing or eliminating the occlusion effect, (c) yielding better sound quality, and (d) reducing or eliminating

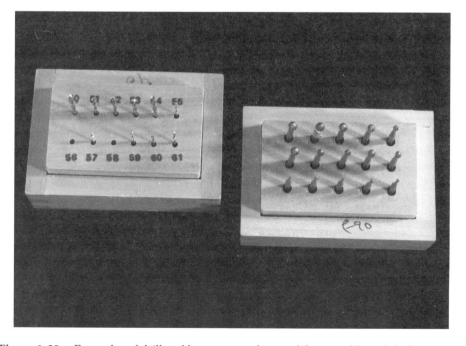

**Figure 6–29.** Examples of drill and burr sets used to modify earmolds and shells.

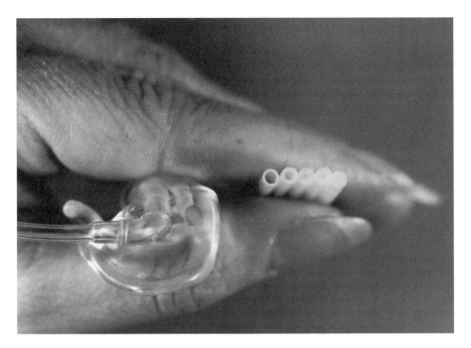

**Figure 6–30.**   Examples of select-a-tube venting.

feedback. This flexibility is permitted by merely inserting different-sized vent plugs (#1 to #5) or tubes that vary in ID and are inserted into a predrilled vent channel.

The SAV comes with a permanently installed clear styrene seating ring and a removable polythylene venting plug, available in a "tree" of five sizes along with a solid plug. The insert channel for the SAV is 4.7 mm deep and 3.6 mm wide. For one manufacturer, the diameters of the SAV inserts are 0.8 mm, 1.6 mm, 2.4 mm, 3.2 mm, and 4.0 mm for inserts #1 through #5, respectively. There is also a #6 insert that is used as a plug to close the vent (see Table 6–8). The SAV is also available from some earmold and hearing aid manufacturers in a mini-SAV format when the sound bore is unusually narrow. For one manufacturer, the diameters of the mini-SAV inserts are 0.5 mm, 0.8 mm, 1.0 mm, 1.6 mm, and 1.9 mm for inserts #1 through #5, respectively. There is also a #6 insert that is used as a plug to close the vent (see Table 6–8). It is important for the reader to understand that the relationship between insert number and the corresponding diameter may be different across manufacturers. In addition, the relationship between insert number and width of the vent may be the reverse from the one described above. That is, in our clinic, the #1 insert has the narrowest diameter and the #6 insert plugs the vent. However, for another manufacturer, the #1 insert may plug the vent and the #6 insert may provide the widest diameter vent.

POSITIVE VENTING VALVE (PVV)

The PVV comes with a permanently installed clear styrene seating ring and a removable polythylene venting plug that is available in a "tree" of five sizes

**Table 6–8.**  Dimensions of Select-a-Vent (SAV), Mini-SAV, and
Positive-Venting-Valve (PVV)

| Type | Inches | mm |
| --- | --- | --- |
| SAV PLUG | | |
| 1 | 0.031 | 0.8 |
| 2 | 0.062 | 1.6 |
| 3 | 0.095 | 2.4 |
| 4 | 0.125 | 3.2 |
| 5 | 0.156 | 4.0 |
| 6 | closed | closed |
| MINI SAV PLUG | | |
| 1 | 0.020 | 0.5 |
| 2 | 0.030 | 0.8 |
| 3 | 0.040 | 1.0 |
| 4 | 0.060 | 1.6 |
| 5 | 0.075 | 1.9 |
| 6 | closed | closed |
| PVV PLUG | | |
| 1 | 0.020 | 0.5 |
| 2 | 0.030 | 0.8 |
| 3 | 0.060 | 1.6 |
| 4 | 0.095 | 2.4 |
| 5 | 0.125 | 3.2 |
| 6 | closed | closed |

Adapted from Microsonic, 1994

along with a solid plug. In comparison to the SAV, the PVV has an insert channel that is shorter and wider (2.5 mm deep and 4.0 mm wide). For one manufacturer, the diameters of the PVV inserts are 0.5 mm, 0.8 mm, 1.6 mm, 2.4 mm, and 3.2 mm for inserts #1 through #5, respectively. There is also a #6 insert, which is used as a plug to close the vent (see Table 6–8). Again, the audiologist needs to be careful because earmold laboratories may offer PVV inserts where the order is reversed (i.e., the smallest number insert has the widest vent size and the largest number insert has the narrowest vent size), and the vent diameters may vary slightly from the diameters provided above.

SAV VERSUS PVV

For both the PVV and SAV systems there is little change in the low-frequency response between inserts #1 to #3. However, some differences in low-frequency reduction will occur between inserts #4 to #5 (Cox, 1979; Lybarger, 1979, 1980, 1985; Valente and DeJonge, 1981; Mynders, 1985; Killion, 1988a). These same researchers favored using the PVV because the PVV uses a shorter and wider insert cup for the vent inserts. These researchers believe that for variable venting systems to work properly, the vent channel must be short and wide so that the vent response will be controlled by the vent hole in the insert rather than the vent channel itself. If the vent channel is long and narrow (i.e., SAV), then changing from one vent insert to another will make little difference in the low-frequency response. It appears that the PVV offers greater low-frequency attenuation because of its shorter and wider insert channel.

Austin, Kasten, and Wilson (1990a; 1990b) reported in separate articles on the differences in real-ear versus 2-cc coupler responses for 47 earmolds with 157 different modifications. They reported that the PVV and SAV revealed very small differences in low-frequency reduction between any insert size and the midfrequency vent-associated resonant peak measured in the coupler was not observed in the real ear. Finally, in agreement with past findings, Austin et al. (1990a and 1990b) concluded that the PVV provides greater low-frequency attenuation than the SAV.

## Additional Issues Associated With Venting

### INTENTIONAL VERSUS UNINTENTIONAL VENTS

The level of the signal reaching the eardrum is a result of combining two paths of sound. One path is the "unaided path" where the signal passes through the vent ("intentional vent") and leaks ("unintentional vent") and reaches the eardrum unaided. The second path is the "aided path" where the intensity level of the signal at the eardrum is provided by the hearing aid. Concurrently, these two paths have some of the amplified sound passing to "the outside" through the same vent and leaks to reduce the sound pressure level at the eardrum in a narrow frequency region. At any frequency in which the intensity of one path exceeds the intensity of other path by 20 dB or more, the path with the lesser intensity has an insignificant effect upon the total intensity at the eardrum (less than 1 dB). However, at any frequency where the two intensities are within 20 dB of each other, the manner in which the two intensities combine depends upon the phase relationship between the two paths. At a frequency where the two paths have equal intensity (often at 250 to 750 Hz), the in-phase addition of the two paths will yield an intensity level that is 6 dB higher than the intensity within each path. At frequencies where the two paths are 180° out of phase, there will be a strong attenuation of the signal. The magnitude of the vent effect is dependent upon the dimensions of the vent, the properties of the ear canal and eardrum, as well as the phase response of the hearing aid. In addition, the presence of vents can sharpen high-frequency resonant peaks so that a rounded response measured in a coupler, with the vent closed, can appear as a sharp peak in the real-ear aided response (Revit, 1994). The degree of "sharpening" of the vent-associated resonant peak from suboscillatory feedback is dependent upon the dimensions of the vent and the ear canal as well as the impedance of the eardrum. One method to reduce the height of the vent-associated resonant peak is to reduce the diameter of the vent.

### SUBOSCILLATORY FEEDBACK

Cox (1982) reported that vented earmolds may cause feedback at lower volume control settings than closed molds. This can prevent the user from achieving the desired gain due to the interference of feedback. In addition, one common practice used by many hearing aid users to adjust the volume control wheel is to rotate the volume control until audible feedback occurs and then "back off" slightly. This strategy may create suboscillatory feedback, which creates a frequency response marked by numerous peaks and troughs. It is clear that the practice of setting the volume control just below the point of audible feedback can have a significant deleterious impact on the frequency response of the hearing aid. If a patient complains that the hearing aid "echoes" or "rings," he is probably experiencing suboscillatory feedback.

ACOUSTIC VERSUS ELECTRONIC LOW-FREQUENCY ATTENUATION

Audiologists can control the low-frequency response via (1) a tone control in combination with a closed mold (electronic tuning) (see Fig. 6–31), (2) use of venting in combination with a hearing aid having a wide-band frequency response (acoustical tuning), or (3) combining strategies 1 and 2 where low-frequency output is controlled by the tone control and the vent may or may not provide additional low-frequency attenuation. The first strategy provides a very efficient way to predict low-frequency attenuation. Use of the second strategy is not as strong in predicting low-frequency attenuation. This second method, as mentioned earlier, adds a midfrequency vent-associated resonant peak and the possibility of altering the frequency response due to audible and suboscillatory feedback, which does not occur with a closed mold.

   Cox and Alexander (1983) recorded speech in KEMAR with a hearing aid coupled to closed molds, vented molds, and open molds with the output from KEMAR matched for the different mold conditions. They used a paired comparison paradigm of sound quality and speech intelligibility judgments for connected discourse presented at 65 dB with signal-to-noise ratios of +5 and +20 dB. They evaluated nine hearing aids, which were divided into 3 groups, depending upon the cutoff frequency (i.e., below 750 Hz, between 750 Hz to 1000, and above 1000 Hz). They evaluated 15 subjects who had normal hearing in the low frequencies and greater hearing loss in the higher frequencies. Results revealed that the subjects had a slight preference for the electronic modification strategy if the cutoff frequency was less than 750 Hz. However, they had a strong preference for the

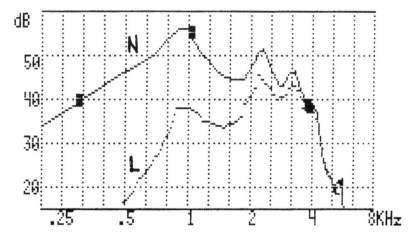

**Figure 6–31.**   Frequency response of a hearing aid when the tone control was rotated for the broadest response (N) and the greatest low-frequency attenuation (L).

acoustic tuning strategy (venting) when the cutoff frequency was between 750 to 1000 Hz and an even greater preference for venting when the cutoff frequency was greater than 1000 Hz. These findings were the same for both signal-to-noise ratio conditions and for sound quality or speech intelligibility judgments.

MacKenzie and Browning (1991) evaluated 83 inexperienced subjects with mild to moderate severe sensorineural hearing loss. When subjects had normal hearing to 1000 Hz, they generally preferred combining venting and high-frequency emphasis to achieve the desired balance between low- and high-frequency amplification rather than only relying on the tone control. For subjects having a flatter audiometric configuration from 250 to 4000 Hz, no consistent preferences were present.

Mackenzie and Browning (1989) reported on real ear measures in 43 ears and found that adjusting the tone control between normal and high-frequency emphasis has less effect in the real ear than in the 2-cc coupler. Adding a 2-mm vent and returning the tone control to the normal position reduced the output by an average of 8 dB at 750 Hz to 1000 Hz. By turning the tone control to high-frequency emphasis and using an earmold with a 2-mm vent, the low-frequency reduction was extended to 10 dB in the same frequency region.

PERCEPTUAL CONSEQUENCE OF VENTS

Lundberg, Ovegard, Hagerman, and colleagues (1992) evaluated nine subjects with normal hearing. They reported no difference in sound quality for vented and unvented earmolds while listening to male and female recordings of connected discourse in quiet and noise. Four subjects reported that the unvented earmolds sounded louder than the vented earmolds, and there was an overall tendency of preferring the sound quality produced by the vented condition.

McClellan (1967), Davis and Green (1975), and Kuk (1991) reported higher word recognition scores in noise when venting was introduced to the earmold. However, Revoile (1968), Hodgson and Murdock (1972), and Northern and Hattler (1970) did not report significant improvement in word recognition scores with the introduction of venting. Kuk (1991) evaluated nine subjects with mild to moderate severe sensorineural hearing loss using unvented and vented (2.2 mm parallel vent) earmolds. Using a paired comparison strategy and a programmable hearing aid, the subjects shaped their preferred real-ear insertion response (REIR) while listening to connected discourse presented at 70 dB SPL. Results indicated that the preferred REIR was similar for the two earmold conditions. However, sound quality for the "clarity" judgment was significantly better for the vented condition. When reading aloud, most subjects preferred the vented condition. No significant differences were found in word recognition scores for W-22 word lists presented at 70 dB SPL. Kuk (1991) concluded that although electronic tuning can be beneficial to assure that measured REIR matches prescribed REIR, venting is necessary to improve user satisfaction.

## Venting in Custom Hearing Aids

Up to this point, the issue of venting has been presented in terms of venting an earmold. Similar decisions need to be made by the audiologist when fitting custom hearing aids. In a custom product, the length of tubing from the output of the receiver to the tip of the shell is typically 10 to 12 mm long and 1 to 2 mm wide (Lybarger, 1985). Preves (1980) described a dual tubing, or stepped bore, arrangement for an ITE that increased the high-frequency response. In this design, the tubing at the receiver is 6.4 mm long and 1.4 mm wide, which increases to a width of 3.6 mm for the second section. In addition, a 2200 ohm fused mesh damper is placed at the receiver to smooth the frequency response. For short bore shells, the 3.6-mm segment of tubing is extended beyond the tip of the shell to maintain the desired acoustic effect. Further increases in the high-frequency response can occur as the diameter of the tubing of the second segment is increased (Staab and Lybarger, 1994). To accommodate the damping needs for ITEs, Knowles Electronics has four dampers that fit into cups with outside diameters of 1.12 mm, 1.25 mm, 1.37 mm, and 1.78 mm to fit inside the narrow ID of tubing used in custom hearing aids from the receiver to the tip of the shell. These dampers are available in acoustic resistances of 330 to 3300 acoustic ohms for the 1.78 mm diameter cup and 680 or 1500 acoustic ohms for 1.25 mm diameter cup. These dampers have a greater effect on smoothing the second peak instead of the first peak, which is common for BTE fittings (Staab and Lybarger, 1994).

Tecca (1991) believes that most of the research on venting for ITEs carefully eliminated slit-leak effects. In actual use, slit leaks are quite common in ITE fittings. He found that the effect of slit leaks are predominantly at 200 Hz (see Table 6–9). He performed real ear measures on 10 subjects whose ear canals had an average ear canal length of 22.6 mm and a mean bore length of 8.2 mm. He used vent diameters of 1.3 mm, 2.0 mm, and 3.0 mm. For the 1.3 and 2.0 mm vents, the attenuation was restricted to below 1000 Hz (see Table 6–9). The attenuation provided by the 3.0 mm vent extended one octave higher (see Table 6–9). When E.A.R. seal rings were used to minimize the effect of slit leak, there was only a slight attenuation of low-frequency gain (see Section B, Table 6–9). In addition, the standard deviation shown in Table 6–9 (0.4 to 4 dB) reveals minimal intersubject variability. Therefore, the ability to predict vent effects for a particular individual is rather good. Finally, as reported before, as vent diameter is increased, there is greater low-frequency attenuation, and the vent-associated resonant frequency increases. Table 6–9 indicates that the vent-associated resonance increased for the 1.3-mm and 2.0-mm vent between the sealed and unsealed conditions, but the effect of sealing was minimal for the 3.0 mm vent.

In another study, Tecca (1992) reported that most variable venting systems for custom hearing aids use vent inserts of varying internal diameters, which are inserted into the lateral end of the vent channel. He evaluated 10 subjects when shells were manufactured having a bore length of 22 mm and vent diameters of 0.45, 0.95, and 1.45 mm. A second condition was where the vent diameter was a constant 2.0 mm and vent lengths were 4.0 mm, 10.0 mm, 16.0 mm, and 22.0 mm. A final condition was where there was a vent diameter of 3 mm and vent length of 4 mm. Results revealed (Section C, Table 6–9) that the degree of attenuation at 200 Hz increased as vent diameter increased from 0.45 mm to 1.45 mm and length was held constant at 22 mm. Minimal attenuation occurred above 200 Hz. When vent diameter was held constant at 2.0 mm, attenuation increased as bore length decreased and the vent-associated resonance increased in frequency. Also,

**Table 6–9.** Mean and Standard Deviation (in parenthesis) of the Real-Ear Vent Effects (dB) for Three Vent Diameters (mm) Relative to the Occluded Condition for ITE Hearing Aids When No Sealing (Section A) or Sealing (Section B) was Placed Around the Shell of the ITE (Tecca, 1991)

| | Frequency (Hz) | | | | |
|---|---|---|---|---|---|
| Diameter | 200 | 500 | 1000 | 1500 | 2000 |
| A. No sealing | | | | | |
| 1.3 mm | –7.1(3.1) | 0.3(2.9) | 1.5(0.7) | 0.5(0.6) | 0.1(0.5) |
| 2.0 mm | –11.1(3.9) | –0.9(3.6) | 1.9(0.9) | 0.7(0.7) | 0.2(0.8) |
| 3.0 mm | –21.9(4.0) | –10.5(3.2) | 3.1(2.8) | 2.6(1.7) | 1.9(0.9) |
| B. Sealing with E.A.R. rings | | | | | |
| 1.3 mm | –6.8(2.2) | 2.8(1.3) | 0.8(0.6) | 0.3(0.4) | –0.2(0.9) |
| 2.0 mm | –12.1(2.5) | 2.2(3.5) | 1.7(0.7) | 0.6(0.7) | 0.3(0.9) |
| 3.0 mm | –25.0(2.6) | –9.8(3.2) | 5.1(2.0) | 2.9(1.4) | 2.0(0.7) |
| C. Diameter (mm) x Length (mm) (Tecca, 1992) | | | | | |
| 0.45 x 22 | –4.9(2.6) | 0.5(2.0) | 0.7(0.8) | 0.1(0.9) | 0.0(0.8) |
| 0.95 x 22 | –9.2(2.0) | 2.8(2.5) | 1.7(0.7) | 0.6(1.1) | 0.5(0.7) |
| 1.45 x 22 | –12.1(2.1) | 1.5(3.9) | 2.3(1.0) | 1.0(1.1) | 0.8(0.7) |
| 2.0 x 22 | –13.9(1.7) | 0.6(4.0) | 2.9(1.3) | 1.4(1.1) | 1.0(0.7) |
| 2.0 x 16 | –15.8(2.3) | –3.7(4.5) | 2.5(1.4) | 0.9(1.2) | 0.3(1.0) |
| 2.0 x 10 | –18.9(2.5) | –7.9(3.7) | 1.8(1.7) | 1.0(1.2) | –0.1(1.5) |
| 2.0 x 4 | –22.6(2.9) | –11.4(4.7) | 0.7(2.0) | 1.5(2.0) | 0.3(1.4) |
| 3.0 x 4 | –24.6(1.8) | –13.4(3.0) | 0.1(2.6) | 2.2(2.2) | 0.9(1.2) |

Section C reports the mean and standard deviation (in parenthesis) of the real-ear vent effects (dB) for five vent diameters (mm) and four lengths (mm) (Tecca, 1992)

differences in the magnitude of low-frequency attenuation between adjacent vent diameters were 3 to 5 dB at 200 Hz and the effect was predominantly below 500 Hz. Recall that Cox and Alexander (1983) suggested using electronic tuning instead of acoustic tuning to enhance user satisfaction when the cutoff frequency was below 750 Hz for venting to result in greater user satisfaction. Finally, Tecca reported that the vent-associated resonance shifted to a higher frequency as vent diameter increased and the mean amplitude varied between 2.0 to 5.1 dB.

Vent diameters for custom hearing aids can also be changed by inserting silicone tubes of different internal diameters into the vent channel (Copeland, Burris, and Griffing, 1986). This, for example, is the method used by ReSound Corporation for their custom hearing aids. This method of venting has the advantage of knowing that the diameter of the selected vent tube is uniform from the lateral to the medial end of the vent channel.

### Miscellaneous

PROBLEMS WITH CERUMEN

One of the most common problems in custom hearing aids is the buildup of cerumen in the tubing from the receiver. The presence of the cerumen will change the electroacoustic characteristics of the hearing aid or attenuate the output so the hearing aid appears "dead." Aside from the need to carefully counsel the patient on this problem and explain preventive measures, several methods have been introduced to help audiologists address this problem.

One recent solution has been the introduction of the Ad-hear™ wax guards (Oliveira and Rose, 1994). These are easy-to-apply disposable filters that stick onto the shell of the hearing aid and are available in three sizes (slim, standard, and large). Between the two adhesive strips is a filter that is placed over the tubing opening from the receiver to prevent cerumen from entering the tubing. Reportedly, the Ad-hear™ wax guards do not change the frequency response of the hearing aid and will last for 1 week before they need to be changed (Oliveira and Rose, 1994). Another solution is a "cerumen filter system." In this case, a small plastic "lid" is pressed into place over the receiver opening. These filters arrive in a pack of 10, and each filter lasts about 1 week.

Audiologists must understand that it is very expensive for manufacturers to replace receivers due to contamination from cerumen. Thus, manufacturers have numerous wax guard options available for audiologists to consider. These options include "wax baskets," "spring dampers," or "element dampers," which are placed in the receiver opening to prevent cerumen from reaching the receiver. These devices are reportedly acoustically transparent in that they do not change the frequency response. However, REIR responses at our facility revealed that using a "wax basket" from one manufacturer decreased the real ear gain around 3000 Hz by nearly 6 dB! Therefore, this facility routinely orders translucent receiver tubing and has it extend 3 mm to 4 mm past the tip of the shell (see Fig. 6–26). This allows the patient to "see" the buildup of cerumen and remove it with a "wax loop" before a buildup creates a problem. In addition, the extended receiver tube places the output from the hearing aid slightly closer to the eardrum. This reduces the volume control setting necessary to achieve a comfortable setting and also reduces the likelihood of feedback.

## Problems and Solutions

Fitting hearing aids can bring pride and satisfaction for audiologists because of the opportunity to make life more enjoyable and satisfactory for their patients. However, the road to successful fittings will not always be smooth and unchallenging. Table 6–10 lists an array of problems brought to our attention from patients. Also provided are some solutions that have been used successfully to address and correct these problems. Sometimes these solutions eliminate the problem and result in greater user satisfaction. Sometimes these solutions only partially solve the problem, but the degree of improvement is sufficient to make the problem less troublesome. On more occasions than we care to admit, the solutions do not solve the problem and the patient feels that the problem is sufficiently great enough to discontinue use of amplification. Also, sometimes the solution to one problem can create a previously nonexistent problem. For example, one solution for eliminating the occlusion effect is to widen the vent. It is entirely possible that this solution could result in feedback. As was mentioned earlier, the road to successful fittings is not always smooth, but it is challenging!

**Table 6–10.**   Trouble-Shooting Chart

| Problem | Possible Solutions |
|---|---|
| 1. Soreness/discomfort | a. Canal/shell modifications<br>b. New impression<br>c. Hypoallergenic material<br>d. Allergy coating (Verglassen) |
| 2. Allergic reaction | a. Coat shell with hypoallergenic nail polish<br>b. Remake impression for Lucite earmold<br>c. Order hypoallergenic material |
| 3. Too tight | a. Grind/buff areas that may be causing the tightness<br>b. New impression |
| 4. Too loose | a. Buildup shell with Addco Addon (soft or hard)<br>b. New impression |
| 5. Hole/crack in shell | a. Patch with polymer–monomer mix |
| 6. Occlusion effect | a. Wider vent diameter<br>b. Provide a deep canal fit<br>c. Bell the bore<br>d. Reduce low-frequency gain<br>e. Use MCT material<br>f. Increase crossover frequency |
| 7. Tinny or harsh | a. Insert filter in receiver or microphone<br>b. Shift high frequencies with a resonant peak control<br>c. Reduce vent and add filter<br>d. Reduce low-frequency gain<br>e. Reduce crossover frequency<br>f. Reduce high-frequency output<br>g. Increase compression ratio<br>h. Reduce high-frequency gain |
| 8. Too much bass | a. Wider vent<br>b. Reduce low-frequency gain<br>c. Increase crossover frequency |
| 9. Too loud | a. Reduce output with output control<br>b. Reduce gain<br>c. Insert filter in receiver<br>d. Widen the vent<br>e. Reduce compression ratio<br>f. Reduce compression kneepoint |
| 10. Too soft | a. Check battery<br>b. Excessive cerumen<br>c. Defective microphone<br>d. Increase overall gain/output<br>e. Increase low-frequency gain<br>f. Increase compression kneepoint<br>g. Decrease compression ratio<br>h. Reduce vent diameter<br>i. Check for excessive battery drain |

**Table 6–10.**  *(continued)*

| Problem | Possible Solutions |
| --- | --- |
| 10. Too soft | j. Check ear canal for debris<br>k. Check receiver tube for debris<br>l. Clean/replace filter in receiver tube<br>m. Check for moisture |
| 11. Windnoise | a. Use windscreen or windhood<br>b. Place foam in the microphone port<br>c. Decrease high-frequency gain or output |
| 12. Internal feedback | a. Check for loose receiver tube<br>b. Check for hole in vent<br>c. Check for pushed-in receiver tube<br>d. Send for repair |
| 13. External feedback | a. Check for excessive cerumen<br>b. Reduce vent size with SAV, PVV, or REVV (tube vents)<br>c. Buildup or lengthen canal<br>d. Coat shell with non-petroleum based oil ("soft seal")<br>e. Use receiver extension tubing<br>f. Add damping<br>g. Reduce canal length because tip may be against canal wall<br>h. Reduce high-frequency output/gain<br>i. Remake the earmold/shell<br>j. Use ER-13R ring seals<br>k. Use ER-13MF microphone filter<br>l. Consider receiver extension tube |
| 14. Distortion | a. Increase high-frequency output<br>b. Lengthen high-frequency release time<br>c. Replace microphone<br>d. Circuit repair |
| 15. Intermittent | a. Replace receiver/microphone<br>b. Replace volume control<br>c. Check for moisture buildup and recommend Dri-Aid kit<br>d. Circuit repair |
| 16. Excessive drain | a. Request lower battery drain from manufacturer<br>b. Reduce gain or output<br>c. Circuit repair |

Riess and Guthier, 1986

Table 6–10 was generated with the hope that some of the suggested solutions would be beneficial for those who face, or will face, these same problems on a daily basis.

## Conclusion

It has been stated more than once that fitting hearing aids is an art as well as a science. It is our belief that greater knowledge of the transmission line's role in shaping the electroacoustic characteristics of hearing aids will help in improving the artistic as well as scientific skills of dispensing audiologists. Hopefully, the information contained within this chapter will provide dispensing audiologists with some of the tools necessary to become better artists and scientists.

## References

Agnew J. (1986). Earmold impression stability. *Hear Instrum* 37(12):8, 11–12.

Agnew J. (1994). Acoustic advantages of deep canal hearing aid fittings. *Hear Instrum* 45(6):22, 24–25.

Alvord LS, Doxey GP, Smith DS. (1989). Hearing aids worn with tympanic membrane perforations: Complications and solutions. *Am J Otolaryngol* 10(4):277–280.

American National Standards Institute. (1987a). Specifications of hearing aid characteristics (ANSI S3.22-1987). New York: ANSI.

American National Standards Institute. (1987b). Preferred earhook nozzle thread for postauricular hearing aids. (ANSI S3.37-1987). New York: ANSI.

Austin CD, Kasten RN, Wilson H. (1990a). Real ear measurements of hearing aid plumbing modifications. Part I. *Hear Instrum* 43(3):18, 20–22.

Austin CD, Kasten RN, Wilson H. (1990b). Real ear measurements of hearing aid plumbing modifications. Part II. *Hear Instrum* 43(4):25–30.

Austin CD, Kasten RN, Wilson H. (1990c). Real ear measurements of hearing aid plumbing modifications. Part III. *Hear Instrum* 43(7):30–35.

Bergenstoff H. (1983). Earmold design and its effect on real ear insertion gain. *Hear Instrum* 34(9):46, 48–49.

Berger K, Hagberg E, Lane R. (1988). *Prescription of Hearing Aids: Rationale, Procedures and Results.* 5th ed. Ohio: Herald Publishing House.

Briskey RJ. (1982). Smoothing the frequency response of a hearing aid. *Hear Aid J* 3:12–17.

Bryant MP, Mueller HG, Northern JL. (1991). Minimal contact long canal ITE hearing instruments. *Hear Instrum* 42(1):12–15.

Burgess N, Brooks DN. (1991). Earmoulds: Some benefits from horn fitting. *Br J Audiol* 25:309–315.

Chasin M. (1983a). Using acoustic resistance in earmold tubing. *Hear Instrum* 34(12):18, 20, 54.

Chasin M. (1983b). Vent modification for added high frequency sound transmission. *Hear J* 6:16–17.

Cockerill D. (1987). Allergies to earmoulds. *Br J Audiol* 21:143–145.

Copeland AB, Burris, PD, Griffing TS. (1986). Open fittings for canal and ITE hearing aids. *Hear Instrum* 37(4):6, 8, 11.

Coogle KL. (1976). NAEL's standard terms for earmolds. *Hear Aid J* 3:5.

Cooper WA, Franks JR, McFall RN, Goldstein DP. (1975). Variable venting valve for earmolds. *Audiology* 14:259–267.

Courtois J, Johansen PA, Larsen BV, Christensen P, Beilin J. (1988). Open molds. In: Jensen JH, ed. *Hearing Aid Fittings. Theoretical and Practical Views. 13th Danavox Symposium.* Copenhagen: Stougaard Jensen, pp. 175–200.

Cox RM. (1979). Acoustic aspects of hearing aid-ear canal coupling systems. *Monogr Contemp Audiol* 1(3):1–44.

Cox RM. (1982). Combined effects of earmold vents and suboscillatory feedback on hearing aid frequency response. *Ear Hear* 3:12–17.

Cox RM, Alexander GC. (1983). Acoustic versus electronic modifications of hearing aid low-frequency output. *Ear Hear* 4:190–196.

Cox RM, Gilmore C. (1986). Damping the hearing aid frequency response: effects on speech clarity and preferred listening level. *J Speech Hear Res* 29:357–365.

*Custom Earmold Manual.* (1994). Ambridge, PA: Microsonic Earmold Laboratory.

Dalsgaard SC. (1975). *Earmolds and Associated Problems. Seventh Danavox Symposium.* Stockholm: The Almqvist & Wiksell Periodical Co.

Davis R, Green S. (1975). The influence of controlled venting on discrimination ability. *Hear Aid J* 27(5):6, 34–35.

Decker TN. (1975). The relationship between speech discrimination performance and the use of sintered metal inserts in the hearing aid fitting. *Audecibel* Summer:118–123.

DeJonge R. (1983). Computer simulation of hearing aid frequency responses. *Hear J* 3:27–31.

Dempsey JJ. (1990). The occlusion effect created by custom canal hearing aids. *Am J Otolaryngol* 11(1):44–46.

Dillon H. (1991). Allowing for real ear venting effects when selecting the coupler gain of hearing aids. *Ear Hear* 12:406–416.

Dillon H. (1985). Earmolds and high frequency response modification. *Hear Instrum* 36(12):8, 11–12.

Egolf DP. (1979a). Fundamentals of acoustics and acoustic wave interaction with the human head and ear. In: Larson VD, Egolf DP, Kirlin RL, Stile SW, Jensen JH, eds. *Auditory and Hearing Prosthetics Research.* New York: Grune and Stratton, pp. 19–37.

Egolf DP. (1979b). Mathematical predictions of electroacoustic frequency response of in-situ hearing aids. In: Larson VD, Egolf DP, Kirlin RL, Stile SW, Jensen JH, eds. *Auditory and Hearing Prosthetics Research.* New York: Grune and Stratton, pp. 411–450.

Egolf DP. (1980). Techniques for modeling the hearing aid receiver and associated tubing. In: Studebaker GA, Hochberg, eds. *Acoustical Factors Affecting Hearing Aid Performance.* Baltimore: University Park Press, pp. 297–319.

Fernandes CC, Cooper K. (1983). Using a horn mold with severe to profound losses. *Hear Instrum* 34(12):6, 54.

Frank T. (1980). Attenuation characteristics of hearing aid earmolds. *Ear Hear* 1:161–166.

Gastmeirer WJ. (1981). The acoustically damped earhook. *Hear Instrum* 32(10):14–15.

Goldstein BA. (1980). Effects of discriminate and indiscriminate placement of sintered hearing aid filters. *Hear Aid J* 3:7, 30, 32, 34.

Green DS. (1969). Non-occluding earmolds with CROS and IROS hearing aids. *Arch Otolaryngol* 89:96–106.

Green DS, Ross M. (1968). The effect of conventional versus a nonoccluding earmold upon the frequency response of a hearing aid. *J Speech Hear Res* 11:638–647.

Griffing TS. (1971). Variable venting of earmolds. *Hear Dealer* 22:23.

Griffing TS, Shields J. (1972). Hearing aid performance and the earmold. *Hear Dealer* 23:6–9.

Gudmundsen GI. (1994). Fitting CIC hearing aids: some practical pointers. *Hear J* 47(7)10, 45–48.

Harford ER, Barry JA. (1965). A rehabilitative approach to the problem of unilateral hearing impairment: the contralateral routing of signals (CROS). *J Speech Hear Dis* 30:121–138.

Harford ER, Dodds E. (1966). The clinical application of CROS: A hearing aid for unilateral deafness. *Arch Otolaryngol* 83:455–464.

Harford ER, Fox J. (1978). The use of high-pass amplification for broad-frequency sensorineural hearing loss. *Audiology* 17:10–26.

Hodgson W, Murdock C. (1972). Effect of the earmold on speech intelligibility in hearing aid use. *J Speech Hear Res* 13:290–297.

Killion MC. (1980). Problems in the application of broadband hearing aid earphones. In: Studebaker GA, Hochberg J, eds. *Acoustical Factors Affecting Hearing Aid Performance* 1st ed. Baltimore: University Park Press, pp. 219–264.

Killion MC. (1981). Earmold options for wideband hearing aids. *J Speech Hear Dis* 46:10–20.

Killion MC. (1982). Transducers, earmolds and sound quality considerations. In: Studebaker GA, Bess F, eds. *The Vanderbilt Hearing-Aid Report.* Upper Darby: Monographs in Contemporary Audiology, pp. 104–111.

Killion MC. (1984). Recent earmolds for wideband OTE and ITE hearing aids. *Hear J* 8:15–18, 20–22.

Killion MC. (1988a). Earmold design: theory and practice. In: Jensen JH, ed. *Hearing Aid Fittings. Theoretical and Practical Views. 13th Danavox Symposium.* Copenhagen: Stougaard Jensen, pp. 155–172.

Killion MC. (1988b). Principles of high fidelity hearing aid amplification. In: Sandlin RE, ed. *Handbook of Hearing Aid Amplification* Vol. 1. Boston: College-Hill Press, pp. 45–79.

Killion MC. (1988c). Special fitting problems and open canal solutions. In: Jensen JH, ed. *Hearing Aid Fittings. Theoretical and Practical Views. 13th Danavox Symposium.* Copenhagen: Stougaard Jensen, pp. 219–228.

Killion MC. (1988d). The "hollow voice" occlusion effect. In: Jensen JH, ed. *Hearing Aid Fittings. Theoretical and Practical Views. 13th Danavox Symposium.* Copenhagen: Stougaard Jensen, pp. 231–242.

Killion MC, Berlin CI, Hood L. (1984). A low frequency emphasis open canal hearing aid. *Hear Instrum* 35(8):30, 32, 34, 66.

Killion MC, Monser EL. (1980). CORFIG: Coupler response for flat insertion gain. In: Studebaker GA, Hochberg J, eds. *Acoustical Factors Affecting Hearing Aid Performance* 1st ed. Baltimore: University Park Press, pp. 149–168.

Killion MC, Revit LJ. (1993). CORFIG and GIFROC: Real ear to coupler and back. In: Studebaker GA, Hochberg J, eds. *Acoustical Factors Affecting Hearing Aid Performance* 2nd ed. Needham Heights: Allyn and Bacon, pp. 65–85.

Killion MC, Tillman TW. (1982). Evaluation of high fidelity hearing aids. *J Speech Hear Res* 25:15–25.

Killion MC, Wiber LA, Gudmundsen GI (1988). Zwislocki was right . . . *Hear Instrum* 39(1):28–30.

Killion MC, Wilson DL. (1985). Response modifying earhooks for special fitting problems. *Audecibel* Fall:28–30.

Konkle DF, Bess FH. (1974). Custom-made versus stock earmolds in hearing aid evaluations. *Arch Otolaryngol* 99:140–144.

Kuk FK. (1991). Perceptual consequences of vents in hearing aids. *Br J Audiol* 25:163–169.

Kuk FK. (1994). Maximum usable real-ear insertion gain with ten earmold designs. *J Am Acad Audiol* 5:41–51.

Leavitt R. (1986). Earmolds: Acoustic and structural considerations. In: Hodgson WR, ed. *Hearing Aid Assessment and Use in Audiologic Habilitation* 3rd ed. Baltimore: Williams and Wilkins, pp. 71–108.

Letowski TR, Burchfield SB. (1991). Study finds greater sound attenuation with silicone than lucite earmolds. *Hear J* 9:18, 20–22.

Letowski TR, Burchfield SB, Hume S. (1991). Perceptual differences between earmold materials. *Hear Instrum* 42(12):14–16.

Letowski TR, Richards WD, Burchfield SB. (1992). Transmission of sound, vibration through earmold materials. *Hear Instrum* 43(12):11–15.

Libby ER. (1979). The importance of smoothness in hearing aid frequency response. *Hear Instrum* 30(4):20–22.

Libby ER. (1980). Smooth wideband hearing aid responses-the new frontier. *Hear Instrum* 30(10):12–13, 15, 18, 43.

Libby ER. (1981). Achieving a transparent, smooth, wideband hearing aid response. *Hear Instrum* 32(10):9–12.

Libby ER. (1982). In search of transparent insertion gain hearing aid responses. In: Studebaker GA, Bess F, eds. *The Vanderbilt Hearing-Aid Report.* Upper Darby: Monographs in Contemporary Audiology, pp. 112–123.

Libby ER. (1990). A reverse acoustic horn for severe-to-profound hearing impairments. *Hear Instrum* 41(12):29.

Lundberg G, Ovegard A, Hagerman B, Gabrielsson A, Brandstrom U. (1992). Perceived sound quality in a hearing aid with vented and closed earmould equalized in frequency response. *Scand Audiol* 21:87–92.

Lybarger SF. (1977). Sound leakage from vented earmolds. *Hear Aid J* 3:8, 28–29, 40.

Lybarger SF. (1979). Controlling hearing aid performance by earmold design. In: Larson, VD, Egolf DP, Kirlin RL, Stile SW, eds. *Auditory and Hearing Prosthetics Research.* New York: Grune and Stratton, pp. 101–132.

Lybarger SF. (1980). Earmold venting as an acoustic control factor. In: Studebaker GA, Hochberg J, eds. *Acoustical Factors Affecting Hearing Aid Performance* 1st ed. Baltimore: University Park Press, 197–217.

Lybarger SF. (1985). Earmolds. In: Katz J, ed. *Handbook of Clinical Audiology* 3rd ed. Baltimore: Williams and Wilkins, pp. 885–910.

Lyregaard PE. (1982). Improvement of the high-frequency performance of BTE hearing aids. *Hear Instrum* 33(2):38, 40, 43, 62.

MacKenzie K, Browning GG. (1989). The real ear effect of adjusting the tone control and venting a hearing aid system. *Br J Audiol* 23:93–98.

MacKenzie K, Browning GG. (1991). Randomized cross over study to assess patient preference for an acoustically modified hearing aid system. *J Laryngol* 105:405–408.

Macrae J. (1981). A new kind of earmold vent-the high cut cavity vent. *Hear Instrum* 32(10):18, 64.

Macrae J. (1983). Acoustic modifications for better hearing aid fittings. *Hear Instrum* 34(12):8, 11.

Macrae J. (1990). Static pressure seal of earmolds. *J Rehab Res Dev* 27:397–410.

Macrae J. (1991). A comparison of the effects of different methods of impression buildup on earmoulds. *Br J Audiol* 25:183–199.

Madell JR, Gendel JM. (1984). Earmolds for patients with severe and profound hearing loss. *Ear Hear* 5:349–351.

McClellan ME. (1967). Aided speech discrimination in noise with vented and unvented earmolds. *J Aud Res* 7:93–99.

Meding B, Ringdahl A. (1992). Allergic contact dermatitis from earmolds of hearing aids. *Ear Hear* 13:122–124.

Meredith R, Thomas KJ, Callaghan DE, Stephens SDG, Rayment AJ. (1989). A comparison of three types of earmoulds in elderly users of post-aural hearing aids. *Br J Audiol* 23:239–244.

Morgan R. (1994). The art of making a good impression. *Hear Rev* 1(3):10, 13–14, 24.

Mueller HG, Hawkins DB, Northern JL. (1992). *Probe Microphone Measurements: Hearing Aid Selection and Assessment.* San Diego: Singular Press.

Mueller HG, Schwartz DM, Surr RK. (1981). The use of the exponential acoustic horn in an open mold configuration. *Hear Instrum* 32(10):16–17, 67.

Mullin TA, Gorlin BH, Lassiter B. (1986). Stethoscopes and earmolds. *Hear Instrum* 37(12):16–17.

Mynders J. (1985). Human acoustic couplers. In: Sandlin RE, ed. *Hearing Instrument Science and Fitting Practices.* Livonia: National Institute for Hearing Instrument Studies, pp. 313–386.

Northern JL, Hattler KW. (1970). Earmold influence on aided speech identification tasks. *J Speech Hear Res* 13:162–172.

Northern JL, Kepler LJ, Gabbard SA. (1991). Deep canal fittings and real ear measurements. *Hear Instrum* 42(9):34–35, 53.

Okpojo AO. (1992). Advances in earmold technology. *J Am Acad Audiol* 3:142–144.

Oliveira RJ, Hawkinson R, Stockton M. (1992). Instant foam versus traditional BTE earmolds. *Hear Instrum* 43(12):22.

Oliveira RJ, Rose DE. (1994). "Keep your wax guard up." *Am J Audiol* 3(1):7–10.

Parker DJ, Okpojo AO, Nolan M, Combe EC, Bamford JM. (1992). Acoustic evaluation of earmoulds in situ: A comparison of impression and earmold materials. *Br J Audiol* 26:159–166.

Peck JE. (1986). The stethomold for hearing aid and stethoscope users. *Hear Instrum* 37(12):17–18.

Pedersen B. (1984). Venting of earmoulds with acoustic horn. *Scand Audiol* 13:205–206.

Preves DA. (1980). Stepped bore earmolds for custom ITE hearing aids. *Hear Instrum* 31(10):24, 26.

Preves DA. (1994). Real-ear gain provided by CIC, ITC and ITE hearing instruments. *Hear Rev* 1(7):22–24.

Revit LJ. (1992). Two techniques for dealing with the occlusion effect. *Hear Instrum* 43(12):16–18.

Revit LJ. (1994). Using coupler tests in the fitting of hearing aids. In: Valente M, ed. *Strategies for Selecting and Verifying Hearing Aid Fittings.* New York: Thieme Medical Publishers, pp. 64–87.

Revoile S. (1968). Speech discrimination with ear inserts. *Bull Prosthet Res* Fall:198–205.

Rezen S. (1980). A research application of innovative hearing aid coupling systems. *Hear Instrum* 31(9):28, 30.

Ridenhour MW. (1988). The effects of shell material on hearing aid performance. *Hear Instrum* 39(9):58–60.

Riess RL, Guthier JD. (1986). In-the-ear modification cookbook. *Hear Instrum* 37(4):18, 21–22, 24, 54.

Robinson S, Cane MA, Lutman ME. (1989). Relative benefits of stepped and constant bore earmoulds: A crossover trial. *Br J Audiol* 23:221–228.

Roesel GW. (1994). CIC + WDRC = A logical combination. *Hear Rev* 1(7):26–27.

Schwartz DM, Surr RK, Montgomery AA, Prosek RA, Walden BE. (1979). Performance of high frequency impaired listeners with conventional and extended high frequency amplification. *Audiology* 18:157–174.

Smolak LH, Iserman BF, Hawkinson RW. (1987). Disposable foam earmolds. *Hear Instrum* 38(12):24–27, 49.

Staab WJ, Finlay B. (1991). A fitting rationale for deep fitting canal hearing instruments. *Hear Instrum* 42(1):6, 8–10, 48.

Staab WJ, Lybarger SF. (1994). Characteristics and use of hearing aids. In: Katz J, ed. *Handbook of Clinical Audiology* 4th ed. Baltimore: Williams and Wilkins, pp. 657–722.

Staab WJ, Nunley JA. (1982). A guide to tube fitting of hearing aids. *Hear Aid J* 9:25–26, 28–30, 32, 34.

Studebaker GA, Cox RM. (1977). Side branch and parallel vent effects in real ears and in acoustical and electrical models. *J Am Audiol Soc* 3:108–117.

Studebaker GA, Cox RM, Wark DJ. (1978). Earmold modification effect measured by coupler, threshold and probe techniques. *Audiology* 17:173–186.

Studebaker GA, Zachman TA. (1970). Investigation of the acoustics of earmold vents. *J Acoust Soc Am* 47:1107–1115.

Sullivan R. (1985a). Part I: An acoustic coupling-based classification system for hearing aid fittings. *Hear Instrum* 36(9):25–26, 28.

Sullivan R. (1985b). Part II: An acoustic coupling-based classification system for hearing aid fittings. *Hear Instrum* 36(12):16, 18.

Sullivan R. (1985c). Part III: An acoustic coupling-based classification system for hearing aid fittings. *Hear Instrum* 36(12):20–22.

Sung GS, Sung RJ. (1982). The efficacy of hearing aid-earmold coupling systems. *Hear Instrum* 33(12):11–12.

Tecca JE. (1992). Further investigation of ITE vent effects. *Hear Instrum* 43(12):8–10.

Tecca JE. (1991). Real ear vent effects in ITE hearing instrument fittings. *Hear Instrum* 42(12):10–12.

Teder H. (1979). Smoothing hearing aid output with filters. *Hear Instrum* 30(4):22–23, 38.

Trychel MR, Hass WH. (1989). Earmold attenuation: The effect on residual hearing. *Hear J* 2:22, 24, 27.

Valente M. (1983). *A Clinically Manufactured Stepped Diameter Earmold for Superior Aided Performance.* Paper presented at the Annual Meeting of the American-Speech-Language-Hearing Association, Cincinnati, OH.

Valente M. (1984a). *Enhanced Aided Listening With a Belled Bore.* Paper presented at the Annual Meeting of the American-Speech-Language-Hearing Association, San Francisco, CA.

Valente M. (1984b). *Interaction of Tubing Insertion and Bore Length Upon the Frequency Response.* Paper presented at the Annual Meeting of the American-Speech-Language-Hearing Association, San Francisco, CA.

Valente M. (1984c). Transmission line acoustics. Unpublished report for the Veterans Administration.

Valente M, DeJonge R. (1981). High frequency amplification. *Audecibel* Fall:168–177.

Vass WK, Mims LA. (1993). Exploring the deep canal fitting advantage. *Hear Instrum* 44(12):26–27.

Walker G. (1979). Earphone termination and the response of behind-the-ear hearing aids. *Br J Audiol* 13:41–46.

Westermann S. (1987). The occlusion effect. *Hear Instrum* 38(6):43.

Williams DE, Gutnick HN. (1990). Hearing instrument performance using earmolds with/without a shell additive. *Hear Instrum* 41(12):8, 10.

Wimmer VH. (1986). The occlusion effect from earmolds. *Hear Instrum* 37(12):19, 57.

# 7

# The Effects of Distortion on User Satisfaction with Hearing Aids

## Francis K. Kuk

## Introduction

Distortion may be one of the least discussed areas among audiologists. Most audiologists feel that the amount of distortion in a hearing aid is predetermined at the manufacturing level. Our general exposure to distortion may be restricted to terms like harmonic distortion and intermodulation distortion. Some audiologists may test a hearing aid for harmonic distortion following the ANSI S3.22-1987 standard when our patients complain that their hearing aids sound distorted. However, distortion occurs more frequently than is indicated from our patients' complaints or revealed from ANSI-S3.22-1987 total harmonic distortion (THD) testing. Indeed, in some hearing aids, distortion occurs with such frequency that their users are urged by the audiologists to accept the distorted sound as typical. Some examples are the "hollowness" perception of one's own voice and poor speech perception in moderately loud noisy situations. An understanding of the different types of distortion that can occur in a hearing aid, their identification, perceptual consequences, and management may help in the proper selection and fitting of hearing aids having minimal distortion.

## What Is Distortion?

An ideal amplification system increases the amplitude of the input signal while faithfully maintaining its temporal and spectral characteristics. In reality, most amplification systems are not ideal. The choice of specific microphone, receiver, amplifier, and battery in hearing aids represents a tradeoff between desirability and acceptability (Cole, 1993). The result is that even an acceptable hearing aid distorts the input sound signal in both desired and undesired manners. Under some conditions, it may also alter the temporal and spectral content of the input signal that it is designed to amplify. Distortion occurs when the output is not an

327

exact replica of the input signal. In cases where additional frequencies (that is, signals at the output that are not present at the input) are generated during the distortion process, such frequencies are called distortion products.

A hearing aid functions by amplifying certain frequency regions of the acoustic input so that the amplified signal can overcome the attenuative effect of a peripheral hearing loss and the degradation in the speech signals caused by interfering noise and distance factors. By definition, a hearing aid distorts the spectra of natural sounds so that they are audible to the hearing-impaired listener. When done properly, this type of distortion is beneficial to the hearing aid wearer. Unfortunately, most distortions do not enhance speech recognition or quality. Indeed, the general effect of distortion is a degradation of the input signal leading to poorer speech quality and/or reduced speech recognition.

## Classification of Distortion

Two classes of distortion can be identified based on the intent of the distortion. Broadly, distortion can be classified into purposeful and nonpurposeful.

### Purposeful Distortion

A linear hearing aid is one that provides the same amount of gain at all input levels. For its operation, it intentionally distorts the acoustic signals so that it can compensate for the loss of sensitivity in the hearing-impaired ear. The spectrum of the wideband input acoustic signal is modified (i.e., frequency shaped) at various stages by the microphone, amplifier, electronic filters, receivers, and tubing to result in a narrower spectrum at the output. Ideally, this modification should result in a frequency–gain response that compensates for the individual's hearing loss. Inappropriate frequency shaping could also lead to poor sound quality and reduced speech understanding. The readers are referred to Valente (1994) for a discussion of the approaches to select and verify optimal settings on a linear hearing aid.

The use of automatic gain control (AGC) or compression in hearing aids also distorts the amplitude relation of the acoustic signals. These hearing aids automatically adjust their gain, depending on the level of the input signals. Typically, a fixed gain is provided when the intensity of the input signal (for input compression) or that of the output signal (for output compression) is below the compression threshold (or knee of compression). When the level of the input (or output) exceeds this knee (which is typically set by the manufacturer or by the audiologists), gain reduces as the intensity of the input signal (or output) increases.

Compression is used for two purposes. Compression limiting is used to limit the output of a signal while avoiding saturation. Typically, hearing aids using this circuitry have high compression thresholds (greater than 75 dB SPL) and high compression ratios (greater than 8:1). Full dynamic range compression is used to restore the "normal" loudness growth in the impaired ear. These hearing aids have low compression thresholds (below 50 dB SPL) and low compression ratios (typically less than 3:1). Like frequency shaping, inappropriate compression settings could result in reduced speech recognition and poor sound quality.

Careful selection of the electroacoustic settings on a hearing aid is important to minimize the undesirable, nonpurposeful outcome of this type of processing. The readers are referred to Chapter 4 for a detailed description of different amplifier types.

### Nonpurposeful Distortion

This type of distortion is generated within a hearing aid as a result of design compromise. Because of this, the type and amount of distortion can vary among hearing aid designs. The types of distortion under this category can be further divided into those that are inherent properties of a hearing aid (extraneous noise, digitization distortion, phase distortion, and temporal distortion) and those that are dependent on the stimulus conditions (saturation distortion).

#### *Extraneous Noise*    *mechanical feedback / Circuit noise*

If a hearing aid is operating below saturation and yet the output contains energy at added frequencies that are not related to the input frequencies, the additional frequencies are said to be extraneous distortion products (Pollack, 1980). Typically, this distortion product takes the form of a broadband noise. The most common cause of extraneous noise is thermal noise, which is generated from resistors, transistors, and other active components through thermal agitation of the free electrons within the electronic components. The total amount of thermal noise in a hearing aid circuit is collectively called circuit noise. In addition, the amount of noise generated by an amplifier is proportional to its gain (i.e., greater gain equals greater noise) (Ballou, 1987). Figure 7–1 shows the spectrum and waveform of a sinusoid superimposed by amplifier noise. The upper two graphs represent the waveform of the sinusoid (left) and the broadband amplifier noise (right). The lower two graphs represent the resulting waveform (left) and spectrum (right) of the sinusoid embedded in noise. Note that the sinusoid is clearly visible temporally (lower left) and spectrally (lower right) as long as its magnitude is greater than that of the noise.

Circuit noise generated from a hearing aid is measured as the overall output sound pressure level from the hearing aid without any acoustic signal present. *EINL* ANSI S3.22-1987 expresses hearing aid circuit noise as the Equivalent Input Noise level (Ln), in dB, which is simply the difference in SPL between the overall noise level in a hearing aid with no input and the amount of gain at that volume control setting. To meet specifications, a hearing aid must have an Ln that is equal to or smaller than the manufacturer's specified tolerance limit with the volume control set at the reference test gain (RTG) position.

Circuit noise in a hearing aid may be irritating and annoying to the wearer. In addition, it may mask low-level signals and interact with incoming signals to create undesirable intermodulation distortions. However, a hearing aid that meets the manufacturer's tolerance limit for Ln may not be acceptable to some wearers either. For the circuit noise to be imperceptible, a hearing aid must have Ln that is lower than the best threshold at any frequency of the impaired ear. For example, hearing aid wearers with 0 dB HL hearing threshold at any test frequencies

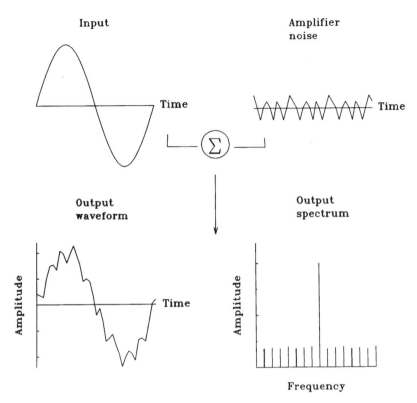

**Figure 7–1.**   Spectrum and waveform of a sinusoid embedded in amplifier noise.

may report hearing "static," or "hisses" from the hearing aid when there is no external input even when the Ln of the hearing aid is below 25 dB SPL, an acceptable value for Ln. In some programmable hearing aids, Ln may exceed 30 dB SPL. It is important to provide proper counselling to the wearers on the nature of this noise, and discuss with the wearer if the benefit of the specific programmable unit outweighs the annoyance caused by the "high" Ln value.

The new ANSI standard (ANSI S3.42-1992) recommends the use of a speech shaped noise to determine electroacoustic properties of a hearing aid. However, no specification is made for the determination of equivalent input noise.

## Digitization Distortion

The application of digital technology to hearing aids suggests that some of the problems associated with digitization (the conversion of an analog signal into binary forms) apply to hearing aids. It is important to stress that digitization distortion only occurs in truly digital hearing aids and not in digitally programmable hearing devices. The types of distortion, or errors as they are frequently called, include aliasing error, quantization error, and imaging error.

In digital processing, an acoustic signal is initially digitized (analog-to-digital conversion, ADC) before it is processed by the central processing unit (CPU).

Digitization Distortion:
- Aliasing error
- quantization error
- imaging error

This involves initial conditioning of the acoustic signal prior to processing through a sample-and-hold stage. The amplitude of the sampled signal is then coded into a series of binary digits (i.e., bits) through a process called quantization so that it can be processed by the CPU. After digital processing, the processed signal undergoes a digital-to-analog conversion (DAC) stage in which the digital signal is reconverted into an acoustic form. The interested readers are referred to Levitt (1987) for a detailed description on this topic.

## Aliasing Error

Aliasing error occurs during the conditioning (i.e., sample-and-hold) stage when the sampling rate of the processor is not sufficient to adequately sample all the frequencies within the input signal. The result is the introduction of unwanted low frequency noise (i.e., an alias) at the output. Figure 7–2 illustrates the generation of an aliasing error, using a sinusoid signal as an example. Suppose that a sampling rate of 20,000 Hz (i.e., sampling period of 0.05 milliseconds) is used to sample an acoustic signal. According to the Nyquist theorem, which states that the sampling rate must be at least twice the highest frequency in the input signal, the highest frequency that could be sampled adequately is 10,000 Hz. If a spurious 15,000 Hz tone is present at the input, this sinusoid will be sampled at every 3/4 cycle of its duration. The waveform that is reconstructed based on the samples will have a lower frequency, that of 5000 Hz (Fig. 7–2a). This is the "alias" signal. In general, the higher the frequency of the spurious signal, the lower is the alias frequency. For example, a 11,000 Hz signal will result in an alias at 9000 Hz and a 18,000 Hz signal will result in an alias at 2000 Hz. A spurious noise band from 11,000 Hz to 18,000 Hz will yield an alias from 2000 Hz to 9000 Hz.

The occurrence of the low-frequency alias error is the unanticipated presence of high-frequency samples in the signal for ADC. To circumvent such occurrence, one can either increase the sampling rate or ensure that the input signal does not contain spurious high-frequency signals. Figure 7–2b shows that a sampling rate of 30,000 Hz would result in accurate sampling of the 15,000 Hz signal. In this case, each cycle is sampled twice during the sampling process. The drawback of this approach is the added size and cost of the ADC process. Typically, an anti-aliasing filter, which is a low-pass filter with a very steep filter skirt, is used at the input stage to contain the signal of interest. Assuming that most of the important speech frequencies are below 6000 Hz, a sampling rate between 12,000 Hz and 14,000 Hz is adequate to prevent aliasing error.

## Quantization Error

Quantization refers to the assignment of a binary digit (i.e., bit) to the voltage of the sampled analog signal (Hauser, 1991). During this process, the value of the sampled voltage is compared to the array of binary representations that best approximate its value through a successive approximation register (SAR). The input voltage is successively compared to subdivisions of the range of binary representations until it is matched to the nearest available digital value. The number of binary representations is determined by the number of bits available

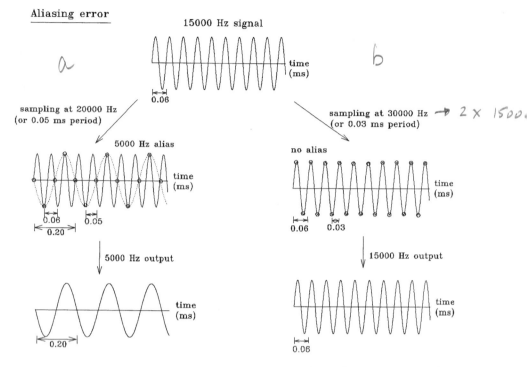

**Figure 7–2.** Generation of aliasing error. Figure 7–2a shows how a 5000 Hz alias is formed. Figure 7–2b shows that the alias will disappear with proper sampling (i.e., at 30,000 Hz rate).

in the digital processor. If there is only one bit, the possible binary representations will be simply 0 or 1. If these representations are used to cover a range of 5 volts, any voltage that is smaller than 2.5 volts will be assigned a value of 0 and any voltage above 2.5 volts will be assigned a value of 1. Thus, the amplitude resolution of a single-bit processor is rather limited. The difference between the actual voltage and the assigned voltage is the quantization error. Resolution improves (or the quantization error decreases) as the number of bits increases. In general, the number of representations is represented by $2^n$, where n is the number of bits within the processor. For example, if there are two bits, the possible representations are 00, 01, 10, and 11 (four altogether). Figure 7–3 shows the digitized waveform of a sinusoid with 4- and 8-bit quantization. Note the smoothness of the sinusoid with the 8-bit quantization in comparison to the 4-bit quantization.

The number of bits available in the ADC process also affects the dynamic range (DR) of the digital system (Hussung and Hamill, 1990; Hauser, 1991). The dynamic range represents the difference between the noise floor and the upper limit of signal representation without distortion. Each bit will increase the DR by approximately 6 dB. Consequently, a 12-bit system will have a DR of 72 dB and a 14-bit system will have a DR of 84 dB.

The number of bits used in a digital processor is a compromise between the acceptable quantization error and the cost, power consumption, and size of the

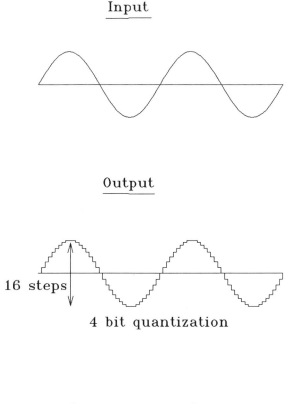

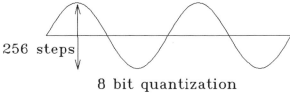

**Figure 7–3.**    Example of a sinusoid quantized at 4- and 8-bit resolution.

device. In general, 11–12 bits are desirable for inaudible quantization errors (Levitt, 1987). This, however, is prohibitively expensive and impractical for hearing aid application. Cudahy and Kates (1993) examined the detectability of quantization errors by removing bits from a 12-bit processor. Their results showed that vowels are more susceptible to quantization errors than consonants. Removal of only three bits led to discernible differences in vowel perception. The effect of bit removal was less marked when fricatives were evaluated. For the phoneme /f/, as many as 10 bits can be removed before subjects experienced a reduction in recognition ability. It is easier to detect distortion in vowels because the periodic harmonic structures in vowels are interrupted. Introducing distortion products to fricatives, because of their already aperiodic nature, is less noticeable to the listeners.

Cudahy and Kates' (1993) findings would suggest a minimum of nine bits in a digital processor for inaudible quantization error. Levitt (1987) suggests using variable quantization intervals to reduce the number of bits and preserve sound quality. Even so, seven bits are still needed. This means that the DR will be restricted to 42 dB (6 dB/bit x 7 bits). Although it would be unacceptable to ears with normal hearing, it may be acceptable to ears with sensorineural hearing loss because of their reduced dynamic range.

Quantization errors affect speech recognition and perceived speech quality differently. Harris, Brey, Chang, Soria, and Hilton (1991) compared the effects of quantization errors on speech recognition and perceived speech quality in 96 normal hearing individuals. Digitized speech was processed to simulate 6-, 8-, 10-, 12-, 14-, and 16-bit integer conversion. No significant difference in speech recognition was noted for 8- to 16-bit conversion. However, speech processed at 12-, 14-, and 16-bit conversion was judged to be superior (subjectively using a paired comparison paradigm) to that processed at 6-, 8-, and 10-bit conversion. Speech processed at a low bit rate was reportedly noisy. These results suggest that subjective tasks may be more sensitive than speech recognition measures to differentiate small differences among hearing aids.

**Imaging Error**

Imaging error occurs at the digital-to-analog conversion stage when the processed digital signal, which looks like the 4-bit sample illustrated in Figure 7–3, is not filtered properly to remove all the "sharp edges." In this case, high-frequency noise will be perceived. An anti-imaging filter, typically a low-pass filter, is used at the output stage of the digital-to-analog converter to minimize this error.

## *Temporal Distortion*

Temporal distortion occurs when a hearing aid is unable to faithfully duplicate the temporal characteristics of input stimuli. The result is an alteration of the intensity relationship among various syllabic structures. A common form of temporal distortion is transient distortion, in which the hearing aid is unable to follow the initial sharp attack or the sudden decay of a sound. This leads to the characteristic "ringing" that one frequently sees on an oscilloscope when a transient signal is amplified by a hearing aid. Transient distortion appears to be related to sharp resonance peaks in the frequency response of the hearing aid (Pollack, 1980) and the limited bandwidth in some hearing aids. Both linear and nonlinear hearing aids can exhibit this type of distortion.

Nonlinear hearing aids, e.g., compression devices, introduce temporal distortion because of the delay in activation and deactivation of the compression circuit. The time (in milliseconds) needed to activate the compression circuit is typically referred to as the attack time. The time taken to deactivate the compression circuit, or the time taken to return to linear amplification, is typically known as the release time. Typically, attack time is short (less than five milliseconds) to prevent loudness discomfort arising from abrupt increases in stimulus amplitude. The optimal release time (also in milliseconds) may depend on different listening backgrounds. If speech is presented in a continuous noise background, a short release time (i.e., less than 50 milliseconds) would lead to noise "fill in" between syllables and give a "pumping" sensation. This happens when the intensity of the linearly amplified noise (between the silent intersyllabic intervals) exceeds the intensity of the amplified, but compressed syllables. Teder (1991) reports that there is an increase in "pumping" with shorter release time. Additionally, the amplitude contrast among syllables is minimized. A longer release time (longer than 100 milliseconds), would decrease this pumping sensation and restore the amplitude contrast. This is because the average interval between syllables is approximately 100 milliseconds (Crystal and House, 1990).

On the other hand, long release times would be undesirable in situations where short but intense interfering noises are present (e.g., dish clanging). In such a situation, a weak syllable following the impulse noise may be significantly attenuated and become inaudible. A shorter release time is necessary in this case. The repeated level alteration in background noise could lead to complaints of noisiness in a hearing aid with compression (Walker and Dillon, 1982). Teder (1991) contends that the optimal release time depends on the stimulus activating the compression circuit. Compression circuits with adaptive release times allow short release time with a short impulsive signal and longer release time with a longer duration signal to maintain an optimal release time in all situations. The readers are referred to Chapter 4 for a more in-depth discussion of compression circuitry.

Kates (1992, 1993) used computer simulation to examine the speech-to-distortion ratio (SDR) as a function of attack and release times on a wide dynamic range compression (WDRC) circuit having a kneepoint or compression threshold at 50 dB SPL and a compression ratio of 2:1. The SDR decreased (i.e., more distortion) as the release time increased. A combination of an attack time greater than 2 milliseconds and a release time greater than 50 milliseconds resulted in a SDR of about 30 dB, a value that is not expected to negatively affect speech intelligibility. Longer release times lead to poorer SDRs. In the same simulation, it was reported that increasing the compression ratio would decrease the SDR. The most significant decrease is noted when the compression ratio is changed from 1:1 to 2:1.

## Phase Distortion

Phase distortion occurs when the timing relationship among input frequencies in a complex signal is altered. Figure 7–4 illustrates an example of phase distortion where a sinusoid is delayed by a quarter of a cycle (i.e., 90° out of phase). However, it is important to realize that phase distortion is not observed during conventional hearing aid tests using single pure tones. The use of complex signal and a two-channel measurement system are required to evaluate phase distortion.

Because of the capacitative and inductive components used in hearing aids, phase distortion occurs in almost all hearing aids. Phase distortion is especially significant in filters with steep roll offs. Anti-aliasing and anti-imaging filters in digital audio applications introduce significant phase distortion (Preis, 1982). Careful filter design (e.g., Butterworth over elliptical filters) and the use of filters

## Phase distortion

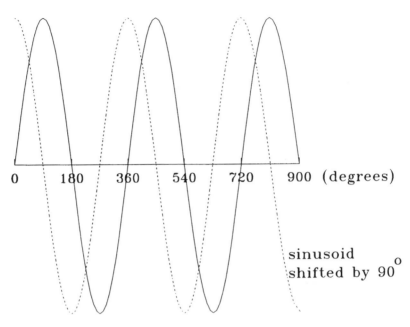

**Figure 7–4.**    Sinusoid with phase distortion (phase shift of 90° is noted).

with flatter slopes could reduce the amount of phase distortion (Preis and Bloom, 1984).

The perceptual consequence of phase distortion is less well known. Deer, Bloom, and Preis (1985) reported that the average listener can detect a phase delay of 2 milliseconds at 2000 Hz. Other authors (e.g., Schroeder, 1975) reported that the ear is relatively insensitive to phase differences for monaural listening to pure tones. At present, it is believed that severe phase distortion may compromise the central auditory system's ability to decode competing sounds in a binaural localization situation (e.g., Moller, 1983). However, in daily situations, the effect of phase distortion is not easily observable because conversational speech is rich in harmonics and transients to mask out the detectability of any minor changes in phase relationship.

The insensitivity of the ear to phase distortion is utilized in speech synthesis. Whereas natural speech has frequency components at various phases, most speech synthesizers use an excitation source with zero phase harmonics (O'Shaughnessy, 1987). Although these synthesized speech signals are fully intelligible, their sound quality may lack "naturalness" (Oppenheim and Lim, 1981). Figure 7–5 shows the contrast between the spectra of natural speech (a), synthesized speech with zero phase (b), and synthesized speech with random phase (c). Compared to (a) and (c), the spectra of synthesized speech with zero phase (b) appeared less well defined with poorer demarcation among its formant structures.

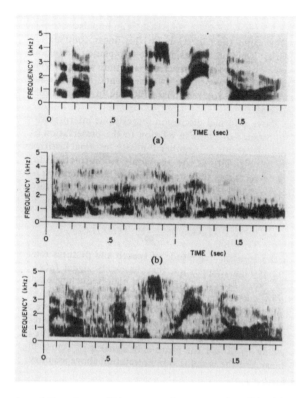

**Figure 7–5.** Spectra of the phrase "Line up at the screen door" in (a) natural production, (b) synthesized form with zero phrase, and (c) synthesized form with unity magnitude (from Oppenheim and Lim, 1981, with permission).

## Saturation Distortion

The most frequently discussed distortion in the hearing aid literature is saturation distortion. Traditionally, this type of distortion has been called amplitude distortion. This nomenclature may be confused with the desired amplitude distortion seen in compression hearing aids. In addition, the term amplitude distortion does not describe the spectral change or source for this type of distortion.

Saturation distortion occurs when the waveform of the output signal (i.e., gain plus input) is clipped when its amplitude reaches the saturation limit of the hearing aid. This is demonstrated in Figure 7–6 using a sinusoidal waveform. In this case, the peaks of the sinusoid are removed (thus, the term peak clipping). Further clipping changes the waveform into a square wave.

### Total Harmonic Distortion

Two types of saturation distortion are commonly known: total harmonic distortion (THD) and intermodulation distortion (IMD). It is important to realize that although these two forms of distortions typically occur at a high input level (i.e., at saturation), both THD and IMD are properties of a physical device reflecting the performance of the device in nonlinear operation (Peters and Burkhard,

## Peak clipping

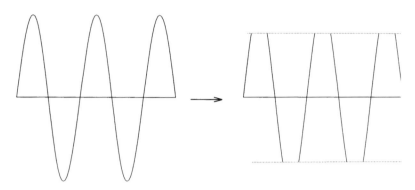

**Figure 7–6.**   Example of peak clipping.

1968). These two types of distortion differ by the stimuli that are responsible for their generation and the distortion products that are generated.

Harmonic distortion occurs when the intensity of the individual sinusoid exceeds the saturation limit of the hearing aid. Each sinusoid generates its own distortion products, which are frequencies that are whole number multiples of the original or primary sinusoid. These are called harmonics and are classified into odd-order and even-order harmonics. For example, a 500-Hz sinusoid generates distortion products at 1000 Hz (second harmonic), 1500 Hz (third harmonic), 2000 Hz (fourth harmonic), and so on. The second and fourth harmonics are examples of even-order harmonics and the third and fifth harmonics are odd-order harmonics. Figure 7–7a shows the harmonics of a signal at frequency $f_1$.

MEASUREMENT OF HARMONIC DISTORTION

Measurement of harmonic distortion is made by hearing aid manufacturers to ensure product quality. The ANSI S3.22-1987 standard specifies that the harmonics generated from 500, 800, and 1600 Hz presented at 70 dB SPL should be measured with the hearing aid set at the reference test gain position. Distortion test at any or all of these frequencies may be omitted when the frequency–response curve rises 12 dB or more between the test frequency and the frequency at its second harmonic. For example, if the output difference between 500 Hz and 1000 Hz is greater than 12 dB, THD testing at 500 Hz may be omitted. Either one of two formulae is recommended for the calculation of percent total harmonic distortion (THD) at each frequency:

$$\%\text{THD} = 100\% \sqrt{\frac{p_2^2 + p_3^2 + p_4^2 + \dots}{p_1^2}} \qquad (1)$$

$$\%\text{THD} = 100\% \sqrt{\frac{p_2^2 + p_3^2 + p_4^2 + \dots}{p_1^2 + p_2^2 + p_3^2 + \dots}} \qquad (2)$$

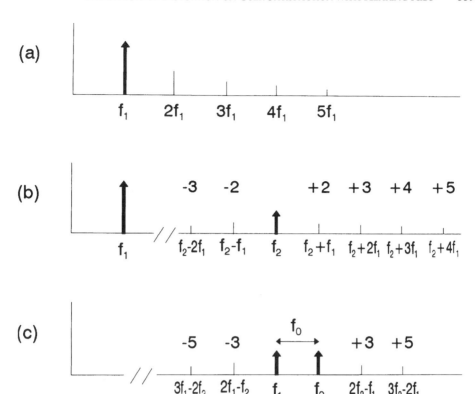

**Figure 7–7.** Spectral relation between primary frequencies (f$_1$ and f$_2$) and distortion products in (a) harmonic distortion, (b) intermodulation distortion, and (c) difference frequency distortion.

where $P_1$ is the sound pressure level of the primary or evoking stimulus, and $P_2$, $P_3$, . . . are the sound pressure levels of the second, third, . . . harmonics generated from the primary stimulus. The measured distortion at each input frequency must not exceed the manufacturer's specification by more than 3% to meet compliance. It needs to be pointed out that different manufacturers have different specifications for maximum allowable distortion. Meeting manufacturer specification does not guarantee acceptable performance for the individual hearing aid wearer.

Equation 1 is a simplified version of Equation 2 on the assumption that the intensity level of $P_2$ is many times smaller than $P_1$. In some applications, only the intensity levels of $P_2$ and $P_3$ are considered in the numerator because the intensity level of the higher order harmonics ($P_4$, $P_5$ . . .) is assumed to be negligibly smaller than that of $P_2$ and $P_3$. The implication here is that the same hearing aid may show different amounts of harmonic distortion if evaluated by different hearing aid test systems. For example, Townsend and Konkle (1982) showed that the different hearing aid measurement systems can show as much as 2% difference in THD with the same hearing aid or 10% false rejection of hearing aids because of excessive THD values. The characteristics of the hearing aid measurement system are important to understand when performing distortion measurement.

The measured THD is affected by the bandwidth of the hearing aid. Specifically, the upper cutoff of the frequency response of a hearing aid limits the detectability of higher order harmonics and the harmonics generated by the higher frequency stimulus (1600 Hz). These harmonics that occur beyond the bandwidth of the hearing aid are rolled off to provide a measure of THD that is smaller than its actual value. Consequently, if an audiologist is interested in measuring both the second- and third-order harmonics in a hearing aid with a high-frequency cutoff at 5000 Hz, s/he has to limit the stimulus tone to lower than 1600 Hz (its third harmonic is at 4800 Hz). If the audiologist is interested in knowing the percent of THD of the second-order harmonic in the same hearing aid, he or she has to limit the primary stimulus to below 2500 Hz. This suggests that harmonic distortion observed in the high frequencies may be lower than that measured in the low frequencies because of its dependence on the upper bandwidth of the hearing aid.

Interaction between the type of hearing aid and the type of hearing aid analyzer may occur to yield inaccurate measurements. For example, a hearing aid with a push-pull amplifier (class B) only yields odd-order harmonics (third and fifth) (Keller, 1984; Agnew, 1988). A hearing aid test system that only measures second- and third-order harmonic distortion products would indicate that the class B amplifier has less distortion than the class A amplifier, which yields harmonics at all multiples of the primary frequency (Burnett, 1967).

LIMITATIONS OF ANSI S3.22-1987 TOTAL HARMONIC
DISTORTION MEASUREMENT

It is widely agreed that the measurement of THD using the ANSI S3.22-1987 standard does not adequately describe the full extent of distortion in a hearing aid. Neither does ANSI S3.22-1987 predict the effect of this distortion on daily use of a hearing aid (Beck, Burnett, Frye, Preves, and Widin, 1993). A hearing aid with high THD may still retain good speech understanding. The fact that ANSI S3.22-1987 measures distortion at only three frequencies (or less) and at one intensity level (70 dB SPL) limits our understanding of the hearing aid only to those discrete frequencies and single intensity level. Information on the interactions among frequencies are unavailable. As Agnew (1994) demonstrated, the amount of harmonic distortion seen at the levels specified by the ANSI-S3.22-1987 standard is not predictive of distortion seen at higher intensity levels. Its dependence on the upper limit of the hearing aid bandwidth argues that its use may be limited to test frequencies below 2000 Hz.

### Intermodulation and Difference Frequency Distortion

Intermodulation distortion (IMD) occurs when 2 or more input frequencies (i.e., primary frequencies) interact to result in distortion products that are the arithmetic sum and difference of the primary frequencies. As an example, if the input signals are 500 Hz ($f_1$) and 2000 Hz ($f_2$), the intermodulation distortion products may be measured at 1500 Hz ($f_2 - f_1$), 2500 Hz ($f_1 + f_2$), 1000 Hz ($f_2 - 2f_1$), etc. It is important to realize that these are just some examples of the possible combinations of intermodulation distortion products produced by $f_1$ and $f_2$. In reality, many more frequencies may be generated. Figure 7–7b shows the spectral relationship among the primary frequencies and the distortion products.

Difference frequency distortion (DFD) is a special case of intermodulation distortion whereby only the distortion products that are the differences between the two primary signals are measured. Using the example of the primary frequencies at 500 and 2000 Hz, difference frequency distortion products at 1500 Hz ($f_2 - f_1$), 1000 Hz ($f_2 - 2f_1$), and so on will be measured (Fig. 7–7c). Both IMD and DFD may occur in daily hearing aid use because speech, as well as many environmental sounds, are complex waveforms that have energy at multiple frequencies.

MEASUREMENT OF INTERMODULATION DISTORTION

Two types of intermodulation distortion (IMD) are common. Modulation distortion is one type and is measured by exciting the hearing aid with a twin-tone stimulus ($f_1$ and $f_2$) that has a fixed intensity difference. Typically, $f_1$ is lower in frequency than $f_2$ and is 12 dB higher than $f_2$. During the measurement, $f_1$ remains fixed in frequency, while $f_2$ is swept across the frequency range of interest.

Difference frequency distortion is another type of IMD and is measured by exciting the hearing aid with a swept twin-tone test signal ($f_1$ and $f_2$) with equal amplitudes (within 1.5 dB) and fixed frequency difference. Different frequency intervals have been used. For example, White (1978) recommended a frequency difference of 160 Hz, while Agnew (1994) reported that 200 Hz separation yielded the largest observable distortion products. The IEC-1983 standard recommends sweeping frequencies between 350 Hz and 5000 Hz at an intensity level of 64 dB SPL and a frequency separation of 125 Hz. In hearing aid measures, typically the second- ($f_2 - f_1$) and third-order ($2f_1 - f_2$) difference frequency distortions are measured. Higher order distortion products decrease rapidly in intensity and do not contribute to the total distortion value (Brockbank and Wass, 1945). The higher frequency ($f_2$) of the twin-tone stimulus is taken to represent the frequency where distortion products are measured (IEC, 1983).

## Similarities and Differences Between THD and IMD

Intermodulation distortion may be more important to consider than harmonic distortion because it represents the interaction of two or more tones. This is a condition that simulates more closely the complex stimuli (e.g., speech, music, sound effects, noise) that hearing aid wearers encounter in their daily environments. In addition, because these distortion products are not harmonically related, they can be more noticeable and more annoying to the wearer (Schweitzer, Causey, and Tolton, 1977; Jirsa and Norris, 1982). In addition, these measurements may more closely reflect the subjective judgments of hearing aid wearers (Agnew, 1988).

Another advantage of measuring intermodulation distortion over harmonic distortion is its reduced dependence on the effective bandwidth of the hearing aid. Higher order harmonic distortion products that are beyond the bandwidth of a "typical" hearing aid are rolled off, thus giving a distortion value that is smaller than its actual value. On the other hand, intermodulation distortion products "fold back" within the bandwidth of the hearing aid and can be measured more accurately. Measurement of the higher order DFD products occurring below $f_1$ may be affected similarly by the lower frequency cutoff of the hearing aid.

Measurements of harmonic distortion and intermodulation distortion determine the amount of nonlinearity of one frequency (or one frequency interval) at a time. Simultaneous interaction among different frequency regions (or at different frequency intervals) is not elicited nor measured. For example, if an audiologist uses a fixed $f_2 - f_1$ interval of 160 Hz in swept frequency intermodulation measurement, he or she would only obtain information at this frequency separation. Information on the interaction between $f_1$ and $f_2$ when they are at different frequency separation, or when they have different amplitude ratios (other than the 0 dB or 12 dB) would not be available. Testing at multiple intensity levels (Agnew, 1994) and using a stimulus that includes energy at all frequency regions are necessary to yield distortion results that reflect simultaneous interactions among frequencies.

Both harmonic distortion and intermodulation distortion can occur at the same time when a complex signal is used. In addition, the harmonics generated with one tone may interact with the difference frequencies of another tone-pair to result in even more distortion products. It is virtually impossible to specify the combination of distortion products present in a complex signal. Because each hearing aid has its own unique frequency response shaping at the input and output stages, a direct relationship between the magnitudes of the distortion products generated from these two types of distortions cannot be made (Olsen, 1971; Thomsen and Moller, 1975).

Intermodulation distortion measurements are not required by the ANSI S3.22-1987 or the ANSI S3.42-1992 standards. Furthermore, they cannot be easily obtained in a clinical setting because of the current need for complex and expensive instrumentation. Using current single microphone hearing aid test systems, an audiologist can qualitatively estimate nonlinear distortion (i.e., harmonic and intermodulation) by examining the "smoothness" of the frequency–response curve of a hearing aid using a random noise signal as the stimulus (Frye, 1986). Figure 7–8a reports the frequency–response curves obtained with a speech-shaped composite noise presented at 65 dB SPL and 85 dB SPL. At 65 dB SPL, the frequency gain curve appears "smooth." At 85 dB SPL, the frequency response curve appears "disorganized and jagged." The gain of the hearing aid has also decreased by approximately 10 dB. This appearance suggests the addition of distortion products from harmonic, and intermodulation distortions from interaction of component frequencies, in the speech input. In contrast, Figure 7–8b shows the output of the same hearing aid at the same setting, but excited with sweep sinusoids presented at 60 dB SPL and 80 dB SPL. The amount of total harmonic distortion (second and third) is also indicated as bars whose values can be read off on the right-hand y-axis (bottom of Fig. 7–8b). Note the increase in harmonic distortion from less than 5% in the upper graph of Figure 7–8b to greater than 40% in the lower graph of Figure 7–8b. Also note the smoothness of the response curve despite the large amount of harmonic distortion at high stimulus level. The absence of interaction among test frequencies resulted in the smooth frequency

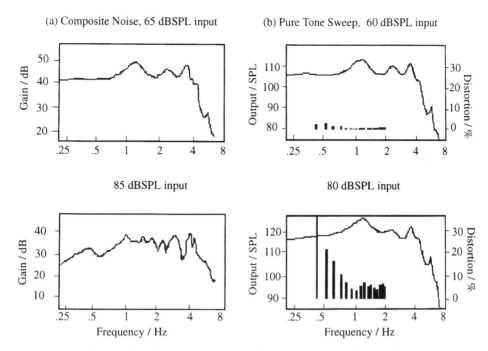

**Figure 7–8.** Coupler (2 cc) responses of a high-gain hearing aid tested at two intensity levels using (a) speech-weighted composite noise at 65 dB SPL and 85 dB SPL and (b) pure-tone sweep at 60 dB SPL and 80 dB SPL. Note high levels of THD at higher input levels.

response. This reinforces the idea that the effect of distortion measures using single frequency may not be easily noticeable on frequency gain response curves.

### Generation of Saturation Distortion

Preves and Newton (1989) cite inadequate "headroom" as the major reason for saturation distortion. "Headroom" is defined as the range of sound pressure level between the maximum undistorted output of the hearing aid and the instantaneous output of the hearing aid. Figure 7–9 is a graphic representation of "headroom" along with the various factors that could affect its value. The SSPL90 setting of a hearing aid is represented by the "ceiling" in the figure. The height of the individual represents the level of the input signal to the hearing aid and the height of the stilts represents the gain on the hearing aid. If "headroom" is defined as the distance between the individual's head and the ceiling of the room, one can see that changing the height of the individual, raising or lowering the height of the stilt, and raising or lowering the height of the ceiling can all have an effect on "headroom." In a simplistic sense, distortion occurs when the person's head bumps the ceiling. This is equivalent to suggesting that the headroom is below zero, or when the instantaneous output of the hearing aid exceeds the maximum undistorted output level of the hearing aid. The amount of distortion increases as the degree of saturation increases. Factors that could affect headroom include:

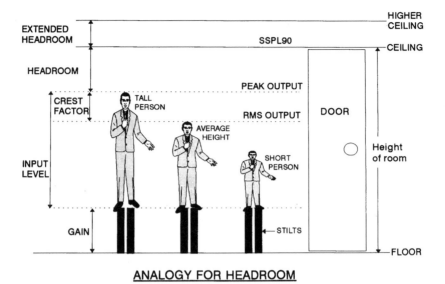

ANALOGY FOR HEADROOM

**Figure 7–9.**   Graphic analogy of the headroom concept.

SSPL90 SETTING

The SSPL90 on a hearing aid (or the ceiling in the room, Fig. 7–9) defines the maximum output of the hearing aid. Consequently, all being the same, the hearing aid with a higher SSPL90 (or higher ceiling) will have a larger headroom than one with a lower SSPL90.

Figure 7–10 reveals the percent total harmonic distortion (at 500, 800, and 1600 Hz) as the SSPL90 setting on a power hearing aid is decreased in 4 dB steps from a peak of 132 dB SPL to 108 dB SPL. A fixed 70 dB SPL swept sinusoid is used as the stimulus, while the gain of the hearing aid is set at 50 dB. It is evident that total harmonic distortion increases as the SSPL90 setting is gradually lowered.

Although it is simpler to regard a hearing aid as distortion free as long as its output is immediately below the SSPL90 setting, a hearing aid is not undistorted up to the SSPL90 output level. Depending on the hearing aid, amplifier design, and frequency response shape, THD and IMD levels of 10% may be measured at about 6 dB below SSPL90 in some parts of the frequency response range (Agnew, personal communication).

GAIN

Higher gain (or taller stilt in Fig. 7–9) leads to higher output. This reduces the available headroom on the hearing aid. On the other hand, Lotterman and Kasten (1967) reported that distortion level was inversely related to the power category of the hearing aid. That is, mild-gain hearing aids yielded more distortion than high-gain hearing aids. This probably reflects the fact that high-gain instruments typically have higher SSPL90. In addition, the bandwidth of these high-gain instruments is narrower in comparison to mild-gain instruments. This

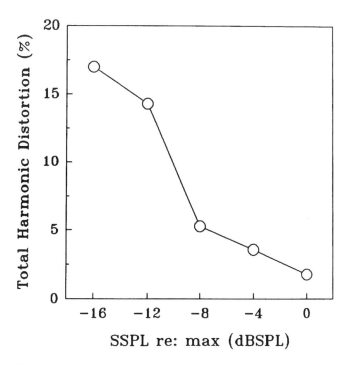

**Figure 7–10.** Percent total harmonic distortion (THD) as a function of SSPL90 setting (re: max SSPL of 132 dB SPL) of a hearing aid.

results in reduced distortion products in the higher frequencies and, thus, lower distortion value.

User gain setting on a hearing aid (i.e., volume control setting) can also influence the amount of headroom on the hearing aid. Figure 7–11 reports the total harmonic distortion (at 500, 800, and 1600 Hz) of a linear hearing aid set at its maximum SSPL90 of 132 dB SPL. A significant amount of harmonic distortion (30%) is noted at the full VC setting. This amount decreases dramatically (less than 5%) at the first 10 dB decrease in gain setting. Further reduction in gain does not lead to any change in total harmonic distortion. Kasten and Lotterman (1967) and Lotterman and Kasten (1967) also showed higher distortion near maximum gain control settings in most (linear) hearing aids.

Today's completely-in-the-canal (CIC) hearing aids are reported to have less distortion than other styles of hearing aids when they are worn. This is because less coupler gain is used to take advantage of the reduced V3 (volume between hearing aid and the tympanic membrane) despite the relatively high SSPL90 of the hearing aid (107 dB SPL or more).

INPUT LEVEL

The output from a hearing aid increases as the input (or the height of the person in Fig. 7–9) to the hearing aid increases at a fixed volume control setting. This will decrease the available headroom and lead to more distortion. Figure 7–12

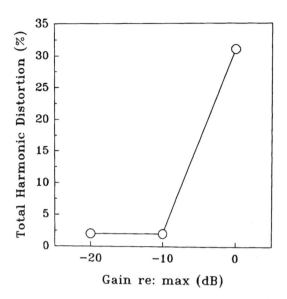

**Figure 7–11.**    Percent THD as a function of gain (re: max gain of 50 dB) on a hearing aid.

reports the total harmonic distortion of a linear hearing aid as the input level is raised in 10-dB steps from 50 dB SPL to 80 dB SPL. Note that THD is only 2 to 3% when the input signal is below 70 dB SPL. However, the percent THD increases drastically (approximately 13%) as the input signal is increased to 70 dB SPL.

An input speech level of 65 dB SPL is used in most prescriptive formulae to select target gain of a linear hearing aid. However, there are numerous situations in which the level of the input signal exceeds 65 dB SPL. For example, during

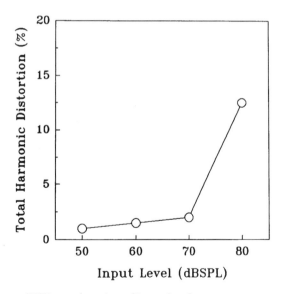

**Figure 7–12.**    Percent THD as a function of input levels.

vocalization, a hearing aid wearer's voice will be 12 to 15 dB more intense when measured at the ear level than when measured at one meter away (Dunn and Farnsworth, 1939; Dunn and White, 1940; Kuk, 1990). Stelmachowicz, Mace, Kopun, and Carney (1993) reported that because of the closer proximity, the speech sound pressure levels measured at the ears of hearing impaired infants produced by their mothers' voices typically exceed 65 dB SPL. These situations raise the possibility that significant reduction in headroom could occur in many daily situations. The readers are referred to the works of Pearsons, Bennett, and Fidell (1977), Teder (1990), Jelonek, Mosher, Lebo, Smith, Schwind, Kurz, Decker, and Krusemark (1993) on the sound pressure levels in various listening situations and for speech at different vocal efforts.

CREST FACTOR

Crest factor refers to the difference in peak SPL and overall root-mean-square (rms) SPL of an acoustic signal (Frye, 1987). The peak SPL is the maximum intensity of the signal during its course, while the rms level of a signal is the intensity of the signal averaged over a specific period of time. An analogy of crest factor may be the difference in height between the tall person and the average person shown in Figure 7–9. Crest factor affects the accuracy with which a hearing aid is tested in the laboratory as well as how easily a hearing aid is saturated in real life.

Sound pressure levels of typical speech elements are reported in overall rms values. However, a hearing aid saturates when the instantaneous peak SPL exceeds the saturation level of the hearing aid. Given the same settings on a hearing aid and the same rms level of the input signal, an input with a higher crest factor will more likely saturate the hearing aid than that with a lower crest factor. Sinusoids typically have a crest factor of 3 dB. A complex signal typically has a higher crest factor. That is, there is greater difference between the peak SPL of a complex signal and its overall rms level. Speech spectrum noise that is used for acoustic measures has a long-term crest factor of 12 dB at 1000 Hz to 1400 Hz and 16 to 17 dB at 300 Hz to 400 Hz (Dunn and White, 1940). This suggests that the long-term spectrum of conversational speech at 65 dB SPL may have peak SPL as high as 82 dB SPL (i.e., 65 dB plus 17 dB), a level that can easily saturate a hearing aid even at a low gain setting.

Recently, Stelmachowicz, Mace, Kopun, and Carney (1993) showed that the short-term crest factor on fricatives measured in a short-time window is significantly greater than 12 dB. As much as 20 to 37% of the measurements revealed a crest factor in excess of 18 dB between 2000 Hz to 4000 Hz.

An example may help clarify this issue. Consider a hearing aid with a SSPL90 setting of 110 dB SPL and user gain setting of 30 dB. This hearing aid setting will not lead to saturation for conversational speech presented at an overall level of 65 dB when the crest factor is 12 dB. This is because the output of 107 dB SPL (i.e., 65 dB + 30 dB + 12 dB) is below the saturation limit (i.e., SSPL90) of the hearing aid. However, as soon as the individual vocalizes, his/her voice will be 77 dB SPL (i.e., 65 dB plus 12 dB) measured at the microphone of the hearing aid (Dunn and White, 1940). This suggests a peak output of 119 dB SPL (30 dB gain + 12 dB crest factor + 77 dB input). This is sufficient to saturate the hearing aid and contribute to the perception of poor quality of the wearer's own voice (Kuk, 1990).

POWER REQUIREMENT

Cole (1993) showed that the maximum SSPL90 on a hearing aid is controlled by the type of hearing aid receiver, its electrical impedance, and the acoustic coupling system. Additionally, the size of the battery also plays a crucial role in limiting the SSPL90. Table 7–1 shows that reducing the size of the receiver (CI in comparison to EH) or reducing the size of the battery (#10 in comparison to #675) will result in lower SSPL90 to achieve 100 hours of battery life. For example, when using a 675 battery and a larger CI receiver, the SSPL90 for 100 hours of battery life is 139 dB SPL. However, if the receiver is reduced to an EH, the SSPL90 for the same battery would be reduced to 125 dB SPL (a difference of 14 dB). On the other hand, if the designer keeps the same CI receiver, but used a #10 battery instead of the #675 battery, the SSPL90 would be reduced from 139 dB SPL to 129 dB SPL. Consequently, SSPL90 can be increased by improving the efficiency of the amplifier or the energy capacity of the battery.

AMPLIFIER TYPE

The type of amplifier used in the output stage of a hearing aid affects the available headroom. The class A amplifier has been used in most hearing aid applications but it has the lowest output voltage. A class B (push-pull) amplifier can provide up to 4 times more output voltage than a class A amplifier, but with a higher current drain. The class D amplifier provides output similar to that of a class B amplifier, but with lower current drain (Preves and Newton, 1989).

Considerable experimental attention has been paid to demonstrate the subjective preference for hearing aids with improved headroom (or reduced distortion) in normal hearing and hearing impaired listeners. Kochkin (1989), Kochkin and Ballad (1991), Fortune and Preves (1992), and Palmer, Killion, Wilber, and Ballad (1995) compared listener preference for class A and class D amplifiers. Higher sound quality ranking was reported for the class D amplifier over the class A amplifier, especially at high presentation levels.

**Table 7–1.** Available HFA-SSPL90 for 100 Hours of Battery Life With Ideal Amplifiers in an ITE Configuration for Four Receivers and Four Battery Types

| Knowles Receiver Types | Receiver Size (cc) | HFA-SSPL90 for 100 Hours Battery Life | | | |
|---|---|---|---|---|---|
| | | #675 | #13 | #312 | #10 |
| CI | 0.29 | 139 | 135 | 132 | 129 |
| EF | 0.19 | 136 | 132 | 129 | 125 |
| ED | 0.08 | 131 | 127 | 124 | 121 |
| EH | 0.056 | 125 | 121 | 118 | 114 |

Cole, 1993; with permission

On the other hand, some investigators did not find preference for the class D amplifier to be universal. Potts, Valente, and Agnew (1994) compared subjective ratings of class A and class D amplifiers when both were matched for undistorted maximum output. A slight preference was noted for the class A amplifier on some subjective scales and equal preference was observed on other scales. Although the number of subjects tested was small (N = 4), the results suggest that class A and class D amplifiers, when matched for undistorted maximum output, may be very similar in distortion performance.

ADAPTIVE GAIN

A hearing aid saturates at an output level that exceeds the saturation limit. If the output can be maintained below the saturation level by decreasing the gain on the hearing aid as the input increases, saturation limit will not be reached and no distortion will be experienced. This can be achieved with the use of compression and adaptive frequency–gain response hearing aids. These devices decrease gain as input level increases to prevent saturation.

Figure 7–13 illustrates the input-output function of a linear hearing aid (1:1) and a hearing aid with a compression ratio of 2:1 and a compression threshold (kneepoint) at 70 dB SPL. Both hearing aids saturate at 120 dB SPL. For the linear hearing aid, saturation is reached at an input of 90 dB SPL. For the hearing aid with a compression ratio of 2:1, saturation is not reached until an input of 110 dB SPL. This extends the headroom by 20 dB! Figure 7–14a shows the 2-cc coupler gain of a compression hearing aid at an input level of 65 dB SPL and 85 dB SPL

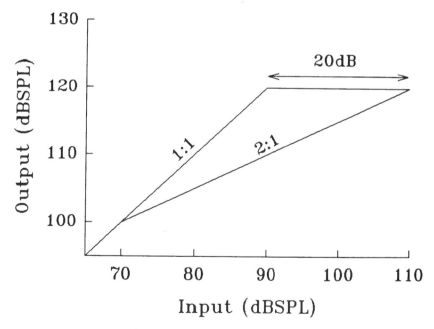

**Figure 7–13.** Input-output function to demonstrate the increase in headroom with compression.

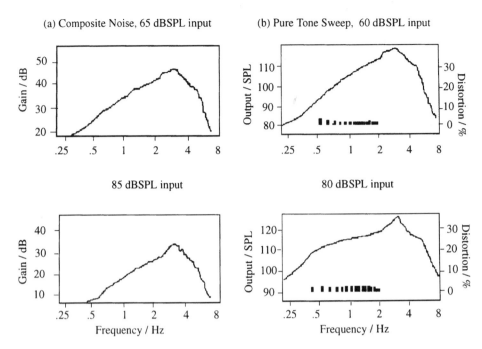

**Figure 7–14.** Coupler (2 cc) output and total harmonic distortion from an input compression hearing aid evaluated at two input levels using (a) speech-weighted composite noise at 65 dB SPL and 85 dB SPL and (b) pure-tone sweep at 60 dB SPL and 80 dB SPL. Note the absence of high percentages of THD at the high input levels.

using speech-shaped composite noise as stimulus. Figure 7–14b shows the coupler output and total harmonic distortion values of the same hearing aid using a 60 dB SPL and 80 dB SPL pure tone sweep as stimulus. Note the smoothness of the frequency gain response obtained at the 80/85 dB SPL condition and that no increase in total harmonic distortion is observed as the input is increased. This is in contrast to the findings for the linear hearing aid (Fig. 7–8). Finally, increasing the compression ratio from 2:1 increases the headroom.

Hawkins and Naidoo (1993) compared the subjective sound quality and clarity between hearing aids with asymmetric peak clipping and compression output limiting. Twelve hearing-impaired subjects listened to connected discourse and music presented under three conditions representing less than 2% to as much as 40% total harmonic distortion. Their results showed that the average subject preferred output limiting compression over peak clipping. Stronger preference for compression output limiting was seen as more saturation was introduced.

These results suggest that the use of hearing aids with compression (both compression limiting and dynamic range compression) is an effective solution to minimize saturation distortion. This may be more effective than adjusting the hearing aid to a higher SSPL90 setting because the SSPL90 setting should typically be set below the wearer's loudness discomfort level (LDL) to avoid discomfort from loud sounds. For those with low loudness tolerance, increasing the SSPL90 to provide for better headroom would necessarily increase the risk of loudness discomfort. Compression hearing aids allow the use of the same low SSPL90 setting while providing sufficient headroom. One needs to remember, however, that amplitude distortion and temporal distortion also occur in compression hearing aids. Therefore, careful selection of compression parameters is necessary. This issue is discussed in greater detail in Chapter 4.

## Perceptual Consequences of Saturation Distortion

The effect of distortion on speech recognition and sound quality depends on the type of the distortion product, the percent of distortion, and the evaluative tool to assess the effect of distortion. It is generally recognized that distortion can affect speech recognition and subjective sound quality of hearing aid processed speech. However, Levitt, Cudahy, Hwang, Kennedy, and Link (1987) commented that the negative effects of distortion may not be noted until the distortion in the signal exceeds the distortion generated in the hearing impaired ear. Although different studies attempted to correlate different forms of distortion with speech recognition or sound quality, it is important to realize that harmonic distortion and intermodulation distortion do occur simultaneously with complex stimuli. Consequently, the mixed relation observed between distortion and perceptual effects could have been the results of simple attempts to evaluate a more complex phenomenon. Additional refinements in evaluative techniques are necessary to establish a more accurate relationship between distortion and its perceptual effects.

### SATURATION DISTORTION AND SPEECH RECOGNITION

Inconsistent findings have been reported on the effect of saturation distortion on speech recognition. Licklider (1946) was probably among the first to report on the effect of peak clipping on speech recognition. This author introduced different forms of waveform alteration to monosyllabic words and required subjects to identify the distorted words. In quiet, neither symmetrical nor asymmetrical peak clipping reduced speech recognition significantly even when the speech waveforms were reduced to a series of rectangular waves. However, in noise, the relative effect of the various kinds of clipping remained similar, although absolute speech recognition scores decreased over the quiet condition. Other investigators (e.g., Corliss, Burnett, Kobal, and Bassin, 1968; Olsen, 1971; Gioannini and Franzen, 1978) also reported that the effect of saturation distortion on speech recognition may be more evident when speech materials are presented in a background of noise.

Thomas (1968) speculated that peak-clipped speech was still perceived as intelligible because of the preservation of the second formant in clipped speech. This author filtered monosyllablic words to remove either the first or second formant. The filtered speech was then clipped, and 10 normal-hearing listeners were asked to identify the filtered, clipped words. A mean speech recognition score of 71% was obtained for clipped speech that retained both the first and second formants, while a mean score of 7.6% was obtained for clipped speech that only retained the first formant.

Thomas and Niederjohn (1968) also argued that at clipping, the first formant of the speech signal would introduce distortion products that could affect the discrimination of higher formants. This suggests that clipped speech with a reduced first formant would be more intelligible than clipped speech without attenuation of the first formant. Their results on 10 listeners revealed that monosyllabic words with reduced first formant amplitude (i.e., filtered) was more intelligible than the unfiltered clipped speech when the signal-to-noise ratio was between +5 and –5 (noise level was 90 dB SPL).

Other investigators reported that saturation distortion significantly affected speech recognition (Harris, Haines, Kelsey, and Clack, 1961; Jerger, Speaks, and Malmquist, 1966; Olsen and Carhart, 1967; Jirsa and Hodgson, 1970; Jirsa and Norris, 1982). However, the effect on speech recognition was minimal until more than 20% of THD was introduced. In addition, the effect of increasing saturation distortion may be less tolerable by hearing-impaired listeners than normal-hearing listeners (Zerlin and Burnett, 1960). The effect of saturation distortion seemed to be most evident in the recognition of phonemes in the word final position (Bode and Kasten, 1971).

Cox and Taylor (1994) correlated the difference in speech recognition scores obtained in an aided and unaided condition with the amount of measured distortion on a hearing aid. The distortion measures included harmonic distortion at 500, 800, and 1,200 Hz, intermodulation distortion at 500, 1000, and 2000 Hz, and transient distortion. These measures were made under three conditions that approximated listening in a quiet living room, a reverberant room, and a party environment. Their results showed a mild, but significant, correlation between speech recognition and harmonic distortion measured in noisy and reverberant environments.

SUBJECTIVE EVALUATION OF SATURATION DISTORTION

The effects of distortion may be more noticeable on sound quality measures before they can be detected on speech recognition measures (Licklider, 1946; Harris et al., 1991; Crain, 1992). Crain (1992) compared the relative sensitivity of speech recognition and sound quality criteria in reflecting the deleterious effects of distortion. This author found that a clipping threshold of 12 dB below the speech peaks resulted in no change in the speech reception threshold (SRT) and virtually no subjective report of unacceptable sound quality. A peak-clipping threshold set to 36 dB below the speech peaks only resulted in a 1 dB decrease in the speech reception threshold. However, over half of the subjects reported unacceptable sound quality at distortion created at this level of clipping.

Agnew (1988) reported that total harmonic distortion of 3 to 6% are common in hearing aids and are not objectionable to the wearers. In addition, he reported that total harmonic distortion in hearing aids is not as objectionable as intermodulation distortion because the former often coincides with the harmonic components present in speech or music. Furthermore, odd-order harmonics (e.g., third, fifth) are said to be more displeasing, while even-order harmonics (e.g., second, fourth) are more harmonious (Agnew, 1988). Langford-Smith (1960) also suggested that harmonics below the sixth order are not displeasing.

Killion (1979) reported that IMD between 6 and 12% may not be noticeable while listening to speech or music. Although the appearance of harmonic and/or intermodulation distortion is associated with reduced subjective preference (Agnew, 1994; Potts et al., 1994), no criterion level can be set to define the limits of acceptability. Individual tolerance to the distortion is just as important as, if not more important than, the magnitude of the distortion in the evaluation of hearing aids.

One frustration in trying to understand the perceptual effect of distortion upon the recognition and quality of speech is the multitude of adjectives that wearers have used to describe distortion. These adjectives include words like "unclear," "unnatural," "tinny," "noisy," "echoic," "hollow," "boomy," "crackling," "static," "hissing," "muffled," "rattling," "fuzzy," and "pumping." These are just some of the many adjectives that have been frequently used to describe the subjective perception of distorted acoustic signals.

Distortion products add to the overall loudness and perhaps annoyance of the acoustic signal. This implies that hearing aids with a higher headroom will less likely saturate and allow higher output levels before reaching an uncomfortable level than devices that have a lower headroom. This concept was evaluated by Fortune and Preves (1992), who compared the real-ear SPL at loudness discomfort levels (LDL) for continuous discourse obtained under headphones and with hearing aids having class A and class D amplifiers. Their results showed higher real-ear SPL at LDL when measured with headphones than when measured with a class D amplifier (100 dB SPL and 98 dB SPL, respectively). Loudness discomfort levels obtained with a class A amplifier was the lowest (93 dB SPL). Subjects in this study also rated the class D amplifier as more "distinct," "clearer," and "brighter." The subjects also reported a greater preference for the class D amplifier. The difference in LDL measures between headphone and hearing aid (class A amplifier) results suggests that one should be cautious in applying headphone data to specify SSPL90 settings on hearing aids, especially those with class A amplifiers.

The perception of distortion may be affected by the magnitude of the distortion. Indeed, it was demonstrated that the perception of distortion grows in a logarithmic manner with increased percentage of distortion. For example, Barry and Kidd (1981) performed magnitude estimation and production of the percent of distortion on speech quality as a function of second-order harmonic distortion. The data obtained from normal-hearing listeners can be fit with a logarithmic function with an exponent of 0.75. This indicates that the perception of distortion grows less rapidly than the physical change in distortion values.

Lawson and Chial (1982) also performed direct magnitude scaling of distortion on normal-hearing and hearing-impaired subjects. They found that speech quality estimates changed more rapidly than the change in percent of total harmonic distortion in normal-hearing subjects. However, the reverse is true for the hearing-impaired subjects. On the other hand, Gabrielsson, Nyberg, Sjorgren, and Svenson (1976) showed that hearing-impaired subjects needed more distortion than normal-hearing listeners to recognize its presence. Crain (1992) reported that normal-hearing and hearing-impaired subjects rated the acceptability of clipped speech in a similar manner.

Kates and Kozma-Spytek (1994) evaluated the subjective change in speech quality as a function of levels of peak clipping. Subjects used a 10-point scale to rate the quality of speech at 4 clipping levels, corresponding to 0.5%, 4%, 10%, and 20% of the time at which sentence materials were clipped. These levels were below the level at which speech recognition was affected. A systematic change in speech quality was noted as the level of peak clipping increased.

The perception of distortion depends on the electroacoustic characteristics of the hearing aid and the phonemes that are clipped. For example, Langford-Smith (1960) reported that 3% THD in a system with a 15,000 Hz bandwidth can become objectionable, whereas one with a 3750 Hz bandwidth may not become objectionable until 12.8% THD is experienced. This is because with the limited bandwidth, most of the higher order harmonics fall beyond the bandwidth of the hearing aid and are inaudible, whereas the system with the wider bandwidth retains the higher order harmonics.

Nakagawa and Levitt (1991) reported that the just noticeable distortion (jnd) index (in percent) for vowels is typically smaller than consonants. As small as 0.1% level of distortion was detectable with the vowel /a/ in isolation. However, as much as 10% distortion was needed before subjects could detect the presence of distortion in the fricative /f/. A hearing aid with a boost in high frequency gain (+12 dB slope) is also associated with a lower jnd than one with a flat frequency response. Distortion from a wideband clipper is easier to detect than that from a narrower band clipper. Cudahy and Kates (1993) examined the jnds for other vowels and consonants and reported similar findings.

### Global Measures of Distortion

Although the measurements of harmonic distortion and intermodulation distortion reveal the electroacoustic performance of hearing aids, these measures fail to predict the effect of such distortion in daily use. Such difficulty may be related to (1) the inherent limitation of harmonic distortion measurement to frequencies below 2000 Hz; (2) the sequential testing of different frequency regions in harmonic and intermodulation distortion, which would prevent the observation of simultaneous interaction among frequency components; and (3) the occurrence of more than harmonic distortion and intermodulation distortion in real life. Other types of distortion discussed in this chapter may occur at the same time. For example, digital hearing aids may show saturation distortion as well as distortion from quantization (Levitt et al., 1987).

Given these limitations, a measure of distortion that tests all input frequencies simultaneously and at multiple intensity levels may more accurately describe the nonlinear behavior of a hearing aid and lead to a better prediction of the effects of distortion on the "real-life" performance of the hearing aid. Burnett (1967), Peters and Burkhard (1968), Frye (1986), Dyrlund (1989), Kates (1989), and Bareham (1990) recommend the use of a broadband noise as the signal source so that all combinations of harmonic and intermodulation distortion can be assessed. However, individual frequencies resulting in distortion cannot be measured easily because they will be embedded within the bandwidth of the original broadband signal. Alternative approaches to quantifying distortion may be needed.

Indices that reflect a general overall measure of distortion have been proposed. The motivation behind a general measure is to quantify the total magnitude of distortion, regardless of its sources. An added objective for this index is to correlate its results with the perceptual consequence of distortion. Williamson, Cummins, and Hecox (1987), anticipating the development of digital hearing aids, proposed a model in which distortion from a hearing aid is simply viewed as the difference between the actual hearing aid output, $y_{(t)}$, and the idealized output from the linear filter, $z_{(t)}$ in response to a complex stimulus, e.g., speech. Distortion from the hearing aid can be represented in a three-dimensional plot with amplitude, time, and frequency as the three dimensions. The merits of this approach are that it consolidates several measures of distortion into one measure and it displays the magnitude of distortion across frequencies and across time. No behavioral data were reported to demonstrate the validity of this measure and its correlation with judgments of sound quality and speech recognition.

Levitt, Cudahy, Hwang, Kennedy, and Link (1987) proposed a distortion spectrum, $D_{(f)}$, to represent the magnitude of the percent of distortion at each test frequency. Simply, $D_{(f)}$ is calculated as the ratio of the signal spectrum at the output to the signal spectrum at the output of an idealized linear spectrum (i.e., one without distortion). The difference between this model and that of Williamson, Cummins and Hecox (1987) is that this model also considers characteristics of the human auditory system in the determination of $D_{(f)}$. This model starts with the magnitude of distortion in each auditory critical band filter. The output spectrum from the filters is then smoothed to approximate the effect of the upward spread of masking. The smoothed distortion spectrum is then averaged across time to approximate integration of the auditory system. The $D_{(f)}$ is calculated as the smoothed, time-averaged distortion across all critical band filters. The application of this model has been evaluated by Levitt, Cudahy, Hwang, Kennedy, and Link (1987), Cudahy and Kates (1993), and Kates and Kozma-Spytek (1994) with fairly positive results.

## Coherence Function

Recently, significant attention has been paid to the quantification of distortion in hearing aids using coherence analysis. Simply, coherence analysis is a method using spectral analysis and Fast Fourier Transform (FFT) to determine the degree of linear relationship between the input signal to a hearing aid and the output signal from the hearing aid measured across many frequencies. A broadband stimulus, usually speech-shaped noise, is used as the input signal to measure coherence. The magnitude of the coherence across frequencies can be presented in a frequency plot called a coherence function. A coherence index can be calculated across the entire frequency display by averaging the coherence measurement across all test frequencies. In mathematical terms, the coherence function at each frequency can be defined as:

$$\gamma^2(f) = \frac{G_{ab}^2(f)}{G_{aa}(f) \cdot G_{bb}(f)} \qquad (3)$$

where $\gamma^2(f)$ is the coherence measure as a function of frequency (f), $G_{ab}(f)$ is the cross-spectrum or the degree to which the same frequency is present in both the input and output signals, $G_{aa}(f)$ is the power spectrum of the input signal, and $G_{bb}(f)$ is the power spectrum of the output signal.

The coherence measure can range from 0 to 1. A value of "1" suggests that the output at a particular frequency or of the whole system is perfectly correlated to the input (i.e., distortion free). A value of "0" suggests that there is no relationship between the input and output signals (i.e., high levels of distortion). A value of 0.5 suggests that there is an equal amount of distortion and noise in the output signal as there is in the input signal.

Introduction of nonlinear distortion and addition of noise can affect the linear relationship between the input and output and, thus, lower the coherence index to a value less than "1."

The advantage of using a broadband signal in coherence measurement is that it allows for simultaneous testing of all frequencies. Coherence measurement is also sensitive to phase fluctuation in the output of the hearing aid (Kates, 1989). In addition, it is a steady-state measurement and is not sensitive to the frequency response of the hearing aid, as long as the internal noise level is significantly lower than the signal level and the saturation level of the hearing aid is not reached (Preves, 1990).

Coherence measurement offers a global assessment of the extent of nonlinearity and noise within the hearing aid at specific stimulus intensities. Unlike harmonic distortion and intermodulation distortion, it does not identify the source of the nonlinearity. It is necessary to interpret the coherence measure in light of the stimulus level at which the coherence function is generated. At a low stimulus level, e.g., 50 dB SPL, low coherence is usually indicative of inherent distortion within the hearing aid, e.g., amplifier noise. At a high stimulus level, e.g., 90 dB SPL, low coherence usually indicates the introduction of harmonic distortion and intermodulation distortion that is produced from the hearing aid in saturation.

Not knowing the source of poor coherence may limit the predictive ability of coherence measurement. For example, a coherence of 0.5 only suggests that half of the product measured at the output is a result of distortion. It does not specify the portion contributed by inherent noise, harmonic distortion, or intermodulation distortion in the total distortion measure. Given that the perceptual consequence of harmonic distortion is different from intermodulation distortion (Agnew, 1988), it is likely that two hearing aids with the same coherence value may yield different perceptual results, depending on the sources of the nonlinearities. Another difficulty is that coherence measure does not include temporal distortion and effects due to noise "fill in" and "pumping." Additional refinement may be needed to use the measured coherence to predict laboratory or real-world performance.

Coherence can also be expressed as a signal-to-distortion ratio (SDR). Dyrlund (1989), Bareham (1990), Preves (1990), and Kates (1992) suggest that the signal-to-distortion ratio can be calculated as:

$$\text{Signal/distortion (SDR)} = \sqrt{\frac{\gamma^2}{1 - \gamma^2}} \qquad (4)$$

$$\text{Percent Distortion} = \frac{100}{\text{SDR}} \qquad (5)$$

where $\gamma^2$ represents the coherent power in the output and $(1 - \gamma^2)$ represents the noncoherent power in the output. This suggests that as the coherent power increases, or as the noncoherent power decreases, the signal-to-distortion ratio improves. For example, if the coherence ($\gamma^2$) is 0.5, the SDR becomes "1"

$$\left( \sqrt{\frac{0.5}{1 - 0.5}} \right)$$

and the percent distortion becomes 100%. Table 7–2 summarizes the percent distortion calculated from different coherence values (Preves, 1994) using Equations 4 and 5.

### Factors Affecting Coherence Measure

The coherence measure reflects the amount of nonlinearity and noise produced by a hearing aid at the stimulus condition in which the hearing aid is tested. Consequently, the coherence index of a hearing aid varies with stimulus conditions and settings on the hearing aid. If one number is needed to represent the coherence of the hearing aid, the hearing aid settings and test conditions must approximate the condition in which the hearing aid is typically used. The following is a listing of the factors affecting the coherence index.

GAIN

Coherence decreases as the overall gain of the hearing aid increases beyond the point where the output exceeds the saturation limit. Figure 7–15 shows the change in coherence values as the gain is increased from 20 dB (a) to 40 dB (c) in a hearing aid with a SSPL90 of 100 dB SPL. White noise presented at 70 dB SPL is used as the input signal. The coherence is "1" at most of the frequencies when the gain is set at 20 dB. Coherence decreases to approximately 0.9 when the overall

**Table 7–2.**  Percentage of Distortion for Selected Coherence Values

| Coherence Value | Percent Distortion |
|:---:|:---:|
| 1.00 | 0 |
| 0.99 | 10 |
| 0.97 | 17 |
| 0.95 | 23 |
| 0.90 | 33 |
| 0.85 | 42 |
| 0.80 | 50 |
| 0.70 | 65 |
| 0.60 | 82 |
| 0.50 | 100 |

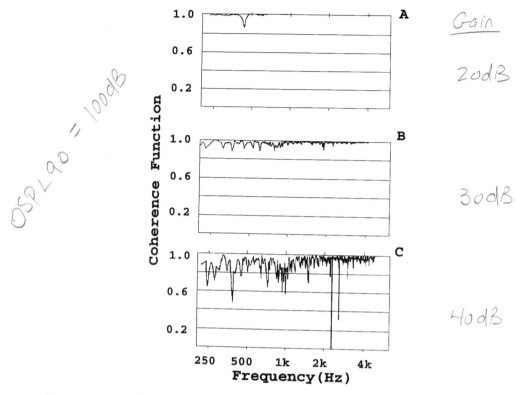

**Figure 7–15.** Effect of gain on measured coherence. Gain values are (a) 20 dB, (b) 30 dB, and (c) 40 dB. A SSPL90 setting of 100 dB is used.

gain is increased to 30 dB. Further deterioration in coherence is noted at the overall gain of 40 dB.

SSPL90 SETTING

A hearing aid set at a low SSPL90 yields lower coherence than a hearing aid in which the output is set at a higher SSPL90. However, this occurs only when the output of the hearing aid is greater than the SSPL90 of the hearing aid. Figure 7–16 shows the increase in coherence as the SSPL90 is increased from 100 dB SPL (a) to 120 dB SPL (c) in 10 dB steps. A 70 dB SPL white noise is used as the input. Note that the coherence improves from approximately 0.8 at the low SSPL90 setting (a) to almost 1.0 at the high SSPL90 setting (c).

INPUT LEVEL

An input level that causes the output to exceed the saturation threshold (SSPL90) of a hearing aid will lead to lower coherence. The higher the input level beyond the saturation threshold, the lower the coherence. Figure 7–17 shows the coherence function as the input to a linear hearing aid (SSPL90 at 100 dB SPL; gain of 40 dB) is changed from 60 dB SPL (a) to 90 dB SPL (d). At the 60 dB SPL input (a),

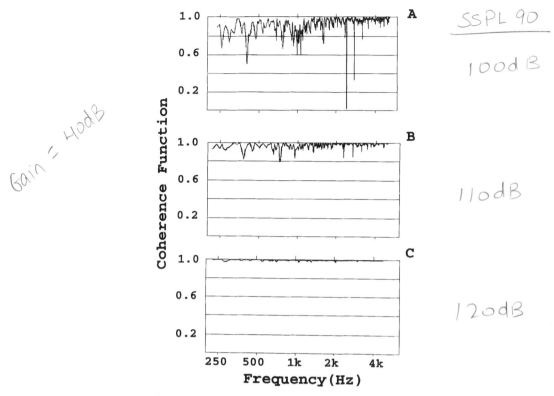

**Figure 7–16.** Effect of SSPL90 on measured coherence. SSPL90 settings are (a) 100 dB SPL, (b) 110 dB SPL, and (c) 120 dB SPL. A fixed gain of 40 dB is used with an input of 70 dB SPL.

coherence is close to "1" across all test frequencies. As the input level increases, greater reduction in coherence is noted from Figure 7–17b–d.

AUTOMATIC GAIN CONTROL (AGC)

A compression hearing aid reduces its gain as the input (or output) levels increase beyond the compression threshold, thereby extending its headroom and minimizing distortion. This is seen in Figure 7–18 where a hearing aid with compression threshold set at 65 dB SPL (SSPL90 is 110 dB; gain is 40 dB) is tested with white noise from 60 dB SPL to 90 dB SPL in 10-dB increments. Note that almost perfect coherence (i.e., 1) is seen at all intensities and frequencies. The appearance of reduced coherence is evident only at an input of 90 dB SPL.

   A hearing aid with a higher compression threshold will saturate sooner than one having a lower compression threshold (at a fixed compression ratio). Dyrlund (1992) also noted that the application of coherence measurement to hearing aids with automatic signal processing (ASP) may be problematic because of the interaction between test signal (a random noise) and the strategy used in the ASP circuitry. Fluctuation in the measured coherence could be experienced

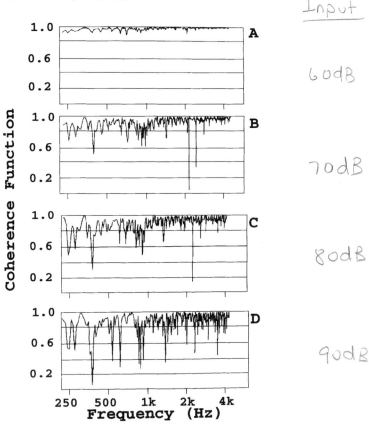

**Figure 7–17.** Effect of input level on measured coherence. Input levels are (a) 60 dB SPL, (b) 70 dB SPL, (c) 80 dB SPL, and (d) 90 dB SPL. A SSPL90 setting of 100 dB is used with a gain setting of 40 dB.

due to the jitter of the random noise. This problem needs to be addressed before a protocol that uses random noise can be formulated for distortion measurement.

INTERNAL NOISE LEVEL

A hearing aid with high internal noise (Ln) will have a high noncoherent output power, thus, low coherence. This is most clearly evident when the input to the hearing aid is low compared to the noise level (e.g., 50 dB SPL).

CREST FACTOR OF TEST SIGNAL

Test signals with a high crest factor will likely saturate a hearing aid at a lower overall input level and lead to a low coherence value. Fortune and Preves (1992) reported the mean coherence detection threshold (CDT, in dB SPL) in four hearing aids as continuous discourse and speech-shaped noise were used as the stimuli (Table 7–3). The CDT reflects the output intensity level (dB SPL) at which the coherence value falls below 0.9. Table 7–3 clearly shows that the use of continuous discourse passage (with a crest factor of 17 dB) led to a lower CDT for all

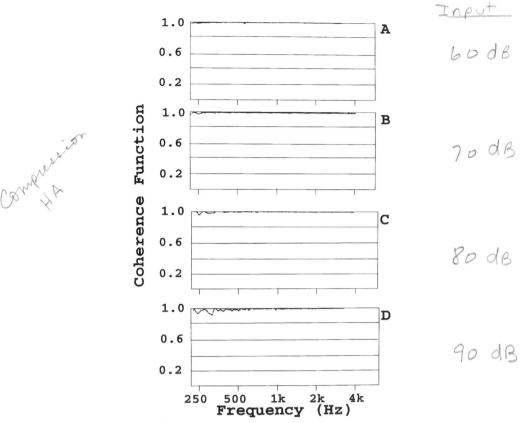

**Figure 7–18.** Effect of input level on measured coherence in a compression hearing aid with compression threshold at 65 dB SPL and a compression ratio of 8:1. Full-on gain of 40 dB and SSPL90 of 110 dB are used. Input levels used are 60 dB SPL to 90 dB SPL from (a) to (d). Note the almost perfect coherence until the 90 dB SPL input is used.

four hearing aids than the use of speech noise (crest factor of 12 dB). Dyrlund (1992) also reported that a speech sample (male speech) with a crest factor of 21 dB gave rise to lower coherence than white noise that had a crest factor of 13 dB.

COHERENCE INSTRUMENTATIONS

Bareham (1990) listed several instrumentation factors that affect the accuracy of coherence measurements. These considerations are beyond the scope of this chapter. Briefly, they include the appropriateness of the time window used to sample the waveform and the compensation (or lack of it) for the delay between the input and output signals. The interested readers are also referred to the work of Kates (1992), who provided a mathematical explanation for these technical issues.

### Perceptual Correlates of a Global Distortion Index

There is some support for the use of coherence to predict perceptual consequences of distortion in hearing aids. Schweitzer, Grim, Preves, Kubichek, and Woodruff

**Table 7–3.** Mean 2-cc Coupler Coherence Deterioration Thresholds (in dB SPL) for Four Hearing Aids Using Continuous Discourse (Crest Factor = 17 dB) and Speech-Shaped Noise (Crest Factor = 12 dB) at an Input Level of 75 dB SPL

| Stimulus Types | Hearing aids | | | |
|---|---|---|---|---|
| | HA#1 | HA#2 | HA#3 | HA#4 |
| Continuous discourse | 112.4 | 109.0 | 87.8 | 84.6 |
| Speech-shaped noise | >119.0 | >114.0 | 95.4 | 94.4 |

Fortune and Preves, 1992, with permission

(1991) compared subjective ranking of 6 hearing aids on different electroacoustic measures. Six normal hearing subjects listened through the hearing aids to a 10-second passage presented at 65 dB SPL. The results showed perfect match between subjective ranking of the hearing aids and results of the coherence measures.

Hawkins and Naidoo (1993) compared the coherence measurement of a hearing aid with asymmetric peak clipping to that of a compression hearing aid with output limiting. The compression hearing aid was judged to provide better sound quality than the peak clipping aid at three levels of total harmonic distortion (from less than 2 to 40%). A coherence index of almost "1" was seen at all three stimulus conditions with the hearing aid incorporating compression, but a coherence index of about 0.5 was seen in the 40% THD condition when the peak-clipping device was measured. This match suggests that the coherence index may have potential to reflect subjective judgments.

Kates and Kozma-Spytek (1994) correlated subjective ratings with the weighted signal-to-distortion ratio (SDR) from seven normal hearing listeners. A correlation index of R = 0.998 was obtained between the weighted SDR and a normalized rating. This supports the potential use of coherence as a predictive tool of real-life effect of distortion products.

### Clinical Management of Distortion

It is evident that a hearing aid may exhibit many forms of distortion. The ability to recognize the types of distortion that are occurring is important for the management of complaints of "distorted" sound. Unfortunately, it is not always easy to identify the types of distortion in a hearing aid because of the following reasons:

1. The hearing aid wearers may not be specific or accurate in their description of the "distorted" sound. A common complaint is that "I don't know what is wrong, but it just doesn't sound right."
2. The adjectives that the wearers use may not be indicative of a specific type of distortion. That is, there is not a specific subjective correlate for each type of distortion. For example, "hazy," "unclear," "muffled" have been used to describe saturation distortion as well as distortion resulting from compression action.

3.  More than one type of distortion may occur within a hearing aid. For example, a compression hearing aid may sound distorted because of amplitude/ temporal distortion or saturation distortion (when the maximum undistorted level is low). A linear hearing aid may sound distorted because of inappropriate frequency–gain response (purposeful distortion) or saturation distortion.

4.  The occurrence of distortion may be condition specific. For example, saturation distortion only occurs when the output of the hearing aid exceeds the saturation limit of the hearing aid. A review of the factors previously listed would suggest that this type of distortion may not be evident unless proper testing condition is used to evaluate the distortion.

5.  There is no objective test that can satisfactorily quantify all the different forms of distortion. The current ANSI-S3.22-1987 standard of measuring harmonic distortion has been criticized for its inadequacy (see previous sections). The use of coherence measurement, although potentially useful as a global indicator of distortion, does not differentiate among distortion types and is still used in a research capacity. Its clinical applicability needs further refinement.

6.  The instrumentation for measuring many of the different types of distortion is expensive and not widely available. For example, the only measurement that one can quantitatively make with current clinical equipment is harmonic distortion, and perhaps attack and release time measurements in some hearing aid analyzers. However, measurement of intermodulation distortion, coherence, and phase cannot easily be made in a clinic.

Despite the apparent difficulties, an audiologist must manage hearing aid distortion to ensure wearer satisfaction. An approach that focuses on the prevention of distortion may be more fruitful than one that corrects for the problem when it occurs. These are the principles we follow in managing patient reports of distortion in our clinic.

First, choose hearing aids that have the least amount of inherent noise (Ln). For conventional analog hearing aids, this means selecting hearing aids with the lowest equivalent input noise levels. Such determination can be easily made on a hearing aid test system. Some programmable hearing aids, unfortunately, have a high Ln. Choice of these devices would require a detailed comparison between the advantages offered by the programmable system and the potential interference of the high Ln. Careful counselling may be needed. For digital hearing aids, information on the number of bits, the sampling rate, and the characteristics of the filters (for aliasing and imaging errors) are important to consider as these factors can affect the sound quality of the processed signal (see section on digitization error).

Second, make sure that the hearing aid characteristics are selected appropriately. An ideal hearing aid purposely distorts the acoustic signal to compensate for the wearer's hearing loss. For optimal performance, settings on the hearing aids must be selected carefully to match the individual wearer's preference and psychophysical abilities. The use of prescriptive formulae to select hearing aid settings, although an efficient starting point, is not sufficient to ensure proper selection without additional verification. Valente (1994) has compiled from several clinicians and researchers ways to verify "optimal" hearing aid fitting.

Along the same line, one may want to select hearing aids that would minimize the occurrence of saturation distortion. Devices with adaptive frequency–gain responses (including ASP and AGC) will extend headroom without increasing the risks of loudness discomfort. However, such devices also introduce temporal and amplitude alterations that may not be accepted by some wearers. Hearing aids with compression limiting may be desirable for these individuals because the intensity relationship among various syllabic structures may be better preserved.

Third, obtain detailed description of the wearer's complaints. Hearing aids that are properly selected may still exhibit distortion under certain conditions and with daily wear and tear. Careful questioning of the conditions in which distortion occurs is needed to identify the problem. For example, is distortion noted at all times or only during specific situations, e.g., vocalization, high intensity noise background, specific speaker, specific volume setting? How does the wearer describe the distortion? Although the adjectives that the wearers use may not be indicative of the specific problem, some adjectives may lead one to suspect one source of distortion over another. For example, "static" generally refers to an increased noise floor; "hollow," "boomy," "echoic," "muffled" generally refer to excessive low-frequency gain; "pumping" generally refers to inappropriate compression release times; "raspy," "blurred," "harsh," "buzzing," and "shrill" may be related to excessive IMD. If the distortion is a natural by-product of amplification, counselling may be the only approach to follow with the patient.

Fourth, obtain verification of the wearer's complaints. Subjective listening tests and objective electroacoustic measures are necessary to better define the complaint. Speech recognition tests may not be sensitive enough to detect small amounts of distortion. Objective tests that are necessary include the measurement of equivalent input noise level to reflect the magnitude of the inherent noise. Measurement of total harmonic distortion (THD) following the ANSI-S3.22-1987 standard, although criticized as noninformative, is still necessary as a means to communicate with hearing aid manufacturers on the extent of distortion in the hearing aid. Another objective measure is to test the suspected hearing aid using a speech-shaped noise at multiple intensity levels (Frye, 1986). This is illustrated in Figure 7–8, where the "roughness" of the frequency–gain response curve indicates the presence of saturation distortion products. Even a "distortion-free" linear hearing aid will reveal a "jagged" frequency–gain response curve at high stimulus levels. Therefore, it is important to note the level when such "jaggedness" occurs and compare that with "distortion-free" devices. Devices that result in the "jagged" frequency response at a low stimulus level should be sent to the manufacturers for repair. In the future, it is hoped that coherence measurement or other alternative approaches to measuring distortion can both describe the distortion and predict its perceptual effects.

## Conclusion

It is evident that different types of distortion can be present in hearing aids to reduce their effectiveness and jeopardize user satisfaction. Although some effort has been spent on the quantification of distortion, there is not yet a single measure or index that has proven to be descriptive (of distortion type and magnitude) and predictive (of its consequences). Additional work must be performed to fill this gap. Meanwhile, one must be attentive to the hearing aid wearers' complaints on the poor or "strange" sound quality of their hearing aids. Testing of distortion with broadband stimulus at multiple intensity levels is necessary to verify these complaints. Sensitive subjective tests are crucial to the understanding of distortion. Such tests still need to be developed and be clinically validated.

## Acknowledgements

Sincere appreciation is expressed to Jeremy Agnew, James Kates, David Preves, and Robert Sweetow for their helpful suggestions during the preparation of this manuscript. Gratitude is also expressed to Tom Victorian at Starkey Laboratories for generating the coherence functions illustrated in this chapter.

## *References*

Agnew J. (1988). Hearing instrument distortion: What does it mean for the listener? *Hear Instrum* 39(10):11–16.

Agnew J. (1994). Measurements of distortion levels in hearing aids: It's not a simple matter. *Hear J* 47(5):25–32.

American National Standards Institute. (1987). Specification of hearing aid characteristics. New York: ANSI S3.22-1987.

American National Standards Institute. (1992). Testing hearing aids with a broad-band noise signal. New York: ANSI S3.42-1992.

Ballou G. (1987). *Handbook for Sound Engineers: The New Audio Cyclopedia.* Indianapolis: Howard Sams & Company.

Bareham J. (1990). Part 2: Hearing instrument measurements using dual channel signal analysis. *Hear Instrum* 41(1):32–33.

Barry S, Kidd G. (1981). Psychophysical scaling of distorted speech. *J Speech Hear Res* 24:44–47.

Beck L, Burnett E, Frye G, Preves D, Widin G. (1993). *New Measures of Hearing Aid Performance Using a Broad-Band Noise Signal: A Tutorial.* (unpublished).

Bode D, Kasten R. (1971). Hearing aid distortion and consonant identification. *J Speech Hear Res* 14:323-331.

Brockbank R, Wass C. (1945). Nonlinear distortion in transmission systems. *J Inst Elec Eng* 92:45–56.

Burnett E. (1967). A new method for the measurement of nonlinear distortion using a random noise test signal. *Bull Prosthet Res* 10:76–92.

Cole W. (1993). Current design options and criteria for hearing aids. *J Speech Lang Pathol and Audiol Monogr Suppl* (1):7–14.

Corliss E, Burnett E, Kobal M, Bassin M. (1968). The relative importance of frequency distortion and changes in time constants in the intelligibility of speech. *IEEC Trans Audiol Electroacoust* 16: 36–39.

Cox R, Taylor I. (1994). Relationship between in-situ distortion and hearing aid benefit. *J Am Acad Audiol* 5:317–324.

Crain T. (1992). The effect of peak clipping on the speech recognition threshold. Unpublished Ph.D. Thesis, U. Minn.

Crystal T, House A. (1990). Articulation rate and the duration of syllables and stress groups in connected speech. *J Acoust Soc Am* 88:101–112.

Cudahy E, Kates J. (1993). Measuring the performance of modern hearing aids. In: Studebaker G, Hochberg I, eds. *Acoustical Factors Affecting Hearing Aid Performance.* 2nd ed. Boston: Allyn and Bacon, pp. 51–64.

Deer J, Bloom P, Preis D. (1985). Perception of phase distortion in all pass filters. *J Audio Eng Soc* 33:782–786.

Dunn H, Farnsworth D. (1939). Exploration of pressure field around the human head during speech. *J Acoust Soc Am* 10:184–189.

Dunn H, White S. (1940). Statistical measurements on conversational speech. *J Acoust Soc Am* 11:278–288.

Dyrlund O. (1989). Characterization of non-linear distortion in hearing aids using coherence analysis: A pilot study. *Scand Audiol* 18:143–148.

Dyrlund O. (1992). Coherence measurements in hearing instruments using different broad band signals. *Scand Audiol* 21:73–78.

Fortune T, Preves D. (1992). Hearing aid saturation and aided loudness discomfort. *J Speech Hear Res* 35:175–185.

Frye G. (1986). High speed real-time hearing aid analysis. *Hear J* 39(6):21–26.

Frye G. (1987). Crest factor and composite signals for hearing aid testing. *Hear J* 40(10):15–18.

Gabrielsson A, Nyberg P, Sjorgren H, Svenson L. (1976). Detection of amplitude distortion by normal hearing and hearing impaired subjects. Karolinska Institute Report TA No. 83.

Gioannini L, Franzen R. (1978). Comparison of the effects of hearing aid harmonic distortion on performance scores for the MRHT and a PB-50/CM tests. *J Aud Res* 18:203–208.

Harris J, Haines H, Kelsey P, Clack T. (1961). The relation between speech intelligibility and the electroacoustic characteristics of low fidelity circuitry. *J Aud Res* 5:357–381.

Harris R, Brey R, Chang Y, Soria B, Hilton L. (1991). The effects of digital quantization error on speech intelligibility and perceived speech quality. *J Speech Hear Res* 34:189–196.

Hauser M. (1991) Principles of oversampling A/D conversion. *J Audio Eng Soc* 39(1/2):3–26.

Hawkins D, Naidoo S. (1993). Comparison of sound quality and clarity with asymmetrical peak clipping and output limiting compression. *J Am Acad Audiol* 4:221–228.

Hussung R, Hamill T. (1990). Recent advances in hearing aid technology: An introduction to digital terminology and concepts. *Semin Hear* 11(1):1–15.

IEC Standards (1983). *International Electrotechnical Commission (IEC): Hearing Aids (Part O: Measurement of Electroacoustic Characteristics).* Publication 118-0. Geneva, Switzerland: Bureau Central de la Commission Electrotechnique Internationale; 1983.

Jelonek S, Mosher E, Lebo C, Smith M, Schwind D, Kurz P, Decker K, Krusemark H. (1993). Restaurant noise: "What was that you said?" *Hear Instrum* 44(10):37–40.

Jerger J, Speaks C, Malmquist C. (1966). Hearing aid performance and hearing aid selection. *J Speech Hear Res* 9:136–149.

Jirsa R, Hodgson W. (1970). Effects of harmonic distortion in hearing aids on speech intelligibility for normals and hyperacusis. *J Aud Res* 10:213–217.

Jirsa R, Norris T. (1982). Effects of intermodulation distortion on speech intelligibility. *Ear Hear* 3:251–256.

Kasten R, Lotterman S. (1967). A longitudinal examination of harmonic distortion in hearing aids. *J Speech Hear Res* 10:777–781.

Kates J. (1989). *A Test Suite For Hearing Aid Evaluation.* New York: Center for Research in Speech and Hearing Sciences, City University of New York.

Kates J. (1992). On the use of coherence to measure distortion in hearing aids. *J Acoust Soc Am* 91:2236–2244.

Kates J. (1993). Hearing aid design criteria. *J Speech Lang Pathol and Audiol Monogr Suppl* (1):15–23.

Kates J, Kozma-Spytek L. (1994). Quality ratings for frequency-shaped peak-clipped speech. *J Acoust Soc Am* 95:3586–3594.

Keller F. (1984). Peak clipping. *Hear Instrum* 35(4):24–26.

Killion M. (1979). Design and evaluation of high fidelity hearing aids. Ph.D. Dissertation, Northwestern University, IL.

Kochkin S. (1989). *Focus Group Results—Dispenser Perception of the EP Receiver.* Itasca, IL: Knowles Electronics.

Kochkin S, Ballad W. (1991). Dispenser sound quality perceptions of class D integrated receivers. *Hear Instrum* 42(4):25–28.

Kuk F. (1990). Preferred insertion gain of hearing aids in listening and reading aloud situations. *J Speech Hear Res* 33:520–529.

Langford-Smith F. (1960). *Radiotron Designer's Handbook.* Harrison, NJ: RCA.

Lawson G, Chial M. (1982). Magnitude estimation of degraded speech quality by normal and impaired hearing listeners. *J Acoust Soc Am* 72:1781–1787.

Levitt H. (1987). Digital hearing aids: A tutorial review. *J Rehab Res Dev* 24(4):7–20.

Levitt H, Cudahy E, Hwang W, Kennedy E, Link C. (1987). Towards a general measure of distortion. *J Rehab Res Dev* 24(4):283–292.

Licklider J. (1946). Effects of amplitude distortion upon the intelligibility of speech. *J Acoust Soc Am* 18:429–434.

Lotterman S, Kasten R. (1967). Nonlinear distortion in modern hearing aids. *J Speech Hear Res* 10:586–592.

Moller A. (1983). *Auditory Physiology.* London: Academic Press.

Nakagawa T, Levitt H. (1991). Clipping distortion in hearing aids. *Proc Int Symposium on Hearing and Speech Sciences.* Osaka, Japan, July 1991, pp. 198–202.

Olsen W. (1971). The influence of harmonic and intermodulation distortion on speech intelligibility. *Scand Audiol* 1:109–125.

Olsen W, Carhart R. (1967). Development of test procedures for evaluation of binaural hearing aids. *Bull Prosthet Res* 10(7):22–49.

Oppenheim A, Lim J. (1981). The importance of phase in signals. *Proc IEEE* 69:529–541.

O'Shaughnessy D. (1987). *Speech Communication: Human and Machine*. Reading, MA: Addison Wesley Publishing Company.

Palmer C, Killion M, Wilber L, Ballad W. (1995). Comparison of two hearing aid receiver-amplifier combinations using sound quality judgments. *Ear Hear* (in press).

Pearsons K, Bennett R, Fidell S. (1977). *Speech Levels in Various Noise Environments*. Canoga Park, CA: Bolt, Beranek, and Neuman, Inc. Prepared for Environmental Protection Agency, Office of Health and Ecological Effects, Washington, DC.

Peters R, Burkhard M. (1968). *On Noise Distortion and Harmonic Distortion Measurements. Project 10350*. Franklin Park, IL: Knowles Electronics, Inc.

Pollack M. (1980). *Amplification for the Hearing-Impaired*. 2nd ed. New York: Grune and Stratton Inc.

Potts L, Valente M, Agnew J. (1994). *Listener Preferences in Class A and Class D Hearing Aids*. Presented at the Sixth American Academy of Audiology Convention, Richmond, VA, 1994.

Preis D. (1982). Phase distortion and phase equalization in audio signal processing—A tutorial review. *J Audio Eng Soc* 30(11):774–794.

Preis D, Bloom P. (1984). Perception of phase distortion in anti-alias filters. *J Audio Eng Soc* 32(11):842–848.

Preves D. (1990). Expressing noise and distortion with the coherence measurement. *ASHA* 32(June/July):56–59.

Preves D. (1994). Future trends in hearing aid technology. In: Valente M, ed. *Strategies for Selecting and Verifying Hearing Aid Fittings*. New York: Thieme Medical Publishers.

Preves D, Newton J. (1989). The headroom problems and hearing aid performance. *Hear J* 42(10):19–26.

Schroeder M. (1975). Models of hearing. *Proc IEEE* 63:1332–1350.

Schweitzer C, Causey D, Tolton M. (1977). Nonlinear distortion in hearing aids: The need for reevaluation of measurement philosophy and technique. *J Am Audio Soc* 2(4):132–141.

Schweitzer C, Grim M, Preves D, Kubichek R, Woodruff B. (1991). *Qualitative Assessment of Hearing Aid Performance by an Expert Pattern Recognition System*. Presented at the Third Annual American Academy of Audiology Convention, Denver, CO.

Stelmachowicz P, Mace A, Kopun J, Carney E, (1993). Long term and short term characteristics of speech: Implications for hearing aid selection for young children. *J Speech Hear Res* 36:609–620.

Teder H. (1990). Noise and speech levels in noisy environments. *Hear Instrum* 41(4):32–33.

Teder H. (1991). Hearing instruments in noise and the syllabic speech-to-noise ratio. *Hear Instrum* 42(2):15–18.

Thomas I. (1968). The influence of first and second formants on the intelligibility of clipped speech. *J Audio Eng Soc* 16(2):182–185.

Thomas I, Niederjohn R. (1968). Enhancement of speech intelligibility at high noise levels by filtering and clipping. *J Audio Eng Soc* 16(4):412–415.

Thomsen C, Moller H. (1975). Swept measurements of harmonic, difference frequency and intermodulation distortion. Application Note 15-098. Bruel and Kjaer, Denmark.

Townsend T, Konkle D. (1982). Comparison of total harmonic distortion measures among hearing aid test systems. *Ear Hear* 3:215–219.

Valente M. (1994). *Strategies for Selecting and Verifying Hearing Aid Fittings*. New York: Thieme Medical Publishers, Inc.

Walker G, Dillon H. (1982). Compression in hearing aids. An analysis, a review, and some recommendations. NAL report No 90, Canberra, Australia.

White P. (1978). Swept measurements of difference frequency intermodulation and harmonic distortion of hearing aids. Bruel and Kjaer Instruments—Application Notes.

Williamson M, Cummins K, Hecox K. (1987). Speech distortion measures for hearing aids. *J Rehab Res Dev* 24(4):277–282.

Zerlin S, Burnett E. (1960). Effects of harmonic and intermodulation distortion on speech intelligibility. *J Acoust Soc Am* 32(A):1501–1502.

# 8

## *Speech Understanding in Background Noise*

### DONALD J. SCHUM

It is almost a cliché at this point to state that individuals with sensorineural hearing loss have difficulty understanding speech in noise, even with the best fit amplification. However, given the severity of the listening difficulties that these patients exhibit, it is extremely important to provide a detailed assessment of our current knowledge of the problem of understanding speech in noise and the state of the art of various technological options available that attempt to mitigate these difficulties. Although Killion (1986) indicated that "there is hope" for the problem of speech in noise, there remains a significant shortfall in actual versus desired performance with the use of hearing aids in such difficult listening environments. The problem of noise interference in the presence of sensorineural hearing loss is not completely understood from the standpoint of basic science. Due to this incomplete understanding of the nature of the problem and, due to some technical limitations in what amplification can currently provide, this problem of understanding speech in noise, unfortunately, will likely continue to be at the forefront of auditory research and clinical science for some time to come.

The ability of an individual with normal hearing to extract meaningful speech information from a background of noise is dependent on a complex interaction of peripheral and central processes. It is often frustrating for individuals with sensorineural hearing loss to fully appreciate the complexities involved in this process of extracting speech from the background of noise. The individual may understand that they have a peripheral sensitivity hearing loss; however, they do not understand how this peripheral sensitivity hearing loss interacts with normal and/or abnormal central processing abilities. (For a discussion of the central auditory system, please see Chapter 9.) The patient and their loved ones often assume that the use of hearing aids to overcome the sensitivity loss will also restore excellent speech understanding ability. Until the audiologist can provide a clear and concise description of speech in noise processing in normal and impaired ears and, until the audiologist can fully elucidate both the benefits and limitations of currently available electronic amplification, the patient is likely to be frustrated with the entire process.

This chapter provides a discussion of why noise is particularly detrimental to speech understanding for persons with sensorineural hearing loss. In addition, current and future electronic techniques that attempt to minimize the effects of background noise will be reviewed. It is hoped that the information provided in this chapter will allow the audiologist to better understand the scope of the problem of understanding speech in noise and provide the information and strategies to the patient in order that they will maximize speech understanding with currently available technology. The better the audiologist is at explaining the complex nature of understanding speech in noise, the more likely it is that all parties involved will deal with the difficulties with realistic expectations.

## The Nature Of Noise

### What Is Noise?

There are a number of definitions of the word "noise" (Webster, 1990). In the past, audiologists have tested speech-in-noise abilities of hearing-impaired individuals using a definition of noise as "composed of several frequencies that involves random changes in frequency or amplitude." In contrast, most hearing-impaired individuals define noise as a background with many other people talking (i.e., babble). This common description on the part of hearing-impaired individuals is far more consistent with a definition of noise being: "Any sound that is undesired or interferes with one's hearing of something." The difference between these two definitions of noise is crucial in considering the poor performance in the past of many of the noise-reduction strategies that have been developed. It is one thing to build a single microphone device that can differentiate the complex waveform of speech from a random electronic noise. It is quite another task to develop a single microphone that can differentiate one voice from others.

A situation where an individual is communicating with one other person while standing next to an air conditioning unit that produces a stable and continuous low-frequency noise is different in nature than when the same listener is attempting to follow one or more talkers in a small group discussion when there are many other people in the room carrying on similar discussions. As the conversation jumps from one talker to another and the levels of the background conversations wax and wane (including laughter and other transient sounds), the listener with a significant hearing impairment is likely to be at a distinct disadvantage. Although hearing aid technologies are currently available that can, to some degree, minimize the effect of the noise produced by the air conditioning unit, there are no currently marketed technologies that can control the levels of other conversations occurring in the room. Even when background noise is not the speech of others, the hearing-impaired person may have little or no control over the level of the noise. Further, some other environmental noises are equally as complex and equally as difficult to minimize electronically as is speech. For example, the level and spectral characteristics of traffic noise are likely to be changing constantly. Although there may be certain predictable characteristics of such a noise, the moment-to-moment fluctuations and the amplitude and frequency characteristics are difficult to predict. Therefore, it is very difficult to develop a noise-cancellation device that would have a significant impact.

At times, the definition of the intended signal versus the unwanted noise can change at a moment's notice. Take, for example, the situation in which a person with hearing impairment is watching television in a quiet room. The person may be experiencing acceptable speech understanding. However, when another person enters the room and attempts to converse with the hearing-impaired viewer, the audio signals from the television may now act as a significant distracting noise. A noise-control system cannot be expected to know that the previous signal-of-interest has now become "noise" (competition).

Figure 8–1 provides data from Lamb, Owens, and Schubert (1983) on rankings by hearing-impaired individuals of the most difficult listening situations. This data represents the responses of 354 hearing-impaired subjects on the revised version of the Hearing Performance Inventory. As can be seen, compared to listening in quiet situations, listening in the presence of other people speaking nearby or other background noises is rated as significantly more difficult.

### Acoustic Characteristics of Externally Presented Noise

Noises and all other sounds can be described in terms of both short-term and long-term spectral characteristics. In considering the problem of speech in noise and the role of amplification in minimizing this problem, both the short-term and the long-term characteristics of noise are relevant. Figure 8–2 provides three different representations of a speech signal. In this figure, and in several subsequent

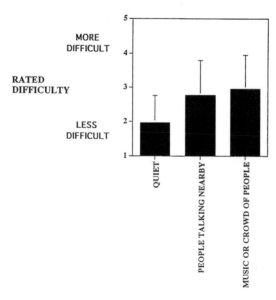

**Figure 8–1.** The rated listening difficulty in three different environments by persons with sensorineural hearing loss. This data is adapted from Lamb et al. (1983).

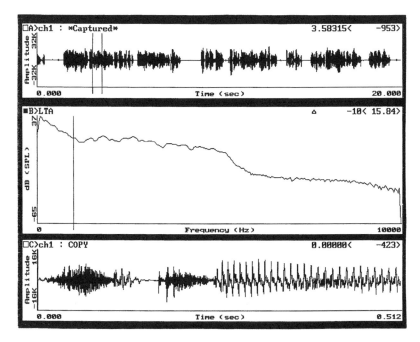

**Figure 8–2.** The acoustic characteristics of a 20-second sample of speech taken from the competing message track of the Synthetic Sentence Identification Test (Jerger et al., 1968).

figures (Figs. 8–1 to 8–12), three panels are displayed. The top panel provides the amplitude waveform of the speech signal over a 20-second time period. The middle panel provides the long-term amplitude by frequency spectrum of the 20-second sample from the top panel. Finally, the lower panel provides the waveform of an approximately 500-millisecond sample drawn from the longer 20-second sample. The cursor in the middle panel is at 1000 Hz (the frequency axis is in a linear, not logarithmic, scale). The two cursors in the top panel reflect the beginning and end points of the approximately 500-millisecond sample provided in the bottom panel.

COMPETING MESSAGE

Figure 8–2 was taken from the single-speaker (male) competing-message track (the Davey Crockett Story) that accompanies the Synthetic Sentence Index test (Jerger, Speaks, and Trammell, 1968). The top panel demonstrates the typical waveform of speech over a 20-second sample. As can be seen, there are periods during the 20 seconds where speech is present and there are also breaks between sentences or phrases. Within the sentences, there are higher amplitude and lower amplitude sections typically corresponding to vowels and unvoiced consonants, respectively. In the expanded section represented in the lower panel, the reader can see a burst of energy, likely representing a consonant, at the beginning of the passage. This initial section represents relatively high-frequency energy, because many zero axis crossings occur in this interval. This section is followed by a break and another high-frequency section, and then by a longer, low-frequency (less zero axis crossings per unit of time) section, most likely corresponding to a vowel or semivowel. The long-term spectra over the 20-second passage (middle panel) is quite consistent with many published long-term spectra of speech (e.g., Pearsons, Bennett, and Fidell, 1977). There is a prominent energy peak in the low frequencies, typically occurring below 500 Hz. This is followed by a gentle rolloff of approximately 5 to 10 dB/octave as frequency increases. Despite the rolloff, there remains significant and important midfrequency energy.

Figure 8–3 represents another 20-second passage from a different (male) speaker. This passage is taken from the Auditec of St. Louis Continuous Discourse Passage. Again, in the upper panel there are silent periods and periods of high amplitude and lower amplitude speech energy. In the bottom panel, again the reader can see passages of both high-frequency and lower frequency speech energy within a single 500-millisecond segment. The long-term spectrum represented in the middle panel again shows a prominent peak in the lower frequencies, but with some significant energy above 1000 Hz. However, the amplitude difference between the low and high frequencies is greater for the talker in Figure 8–2 than for the talker in Figure 8–3.

Again, this characteristic of significant low-frequency energy, but also mid- to high-frequency energy is quite typical of what is known about the long-term spectrum of human speech. As will be seen in subsequent figures, there are a variety of noises, both nonspeech and speech competition, that mask energy in either the low frequencies and/or the mid- to higher frequencies. The likelihood

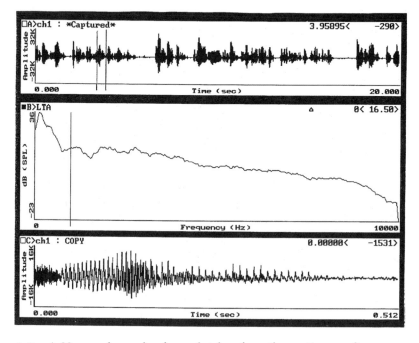

**Figure 8–3.** A 20-second sample of speech taken from the continuous discourse passage in the Auditec of St. Louis tape series.

of overlap between the intended speech target and a variety of potential competition noises is high. This is the heart of the difficulty of designing a noise-reduction system that effectively can separate speech from background noise.

ENVIRONMENTAL NOISES

Figure 8–4 provides acoustic data on noise from a cooling fan on the back of a laboratory computer. As shown in the top panel, the waveform of the acoustic output of this fan is relatively constant in amplitude over time. This is confirmed by viewing the shorter time sample indicated in the lower panel. The long-term spectrum of this fan noise (middle panel) is somewhat similar to the previous representations of long-term speech spectra. There is a significant amount of energy in the lower frequencies; however, there continues to be energy even in the region from 1000 to approximately 3000 Hz. Given that important speech cues fall within this mid- to high-frequency region, it is clear that this particular environmental noise may have a significant masking effect on speech.

Figures 8–5 and 8–6 provide acoustic data on 2 machinery-induced noises. Both were taken from the Widex recordings of environmental noise tapes. Figure 8–5 shows a 20-second sample of the noise produced by a bandsaw. Figure 8–6 shows a sample of the noise produced by an air compressor blowing compressed air. In contrast to the noise from the computer fan represented in Figure 8–4, there are significant variations in overall amplitude of these noises over the 20-second time period (and over the 500 millisecond sample). There are periods of relatively low amplitude or essentially no background noise followed by rapid increases in amplitude. The long-term spectra (middle panels) are slightly differ-

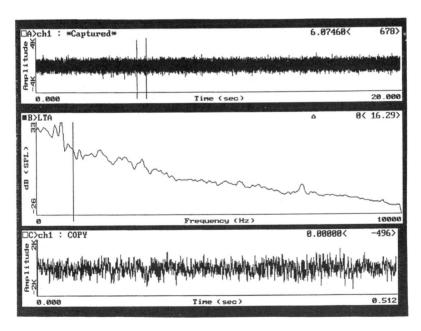

**Figure 8–4.**   A 20-second sample of the noise produced by the cooling fan on the back of a laboratory computer.

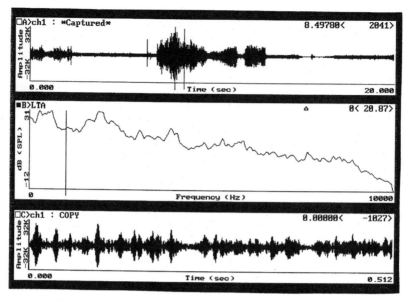

**Figure 8–5.** A 20-second sample of the sound produced by a bandsaw taken from the Widex series of environmental sounds.

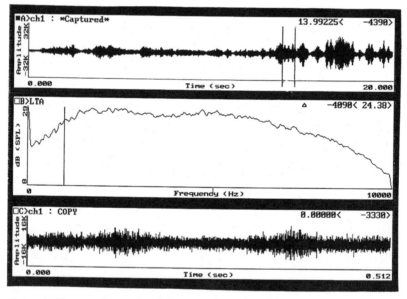

**Figure 8–6.** A 20-second sample of the sound produced by an air compressor blowing compressed air taken from the Widex series of environmental sounds.

ent for the two different noises. In Figure 8–5, the bandsaw, both low- and mid-frequency noise energy is present. In Figure 8–6, the air compressor, the noise energy is confined to the higher frequencies. In either case, these noises would be expected to have a significant masking effect on relevant speech cues as they are generally in the same frequency range.

TRAFFIC NOISE

Figure 8–7 illustrates the spectrum of a passage of traffic noise as recorded on the 3M environmental noise tape series. Again, there are changes in amplitude over this passage. However, there are no significant quiet periods. There is always some ambient level of noise with sections of higher amplitude superimposed. The long-term spectrum of this noise, again, is quite similar to published representations of the long-term spectrum of speech with significant energy below 1000 Hz and a gradual rolloff in the higher frequencies. Therefore, as can be seen in Figures 8–5 to 8–7, even nonspeech, environmental-type noises can still occupy frequency ranges that would be expected to interfere with the understanding of speech.

Many background noise situations will include both speech and nonspeech sound energy. Figures 8–8 to 8–11 provide four examples of such environments. Figures 8–8 and 8–9 are taken from the Widex tape series. Figure 8–8 represents a "party" environment. Figure 8–9 represents an office environment. Figure 8–10 is from the 3M series and also represents an office listening environment. Finally, Figure 8–11 is from the Auditec tape series and represents cafeteria noise. For all four sound environments there is a mixture of both speech and nonspeech background noise, but there is some variation in the degree of amplitude fluctuation across time. Figures 8–8 and 8–11 show relatively stable amplitude, as indicated by small variations in the maximal versus minimal vertical excursions in the top panels. Figures 8–9 and 8–10 demonstrate situations in which the overall amplitude of the noise changes quite dramatically over the 20-second time period. The long-term spectra of these four environments, again, are relevant when considering

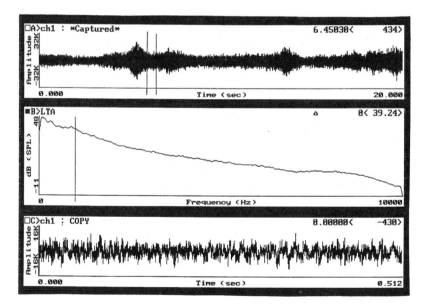

**Figure 8–7.**  A 20-second sample of traffic noise as provided by the 3M series of environmental sounds.

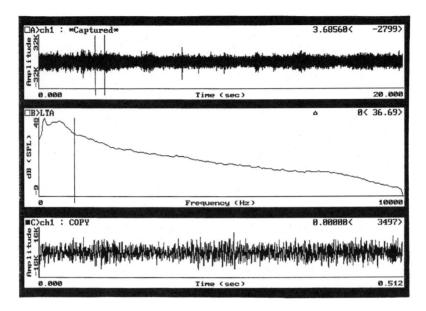

**Figure 8–8.** A 20-second sample recorded in a party environment taken from the Widex series of environmental sounds.

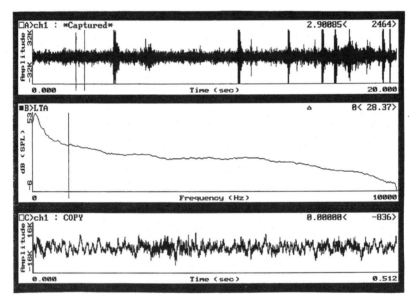

**Figure 8–9.** A 20-second sample recorded in an office environment taken from the Widex tape series of environmental sounds.

potential masking effects on speech. For all four environments there is a significant low-frequency peak in the energy, with gradual rolloff through the mid- to high frequencies. A significant amount of energy remains in the vicinity of important high-frequency speech information.

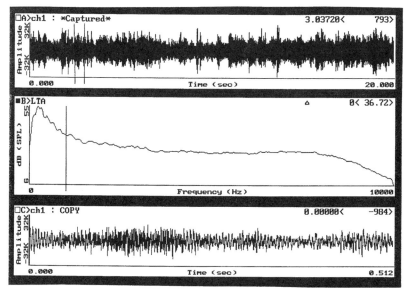

**Figure 8–10.**    A 20-second sample recorded in an office environment taken from the 3M series of environmental sounds.

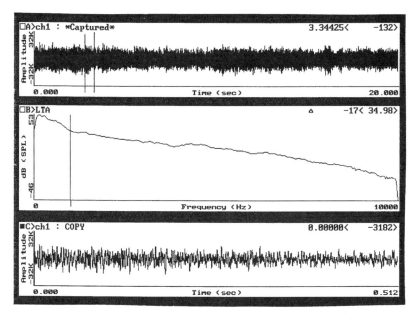

**Figure 8–11.**    A 20-second sample of cafeteria noise taken from the Auditec of St. Louis tape series.

SPEECH BABBLE

Recordings of speech babble are often used as background noise during audiological testing. Babble is a mixture of more than one voice speaking at the same time. After more than three or four voices are present in the recording, it is very difficult to meaningfully follow the speech of any one of the talkers for more than a moment or two. The overall effect is a background of speech-like sound without significant linguistic meaning.

Figure 8–12 shows 5-second samples from each of four different babble recordings (D–E). For comparison purposes, the top panel (A) shows a second passage from a single speaker (taken from the SSI Competing Message). Notice the amplitude fluctuations and the presence of gaps, as expected. The second panel (B) shows a second passage from the Auditec four-talker babble recording with only four talkers. There are times when no sound energy is present. In this second passage, there are two silent gaps, and significant observable amplitude changes over time. The third panel (C) shows a passage from the Auditec multitalker babble recording. This recording contains 20 different talkers. As the number of talkers increases to 20, the likelihood of a "dead spot" or a "gap" in the babble is reduced and amplitude fluctuations are also somewhat reduced. The fourth panel (D) shows a passage of the competing speech babble from the Connected Speech Test (Cox, Alexander, and Gilmore, 1987). This competing babble contains six different talkers. There are no significant "dead spots," and a degree of amplitude fluctuation that is clearly reduced compared to the single speaker (top

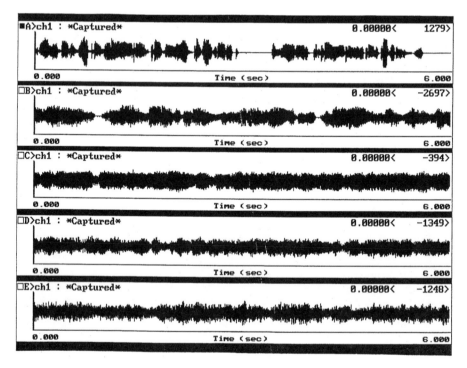

**Figure 8–12.** Twenty-second sample of a speaker taken from the single-talker competing message of the Synthetic Sentence Identification Test (top panel; A), four-talker babble taken from the Auditec of St. Louis tape series (second panel; B), multitalker babble taken from the Auditec of St. Louis tape series (third panel; C), competing speech babble taken from the Connected Speech Test (fourth panel; D), and speech babble taken from the SPIN test (fifth panel; E).

panel). Finally, the fifth panel (E)in Figure 8–12 shows the competing babble from the Speech Perception In Noise (SPIN) test (Kalikow, Stevens, and Elliott, 1977). This babble contains 12 different talkers. Again, there is less amplitude fluctuation than with the single talker, but still there is not a perfectly constant amplitude across time.

As would be expected, the long-term spectrum of speech babble typically corresponds quite closely to the long-term spectrum of speech from any given single talker. Figure 8–13 provides the long-term of the speech materials from the Connected Speech Test (CST, Cox et al., 1987) (thick solid line), the Rainbow Passage recording from the Auditec compact disk (thin solid line), and the babble track from the CST (dashed line). In general, all three spectra have a similar overall shape. This observation is not unique to this writing. For example, Kalikow et al. (1977) present the long-term spectra of the speech material from the Speech Perception in Noise test along with the competing babble from that test. Again, the long-term spectra of the speech material from the single talker from the SPIN test matches closely the spectra of the babble.

OVERALL LEVEL OF NOISE

Another relevant acoustic characteristic of noise is its overall level in dB SPL in a listening environment. The absolute noise level is important, but the more relevant issue is the level of the noise in comparison to the level of the speech that the listener is attending to: i.e., the signal-to-noise (S/N) ratio.

In a landmark study, Pearsons et al. (1977) measured levels of speech and noise in a variety of different listening environments. This study was commissioned by the Environmental Protection Agency (EPA) in an attempt to assess acoustic characteristics of non-laboratory (or "real life") communication environments. Settings evaluated included homes, schools, transportation vehicles, and other public places.

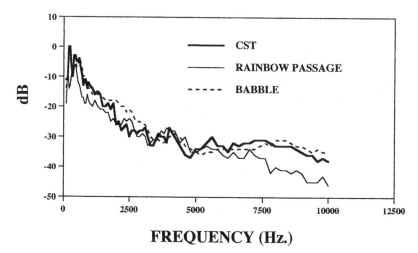

**FREQUENCY (Hz.)**

**Figure 8–13.** The long-term spectra of the speech from the Connected Speech Test (CST) (thick solid line), the Rainbow Passage from the Auditec compact disc (thin solid line), and the babble from the CST (dashed line).

Pearsons and his colleagues reported that, for relatively low background noise levels [48 dB(A) or less], talkers produce levels of, on average, 55 dB(A). Therefore, the typical low-noise communication situation has a S/N ratio of about +7 dB. As background noise levels increase from 48 to 70 dB(A), typical talkers raise their voices at a rate of 0.6 dB for each one dB increase in the background noise level. Thus, for a background noise level of 70 dB(A), the typical talker produces speech at only 67 dB(A), yielding a –3 dB S/N ratio. As might be expected, overall noise level was found to vary by type of environment. Figure 8–14 is a graphical representation of the data from Pearsons et al. (1977). In each of the 8 environments described, the left bar graph (diagonal line) represents the average noise level and the solid black bar graph represents the typical conversational speech level measured at a distance of 2 meters from the talker. In homes, schools, and patient rooms in a hospital, the background noise levels are relatively low, thus resulting in relatively high S/N ratios. As the reader moves to the more noisy settings such as a hospital nurses' station, department store, and in transportation vehicles, the average levels of the background noises increase. In addition, the S/N ratios decrease reaching negative values in those situations with the highest levels of background noise (transportation vehicles).

## Performance in Background Noise

### Subjective Performance in Noise

Given that communication often takes place in situations where the noise level is not significantly lower than the overall level of speech, it is important to evaluate

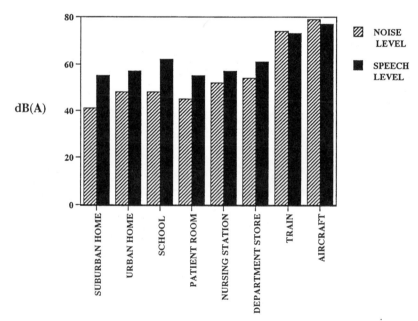

**Figure 8–14.** Average noise and speech levels measured in different settings. This data was adapted from Pearsons et al. (1977).

how persons with sensorineural hearing impairment perceive their performance in such situations. Figure 8–15 is from a study by Schum (1994), in which 69 potential hearing aid users were surveyed on a variety of issues including the listening difficulty experienced in a variety of communication environments. The author adapted the questions from the Hearing Aid Performance Inventory (Walden, Demorest, and Hepler, 1984). Questions were rephrased to describe a given listening situation and the respondent was asked to rate the severity of listening difficulties on a scale from one to three. A response of one corresponded to *very much listening difficulty,* a response of two corresponded to *some listening difficulty,* and a response of three corresponded to *very little listening difficulty.* Similar to the data of Lamb et al. (1983) provided in Figure 8–1, the mean results from these patients indicated a significant difference between rated difficulty for listening to speech in background noise (the first column in Fig. 8–15) as compared to listening to speech in quiet (the second column). Listening to speech in noise is rated at a similar difficulty level as listening to speech without visual cues (the third column). Listening to nonspeech signals (such as warning or alerting signals) is rated as the easiest type of situation. Although there is significant variation around the mean scores (bars indicate ±1 SD), only 7% of the respondents rated quiet situations as being more difficult than noise situations.

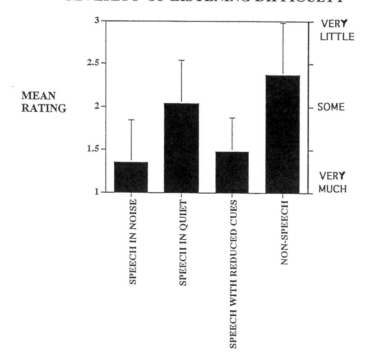

**Figure 8–15.** The reported severity of listening difficulty in several different listening environments by 69 potential hearing aid users as reported by Schum (1994).

### Objective Performance

The reported speech-in-noise difficulties of persons with hearing impairment confirmed with objective data available in the audiologic literature for nearly 25 years. Examples include work by Groen (1969), Carhart and Tillman (1970), Cooper and Cutts (1971), Gengel (1971), Cohen and Keith (1976), Suter (1985), and Crandell (1993). Although performance in noise compared to normally hearing listeners varies, depending upon the type of speech material used, the type of background noise, and the specific listening task, the overwhelming conclusion that can be drawn from the accumulated data is that persons with sensorineural hearing loss are at a distinct disadvantage in situations where background noise is present.

A classic example of research in this area is a study conducted by Dirks, Morgan, and Dubno in 1982. These authors adaptively varied the level of a background random noise (which was shaped to match the long-term characteristics of speech; i.e., speech spectrum noise) to determine the signal-to-babble (S/B) ratio necessary to identify 50% of the speech material. The investigators used spondee words and monosyllabic words from the NU-6 test. Figure 8–16 presents results for the spondee words, and Figure 8–17 presents results for NU-6 monosyllabic words from the Dirks et al. (1982) study. In both figures, the results

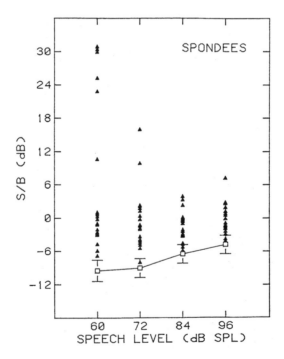

**Figure 8–16.** The signal-to-babble ratio necessary to identify approximately 50% of spondees presented in a background of speech spectrum noise. The triangle represents the data from 20 individual subjects with sensorineural hearing loss. The square represents mean performance from normally hearing individuals, the [ ] indicates ±2 standard deviations. This figure is from Dirks et al. (1982). (Used with permission.)

from normal-hearing listeners are the open boxes with brackets indicating ±2 SD, and results from 20 subjects with sensorineural hearing loss are indicated by closed triangles. Note that higher S/B ratios indicate poorer performance.

Several observations can be made from these figures. First, the intersubject variability for the normal hearing group was less than 5 dB. In contrast, the performance range for the hearing-impaired subjects was significantly greater, especially for the monosyllabic words. This greater intersubject variability for persons with sensorineural hearing loss is consistent with results of many previous investigations using both speech and nonspeech signals. In fact, performance can vary greatly even within a group of patients with very similar audiometric thresholds, suggesting that difference in suprathreshold processing abilities are a factor in speech recognition, as well as audibility.

A second observation that can be made from these figures is the greater variability within the group of hearing-impaired subjects for the monosyllabic words as opposed to the spondees. The explanation for this phenomenon is that spondee identification requires less high-frequency integrity in the auditory system because the important region for identifying spondees is in only lower frequencies. In contrast, the ability to identify open-set monosyllables requires good high-frequency processing efficiency, which is often not present with sensorineural hearing loss.

The results from the Dirks et al. (1982) study can be compared to the data presented by Pearsons et al. (1977). Recall that Pearsons et al. indicated that the S/N ratio of typical listening situations varies from +7 to –3 dB. Evaluation of Figures 8–16 and 8–17 indicates that most subjects with normal hearing can still perform adequately at those S/N ratios. However, it is far more likely that the person with sensorineural hearing loss will require a significantly better S/N ratio to obtain even a minimal level of performance.

One other aspect of note in the data of Dirks et al. (1982) is that there were typically only moderate correlations between the hearing-impaired subjects' performance in quiet and their performance in noise (depending on presentation level). The implication is that it is difficult to predict how much difficulty a listener will have in background noise situations based only on the amount of sensitivity loss.

A similar observation was made by Schum, Matthews, and Lee in 1991. In that investigation, the articulation index (AI) was used to compare predicted performance to actual performance with sensorineural hearing loss listening under conditions of quiet and noise on word recognition tests. Speech recognition testing was performed at levels at least 30 dB above the patient's speech reception threshold. Results from that study are presented in Figures 8–18 and 8–19. Figure 8–18 shows the results for understanding speech (NU-6 word lists) in quiet. The X axis indicates deviations in speech recognition performance from the AI-predicted values (which are based on audibility of the speech material). In other words, a score of 0 indicates that the patient actually understood as much speech material as was expected based on how much of the speech energy was above the person's threshold. The Y axis provides the number of subjects providing the indicated score. Figure 8–19 shows the results for speech understanding (low predictability items from the SPIN test) in a background of speech babble noise. Figure 8–18 clearly shows that, in the quiet situation, most listeners' speech understanding

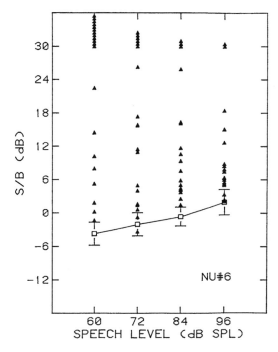

**Figure 8–17.**    The results from the Dirks et al. (1982) study for monosyllabic words. (Used with permission.)

performance was limited only by the audibility of the speech material. In other words, the higher above-hearing threshold that the speech material was presented, the more likely they were to understand the material. In contrast, Figure 8–19 shows that listeners typically perform significantly poorer in background noise than would be expected based on the amount of speech information above threshold and above the background noise. Schum et al. (1991) reported that the correlation coefficient between performance in quiet and performance in noise was only 0.52. Again, the implication of these results is that the ability to predict performance of understanding speech in noise is not strongly related to performance in quiet.

### The Effects of Specific Types of Noises

The effect of one type of background (masking) noise will be different from the effect of other types of noises. There are several general principles that have been reported in the literature. First, the greater the similarity in the spectrum of the masker to the speech material, the more effective will be the masking noise in disrupting the understanding of the speech material. In other words, understanding an open set of monosyllabic words or understanding words loaded with high-frequency consonant sounds, or understanding nonsense syllables will be more difficult if the masking noise emphasized the high-frequency region. In this case, a band of noise limited below 500 Hz will be less effective in

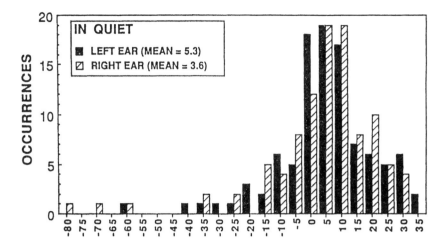

ACTUAL SCORE MINUS PREDICTED SCORE (RAU)

**Figure 8–18.** The deviation from expected performance in quiet listening for hearing-impaired individuals, based on an articulation index analyses. This figure is taken from Schum et al. (1991). (Used with permission.)

masking those speech materials than if a wide-band or a speech-shaped noise were used. As the speech materials become less difficult and/or typically more redundant (such as a closed set of spondee words or common everyday sentences), there is less need for the clear perception of high-frequency information. The listener can tolerate greater levels of masking noise limited to the higher frequencies.

CONTINUOUS VERSUS FLUCTUATING NOISE

The second important factor in determining the effectiveness of various types of masking noises is how temporally constant they are in the amplitude domain. If speech understanding performance is compared for a constant background noise versus one that is amplitude modulated, performance will be better for the modulated noise (Carhart, Tillman, and Greetis, 1969). The assumption is that the listener has a greater likelihood of perceiving speech information that occurs during the low amplitude gaps of the masking noise. However, if the modulations are designed to mimic the envelope of speech, the modulated noise may be more disruptive than steady-state speech-shaped noise (Souza and Turner, 1994).

The third factor in determining the effectiveness of the masking noise is the linguistic similarity between the masking noise and the speech signal. Although the results from the literature on this point are mixed, several investigators have observed that if maskers are used that contain linguistically significant and identifiable material, they may have a greater masking effect on a speech signal than materials lacking linguistically meaningful passages (Trammell and Speaks, 1970; Papso and Blood, 1989; Souza and Turner, 1994). For example, a masking noise comprised of several talkers presented in the normal (or forward) condition has

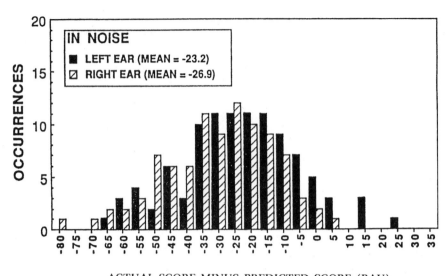

**ACTUAL SCORE MINUS PREDICTED SCORE (RAU)**

**Figure 8–19.** The results from the Schum et al. (1991) study for word recognition performance in a background of speech babble. (Used with permission.)

been observed to be a more effective masker than the same material played backwards. When the material was played backwards, the linguistic information of the masker was no longer identifiable. However, data from Dirks and Bower (1969), Lewis, Benignus, Muller, Malott, and Barton (1988), Hygge, Rünnberg, Larsby, and Arlinger (1992), and Larsby and Arlinger (1994) have suggested that this effect may not be consistent. If linguistic interference does occur, it implies that the babble of a few individuals has a greater masking effect than a babble in which many speakers are present and meaningful linguistic information cannot be observed. This finding contradicts the effect of amplitude consistency that was reported in a previous section of this chapter. As reported in Figure 8–12, the greater the number of speakers in the babble, the more that amplitude fluctuations are reduced. However, as more speakers are added, there is also a decreasing likelihood of the listener identifying meaningful linguistic material in the babble. Given this conflict, the precise effect of adding more and more speakers to the competing signal is yet to be fully understood.

It was common practice in audiology clinics to use very stable background noises, such as white noise (flat spectrum) or speech-shaped noise (spectrum falling at a rate of approximately 6 dB/octave), when testing speech understanding in a background of noise. However, in an attempt to use background noises that are more representative of real-life situations, the use of speech babble and cafeteria noise has increased significantly in audiology clinics as the competition of choice during testing of speech in noise. One notable exception is the competition "noise" used for the Synthetic Sentence Identification Test (Jerger et al., 1968), which has always used a single talker. Further, the speaker for the competing message is the same speaker who recorded the test materials. This situation increases the likelihood of confusion between the competition and the speaker. For this test, the authors specifically intended that the competing message be very difficult so that the test would be sensitive to central influences on speech understanding.

## Why is Noise a Problem?

It should be clear by now that a person with sensorineural hearing loss may have a substantially reduced ability to understand speech in background noise. A variety of explanations for this increased difficulty have been advanced. It is likely that for any given person with sensorineural hearing loss, a combination of factors is probably at play.

### AUDIBILITY

One explanation that is often overlooked when attempting to explain the problems of understanding speech in noise for patients with sensorineural hearing loss is a simple audibility-based explanation (Humes, 1991). That is, when one carefully accounts for the simple masking effects of the background noise in combination with the effect of the audiometric configuration, much of the performance deficit in noise can be explained. For example, when faced with a low-frequency environmental noise, a person with normal hearing has the option of searching in the higher frequencies for necessary cues to identify the speech material. However, a patient with a sloping sensorineural hearing loss does not have this option. In this hearing-impaired listener, noise acts as a significant masker in the lower frequencies, yet the pure-tone hearing loss acts to reduce audibility of high-frequency consonant sounds. Therefore, in the same magnitude of noise, the person with a sloping hearing loss is at a significant disadvantage compared to the person with normal hearing. In some investigations, no additional information about the effect of the hearing loss other than the decreased hearing sensitivity was necessary to explain performance differences in noise (e.g., Zurek and Delhorne, 1987).

There is a limit, however, to which this observation can be used to explain all the problems associated with understanding speech in noise. In situations where speech is presented in the presence of a masker with similar long-term spectral characteristics, it is often observed that a subject with sensorineural hearing loss is at a greater disadvantage than a person with normal hearing even though equally audible amounts of speech information are present for both groups. In the Schum et al. (1991) study and in several other studies using AI analyses (e.g., Kamm, Dirks, and Bell, 1986), the effects of the configuration of the hearing loss and of masking noise were taken into account. Yet the subjects with sensorineural hearing loss still had increased difficulty understanding speech in the background of noise. Thus, the simple audibility explanation for problems of understanding speech in noise does explain several of the observed difficulties that subjects with sensorineural hearing loss may have. However, this explanation does not completely account for all of the observed performances.

SQUELCH EFFECT

Another explanation that has been advocated to explain the problem of understanding speech in noise for subjects with hearing impairment is the loss of the binaural "squelch" effect. When a normal hearing listener is given the opportunity to
listen binaurally in a background of noise compared to monaural listening, a significant speech-in-noise advantage is obtained. Carhart (1965) reported a squelch
effect of improving the S/N ratio by 3 dB or more. The explanation for the squelch
effect is that the brain compares the input from each ear and utilize the slight differences in the spectral content between the messages received in the two ears. The
slight spectral differences can serve to identify and separate the speech signal from
the background of noise. This "figure-ground" effect is not restricted to just the
auditory system. There are a variety of examples of visual processing abilities that
are dependent on binocular input. The viewer is able to pick out an object from a
complex background based on slight image differences in one eye versus the other.

In the presence of binaurally asymmetrical hearing loss, the brain does not
have access to the same sort of information coming from the two auditory
peripheries. Even in the presence of bilaterally symmetrical hearing loss, much of
the squelch effect appears to be lost (Bronkhorst and Plomp, 1990; Ter-Horst,
Byrne, and Noble, 1993). Apparently, squelch ability is dependent on normal
auditory information advanced by the peripheral sensory system. Therefore, the
ability of a normal hearing individual to extract meaningful speech information
in a 0 dB signal-to-noise listening situation is quite dependent on the ability to
listen with two ears. When the normal binaural input is disrupted, the speech
target is more likely to be lost in the background of noise.

UPWARD SPREAD OF MASKING

Another effect of sensorineural hearing loss that is known to take place is the
phenomenon of upward spread of masking. It has been observed that there are
some masking effects outside of the pure physical bandwidth of a masking stimulus, even in normal ears. The assumption is that the auditory system is susceptible
to activation of nerve fibers arising from one frequency region by off-frequency
maskers. Further, even in the normal ear, the ability of a low-frequency masker
to affect high-frequency hearing is greater than the ability of a high-frequency
masker to affect low-frequency hearing. For many patients with sensorineural
hearing loss, there is an upward spread of masking that is significantly greater
than reported for listeners with normal hearing (Jerger, Tillman, and Peterson,
1960; Rittmanic, 1962; Martin and Pickett, 1970; Gagné, 1988). Figure 8–20 is data
from Klein, Mills, and Adkins (1990). In this study, the authors had normal-hearing
and sensorineural hearing-impaired subjects track their auditory thresholds
using Bekesey audiometry while listening in quiet and in the presence of a low-
frequency noise. The filled circles represent the mean normal threshold in the
presence of a low-frequency masker. The crosses represent the thresholds of a
given subject with hearing impairment in quiet. The open squares represent the
thresholds in the presence of the low-frequency noise for the same hearing-
impaired listener. The filled region in this Figure 8–20 represents the amount of
excess threshold shift for one hearing-impaired subject that cannot be explained

**ELDERLY WITH OVERMASKING**

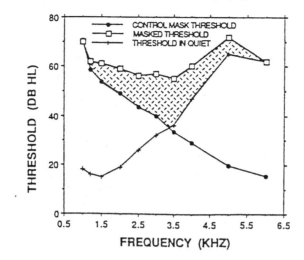

**Figure 8–20.** The masked and unmasked thresholds from one hearing-impaired individual in the presence of a low-frequency noise. This figure is taken from Klein et al. (1990). (Used with permission.)

simply by the masking effect of the band of noise (as referenced to performance of the normal-hearing subjects in the presence of the same band of noise), or by the subjects' thresholds in quiet. This region of excessive masking demonstrates the dramatic effect of upward spread of masking present for this particular subject. Klein and his colleagues, as well as several other investigators, observed that the effect of upward spread of masking is quite variable from one patient to another. In fact, Klein et al. (1990) reported that some of the subjects with sensorineural hearing loss had an "undermasking" effect. This means that the masked thresholds were actually better than those reported for the normal hearing group. Van Tasell (1980) also noted significant intersubject variability concerning susceptibility to the effects of upward spread of masking.

The effect of upward spread of masking is thought to partially explain the problem associated with understanding speech in noise seen in persons with sensorineural hearing loss. As indicated in Figures 8–2 to 8–13, most masking noises in the environment have a significant amount of low-frequency energy. It is assumed that for many persons with sensorineural hearing loss, this significant low-frequency energy has the effect of masking mid- and high-frequency auditory thresholds. This masking of thresholds is greater than would be expected for a normal-hearing individual listening in the same background noise. The effects may even occur within average conversational speech; that is, the more intense lower frequency sounds (vowels) may interfere with the perception of the high-frequency segments (consonants) (Danaher and Pickett, 1975; Hannley and Dorman, 1983). This phenomenon forms the basis of many current attempts in hearing aids to reduce the effects of noise. That is, apply strategies that reduce low-frequency amplification when the listener is surrounded by background noise.

TEMPORAL SMEARING

A final explanation to be considered for poor performance in noisy situations is the effect of temporal smearing. It has been observed that subjects with sensorineural hearing loss perform more poorly on tests of psychoacoustic abilities (for reviews, see Humes, 1982; Scharf and Florentine, 1982; Tyler, 1986). The strongest correlations between speech understanding and psychoacoustic abilities have been observed for temporal-based psychoacoustic tasks (Tyler, Summerfield, Wood, and Fernandes, 1982). It is assumed that persons with sensorineural hearing loss, because of the pathological changes in the auditory system, do not have as fine a discrimination between the timing of auditory events (Fitzgibbons and Wightman, 1982; Bacon and Viemeister, 1985). In a situation where a listener with normal hearing is attending to a "wanted" speech signal in a background of other "unwanted" speech signals, there is a higher likelihood that the timing of the "wanted" speech signal can be discriminated from the other random events in the "unwanted" speech signal. In the case of sensorineural hearing loss where temporal abilities have declined due to poor resolution within the auditory system, there is a greater likelihood of an effective temporal overlap between the speech signal and events in the background competition.

## Current Noise Reduction Approaches

There are a variety of techniques currently available to help reduce the effects of background noise on understanding speech for the hearing aid user with sensorineural hearing loss. These techniques include both clinical strategies for the selection and fitting of hearing aids and specific circuitry designed in an attempt to electronically reduce the deleterious effect of background noise on the understanding of speech.

### Clinical Strategies

BINAURAL AMPLIFICATION

There are three basic strategies that can be used in the selection of a conventional hearing aid to maximize the understanding of speech in background noise. First, the audiologist has the option of providing a binaural fitting. As previously indicated, a normally functioning binaural system affords the listener a significant advantage when listening in a background of noise, due to binaural squelch. Although the selection and fitting of binaural hearing aids does not guarantee a complete recapturing of the normal binaural squelch effect, there is evidence to suggest that listeners fit binaurally perform somewhat better in noise than when fit monaurally. This evidence can be drawn both from subjective patient reports (e.g., Brooks and Bulmer, 1981; Erdman and Sedge, 1981), and from the results of clinical studies on the advantage of binaural amplification when listening to speech in the background of noise (for a review, see Byrne, 1980). It should be noted, however, that even with a well-fitted set of hearing aids, some hearing-impaired listeners do not perform as well as normal-hearing listeners in understanding speech in noise (e.g., Hawkins and Yacullo, 1984). As indicated earlier, there are issues other than audibility that likely reduce speech understanding in noise. Further, some investigators (e.g., Festen and Plomp, 1986) have found limits on the benefits of binaural amplification for understanding speech.

REDUCTION OF LOW-FREQUENCY AMPLIFICATION

The second strategy available in selecting hearing aids is to set tone controls to emphasize a high-frequency region. The assumptions behind providing a higher-pass frequency response to provide better understanding of speech in noise are that: (1) a significant amount of environmental noise is centered in the low-frequency region, and (2) many patients with sensorineural hearing loss show an excess effect of upward spread of masking that was discussed earlier. By reducing low-frequency amplification as compared to a broader frequency response, the audiologist is increasing the likelihood that the more intense low-frequency environmental sounds will not be amplified and that the effects of the upward spread of masking will be reduced. For example, Figure 8–21 provides a broadband prescriptive target for a patient with a gently sloping hearing loss as specified by the Revised National Acoustics Laboratory Fitting Procedure (Byrne and Dillon, 1986). Also shown is a real-ear insertion response (REIR) designed to match the low-frequency slope of the NAL-R target and an REIR from the hearing aid adjusted to present a high-frequency response. Below 1000 Hz the high-frequency setting provides a significant reduction (5 to 15 dB) in the REIR, despite the fact that measurable hearing loss is present below 1000 Hz.

Fitting high-frequency emphasis amplification to minimize the effects of noise has been criticized by pointing out that the S/N ratio in any given frequency region has not been modified when using this approach. Further, it has been argued that significant speech information is present in the lower frequencies,

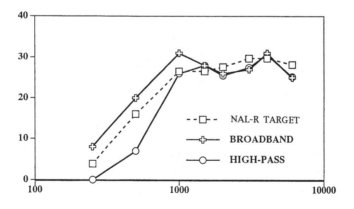

FREQUENCY (Hz.)

**Figure 8–21.**   The real-ear response of a hearing aid providing a broadband (indicated by the +), and a high-pass (indicated by open circle) frequency response in relation to the NAL-R prescribed target for a listener with a gently sloping mild-to-moderate hearing loss.

which should not be attenuated or eliminated. Whereas these criticisms are accurate, there appears to be benefit from reducing low-frequency amplification for at least some patients (e.g., Gordon-Salant, 1984).

It is true that high-frequency amplification does not improve the S/N ratio in any given band and that significant speech information is in the lower frequencies. It can also be argued, however, the speech information in the low-frequency band should only be amplified when there is an overwhelming drawback to its presence. If a patient is prone to the effects of upward spread of masking, then some of the speech information in the lower frequencies may need to be reduced to ensure better perception of more important higher frequency cues. Although the actual S/N ratio in any given band may not change, the "effective" S/N ratio (that is, the level of noise that is tolerated to achieve a certain level of performance) may be improved if the patient is prone to the effects of the upward spread of masking.

INCREASED HEADROOM

The third strategy to improve the understanding of speech in noise is to increase the "headroom." Some hearing aids use peak clipping to limit the output of the hearing aid. In situations where speech is presented in a background of noise, the speech peaks may rise above the overall level of the noise clipped and the peaks of speech will be clipped. The clipping of the speech peaks will result in the level of the speech to be reduced relative to the overall level of the noise. In other words, peak clipping will result in a poorer S/N ratio as well as providing a more distorted signal. The use of peak clipping as a method of output control has been common for many years. However, it is likely that the use of peak clipping will be reduced in the years ahead as more is known about the relative benefits of a less distorted output signal. Historically, the methods of peak clipping have been used in hearing aids for two reasons. First, a hearing aid can be placed into saturation if the output is adjusted too low when compared to the gain applied to typical input levels. This situation occurs frequently in hearing aids using the older Class A amplifier. However, this situation is not as common when using Class B or Class D amplifiers. The second reason why a hearing aid may be forced into saturation is that the maximum output of the hearing aid is adjusted to a low setting to prevent effects of loudness. Although a circuit may have the potential to produce an output of 120 dB SPL or more, the audiologist may choose to reduce the maximum output in an attempt to avoid loudness discomfort complaints.

Increasing the headroom by increasing the maximum output can certainly decrease the likelihood of clipping for speech peaks. Hearing aids with Class B or Class D amplifiers can provide the extra headroom needed to avoid peak clipping-induced distortion and decreased signal-to-noise ratios (see Chapters 3 and 4). However, the technique of increasing headroom (i.e., output) to avoid the distortion results from peak clipping is counter to the common fitting philosophy of adjusting the maximum output to avoid loudness discomfort.

There is some evidence to suggest that patients will tolerate higher maximum output levels as long as signal distortion is kept to a minimum (Fortune and

Preves, 1992a; 1992b). Therefore, hearing aids with Class B or Class D amplifiers that allow for higher levels of output without saturation-induced distortion may allow the patient to tolerate a higher maximum output level without discomfort. However, there are many situations where patients may have a loudness discomfort level that is below the average maximum output provided by many Class B and Class D amplifiers. The use of an amplifier with increased headroom is potentially a useful strategy to improve the understanding of speech in noise if the audiologist is not concerned with loudness discomfort. In cases where potential loudness discomfort is a problem, increasing the headroom may reduce the likelihood of saturation-induced distortion; however, the user may still be forced to adjust the volume control to provide less gain than is optimal in an attempt to avoid excessively and uncomfortably loud output levels.

## Circuitry Designed to Reduce Noise Effects

For a number of years, hearing aid manufacturers have been attempting to design hearing aid circuitry that will reduce the effects of background noise. These approaches have met with mixed success.

### USER TONE CONTROL

One of the earliest attempts to reduce the effects of background noise was to provide the hearing aid user with a two-position tone control. The switch allows the user to adjust the amount of amplification in the lower frequencies from a more broadband to a high-pass response. As indicated previously, the selection of a high-frequency response in hearing aids will allow, for some patients, better performance in certain noise backgrounds. The disadvantage to having a single high-frequency response is that there tends to be a preference for broader frequency response when listening in quiet situations (e.g., Punch and Beck, 1980, 1986). Therefore, to have the dual benefit of high-frequency amplification in noisy situations and broadband amplification in quieter listening situations, some manufacturers provide the option of a two-position tone control that the user can activate at any time. If the patient feels that there is sufficient background noise present, he can manipulate a switch to change the frequency response from a broadband response to a high-frequency response. The disadvantage is that it takes time for the patient to activate the switch. In a situation where the background noise is varying quickly, the patient may prefer not to make frequent adjustments to the hearing aid. However, if the background noise level is relatively stable, or if the patient is willing to tolerate a high-frequency response during the quieter periods, a user-activated tone control is certainly a reasonable option. The reader is referred to Chapter 5 for more information concerning user tone controls.

### DIRECTIONAL MICROPHONES

Another feature that has been available is the use of directional microphones. Most microphones used in hearing aids are omnidirectional. This means that they are equally sensitive to sound arriving from all directions, but many hearing aids (primarily behind-the-ear models, but also some in-the-ear models) offer directional microphones. A directional microphone has a front and rear sound port. The input signal arrives at the rear port delayed in time and phase shifted 180° relative to the input signal arriving at the front port. The time delay is such that any sound from behind the patient entering the rear port will reach the diaphragm of the single microphone at the same time as sound entering the front port. By having the two microphone ports 180° out of phase, such competing sounds are cancelled. The microphone is designed to be most efficient when the desired speech is in front of the patient, and the "unwanted" background noise arrives from behind the patient. Therefore, the background noise from behind will be cancelled with no deleterious effect upon the speech signal arriving from the front.

Directional microphones have been demonstrated to provide over 10 dB of suppression in certain frequency regions for sounds arising from the rear in optimal listening situations (Studebaker, Cox, and Formby, 1980). The benefit of directional microphones, however, is reduced in reverberant listening situations or when the noise arises from some other azimuth. However, directional microphones have been demonstrated to continue to provide at least some advantage in realistic listening environments (Hawkins and Yacullo, 1984).

WIDER BANDWIDTH

As indicated earlier, one of the most straightforward explanations for poor perception in noisy situations by persons with hearing impairment is the simple audibility effect of the hearing loss combined with the presence of background noise. One approach to improve performance in noise is to provide a wideband frequency response. As time has gone by, the frequency responses of hearing aids have become smoother and have been extended into the higher frequency region (see Chapter 6). One of the basic advantages of such a filter is to improve the recognition of the weak high-frequency consonant sound. For the typical situation where a patient cannot recognize speech because of the presence of noise and a high-frequency hearing loss, a hearing aid with an extended high-frequency response should improve the audibility of the high-frequency consonant sounds.

A modification of this approach is the K-AMP (Preves, 1992; Killion, 1993). With this amplifier, the frequency response changes with different input levels. For soft input levels, the amplifier provides a significant amount of high-frequency gain. As the input level increases, the amplifier provides a broader response with decreasing gain. In the fully described application, a hearing aid with a K-AMP amplifier will provide useable gain beyond 4000 Hz. One of the reported advantages of the K-AMP is improved audibility for the weaker high-frequency consonant sounds. The reader is referred to Chapter 4 for more information concerning the K-AMP.

Although the K-AMP makes no attempt to reduce the noise, the assumption is that as long as the patient has better audibility of the soft high-frequency consonants, overall performance in background noise will improve. In contrast to previous hearing aids that often could not provide useable gain above 2000 Hz, many current hearing aids can provide significant high-frequency gain beyond 6000 Hz. Despite the fact that some evidence existed that new hearing aid users may learn to better use aided sound over the first few months (Cox and Alexander, 1992; Gatehouse, 1992), clinical studies have demonstrated that speech understanding in noise improves with experience when listening with a hearing aid having a broader frequency response.

## AUTOMATIC LOW-FREQUENCY REDUCTION

In the mid-1980s, a new class of circuitry was introduced that "automatically" reduced low-frequency amplification as the input signal increased in intensity. This technology has been described as "automatic signal processing (ASP)," "adaptive frequency response (AFR)," and "bass increase at low levels (BILL)." Although the term automatic signal processing (ASP) can be applied to any number of currently available amplifiers, the term ASP has often been used to specifically describe automatic low-frequency reduction. These types of hearing aids are designed to provide the same benefits described earlier for static high-frequency amplification when listening in noisy situations. In addition, ASP circuits reportedly avoided the presumed disadvantages of eliminating a broadband frequency response that is better for listening in a quiet situation. The ASP circuit also did not require the patient to change a switch every time the listening environment changed. The positive effect of such circuits is presumed to be based on the assumed advantages of reducing the effects of the deleterious low-frequency environmental noises and minimizing the effect of the upward spread of masking.

Despite the widespread clinical use of this technology, the number of controlled studies to demonstrate its usefulness has been limited. Several authors have reported an advantage to use of such circuitry (Ono, Kanzaki, and Mizoi, 1983; Dempsey, 1987; Sigelman and Preves, 1987; Stach, Speerschneider, and Jerger, 1987; French-St. George, Engebretson, and O'Connell, 1992; Hogan, Walton, Frisina, Frisina, and Bancroft, 1993), but other investigators have found no demonstrable advantage for such circuitry (e.g., Tyler and Kuk, 1989; Horwitz, Turner, and Fabry, 1991; Bentler, Neibuhr, Getta, and Anderson, 1993a, 1993b). Still others have reported mixed results, with some patients revealing no benefit of an actual device in performance when using such a circuit, whereas other patients within the same study revealed a significant improvement (e.g., Kuk, Tyler, and Mims, 1990; Schum, 1990; Gordon-Salant and Sherlock, 1992).

Again, the major criticism of such an approach to noise control is that the S/N ratio in any given frequency band is not improved (Fabry and Van Tasell, 1990). Therefore, the notion that this circuit will "eliminate background noise" cannot occur. However, the evidence is still unclear whether or not progressive reduction of low-frequency amplification for some patients in some background noises will lead to an overall improvement in the understanding of speech due to reducing the effects of upward spread of masking.

## MULTIMEMORY HEARING AIDS

Over the past several years a number of manufacturers have offered hearing aids with programmable multimemories. In these devices, several memories containing different electroacoustic characteristics can be stored either in the hearing aid or a remote control. The user can then choose the preferred memory for different listening situations. Although some manufacturers include sophisticated forms of nonlinear signal processing, others have produced multimemory hearing aids with straightforward linear amplification.

The fitting strategies advanced for setting the multimemories often revolve around reducing low-frequency amplification for those memories designed for listening in background noise. Numerous adaptive strategies are available to adjust the various features in both programmable and nonprogrammable hearing aids (Kuk, 1993), and to modify compression characteristics in multiple memory hearing aids containing the sophisticated signal processing (e.g., ReSound, 1993; Stypulkowski, 1993). However, programmable multiple memory hearing aids with linear circuitry will often be simply adjusted by reducing low-frequency amplification for those memories designed to be used in noisy situations. This strategy is again consistent with the assumption that low-frequency amplification should be reduced in situations where excessive noise is present. As with the previously discussed example of the frequency static high amplification or user-activated tone control or automatic low-frequency reduction approaches, there is no strong evidence to prove benefit using such a strategy. However, some investigators have noted that some patients report better performance when choosing these memories while listening in noisy situations. For example, Fabry and Stypulkowski (1992) fit a group of patients with sensorineural hearing loss with multiple memory hearing aids. Two frequency responses were programmed into each hearing aid. One memory had a broad response; the other memory contained a frequency response that emphasized the high frequencies. These investigators found that patients preferred using the memory with the high-frequency emphasis response when listening in noise. Similar results have been noted by Ricketts and Bentler (1992). Unfortunately, some other investigators reported minimal differences in the shape of the frequency response chosen by hearing-impaired listeners while listening in different backgrounds of noise (e.g., Stelmachowicz, Lewis, and Carney, 1994).

COMPRESSION

Among other reasons, compression in hearing aids is often used to maximize audibility of speech within the limited dynamic range (the range from hearing threshold to UCL) that is often present in conjunction with sensorineural hearing loss. However, there may be advantages to using compression amplification when listening in a background of noise. As mentioned earlier, peak clipping can reduce or eliminate the higher amplitude segments of the speech signal and reduce the S/N ratio. Figure 8–22 provides a schematized version of such an effect. The left panel demonstrates the speech peaks rising above the level of the background noise. In the middle panel, the speech peaks have been "clipped" because they exceeded the clipping threshold. The waveform has been altered significantly and S/N ratio has been reduced because of the reduction in the speech peaks without reducing the level of the noise (which did not reach the clipping threshold). The right panel represents a situation where wideband compression is present. In this situation, the higher amplitude speech peaks activate the compression circuit. The overall gain is reduced so that the speech waveform retains its form and the S/N ratio is maintained. In this case, there is no reduction in the S/N ratio. It has not been improved but, by the same token, it has not been reduced, as was the case with peak clipping. In addition, this method of limiting does not generate distortion, as is the case with peak clipping. This latter factor will usually yield an amplified speech signal with higher sound quality ratings as compared to the sound quality rates for clipped speech.

Compression can currently be accomplished in single or multiple bands. For hearing aids with multiple band compression, most systems have 2 bands and one has three bands. Hearing aids have been available in the past with many more frequency bands; however, as mentioned earlier, the most current applications include two or three bands in which the compression characteristics can be adjusted independently.

A potential disadvantage to single band compression is shown in Figure 8–23. In the top panel, the unaided spectrum of the vowel /i/ is shown plotted in dB SPL. Also shown are the hearing thresholds (dB SPL) for a patient with a moderate, gently sloping hearing loss. As can be seen, the first formant (i.e., the first peak) is audible, and the second through fourth formants (i.e., the three peaks) are inaudible. In the second panel, the effect of linear amplification is demonstrated. In this situation, the appropriate gain has been applied. The first formant is now well above threshold. In addition, the second through fourth formants are also audible. However, if the intensity level of the vowel placed the single-band hearing aid into compression, the effect would be that shown in the third panel. In this case, 10 dB of compression has been added to the signal. This magnitude of compression lowered the gain and placed the second through fourth formants below the threshold level. Therefore, single-band compression had a deleterious effect on the audibility of high-frequency formants of the vowel.

However, if the same vowel has been processed using two-channel compression with a crossover frequency adjusted to 1000 Hz, the effect can be demonstrated in the lower panel. The compression characteristic of the low-frequency channel reduced the gain of the first formant, although it is still audible. However, compression is not activated in the higher frequency channel, which

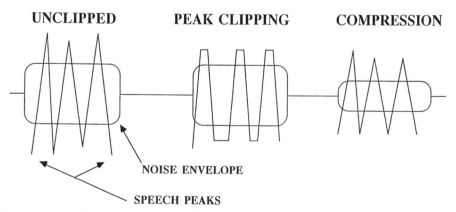

**Figure 8–22.** Schematized example of the negative effects of peak clipping on the signal-to-noise ratio.

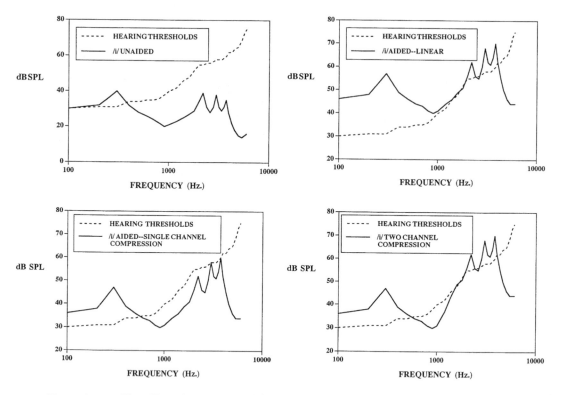

**Figure 8–23.**   The effect of various amplification modes on the spectrum of the vowel /i/ in relation to an individual's hearing thresholds.

has a higher compression threshold, thus allowing the second through fourth formants to remain audible. The advantage of multiple compression can also be useful to provide adequate amplification of high-frequency consonant sounds, which occurs in close temporal proximity to an intense low-frequency vowel sound. If the time constants of a single-channel system are relatively long, the less intense high-frequency sound may be compressed due to the occurrence of the previous intense low-frequency vowel sound. A two-channel system may have avoided this effect.

Older research on the advantage of compression amplification in improving the understanding of speech in noise was generally negative, even for the multiple band hearing aid systems (Walker, Byrne, and Dillon, 1984; Plomp, 1988; Peterson, Feeney, and Yantis, 1990). However, reports surfacing over the past several years have demonstrated some benefits from multiple-band compression in comparison to linear and single-band compression (Moore, 1987; Kiessling and Steffens, 1991; Van Dijkhuizen, Festen, and Plomp, 1991; Maré, Dreschler, and Verschuure, 1992). The benefits of multiple-band compression seem to maintain even when speech is presented in a background of noise. For example, Moore, Johnson, Clark, and Pluvinage (1992) reported improved understanding of speech babble for a two-channel input compression hearing aid when compared with linear amplification in the same listening situations.

Most advances in hearing aid circuitry that are likely to occur in the very near future will involve programmable multiple compression. The recent success of such signal processing in a variety of listening situations has seemed to have the effect of encouraging even more manufacturers to enhance and expand upon multiple band technology. Evidence has been accumulating in the literature (e.g., Moore et al., 1992) to suggest that this approach may hold promise of improving performance of persons with sensorineural hearing loss for listening to speech in noise.

## Future Expectations

A significant amount of work is being conducted on designing new circuits specifically targeted at improving speech understanding for individuals with sensorineural hearing loss. These technologies are several years away from commercial use, but theoretically hold significant promise for improving performance. Audiologists can expect to see some radical changes in available hearing aid technology within the next decade.

There are three particularly encouraging areas of investigation. However, most of the proposed changes in fundamental hearing aid circuit designs, especially as related to speech understanding in noisy situations, depend on the availability of a "true" digital hearing aid (digitization of the incoming signal).

### Consonant Enhancement

The first area involves identifying and enhancing the amplitude and perhaps temporal characteristics of consonant sounds. It is well known that consonants carry the information burden of speech. However, consonant energy is most often inaudible for persons with sensorineural hearing loss. The traditional way to try to improve consonant perception is to simply boost the frequency response of the hearing aid in the higher frequencies. However, there are some disadvantages to emphasizing the high-frequency response to improve consonant perception. These include tolerance problems resulting from an overemphasis of high-frequency output due to the usual reduced dynamic range in the high frequencies. Also, consonants can have significant energy present in the lower frequency regions. Techniques have been proposed that would allow an electronic "sensor" to automatically identify the presence of a consonant sound and make specific changes in the waveform, such as increasing amplitude and perhaps temporal lengthening changes. The major reason why this technology has not yet been applied in commercial application is the difficulty in designing a computer algorithm to accurately and consistently identify the presence of a consonant from any given speaker in any background noise. When such consonant manipulation is performed offline using digital editing procedures, significant improvements in speech intelligibility have been demonstrated by Gordon-Salant (1987) and Montgomery and Edge (1988).

### Spectral Shaping

A related approach is that of spectral sharpening or spectral enhancement. It is well known that persons with sensorineural hearing loss have poorer frequency resolution than normally hearing individuals. Attempts have been made to emphasize the spectral peaks of speech in an attempt to improve speech recognition. Stone and Moore (1992) found that a spectral sharpening scheme resulted in higher subjective ratings of sound quality and speech intelligibility in noise by persons with sensorineural hearing loss.

## Noise Estimation Technique

Procedures are being developed by which the spectral characteristics of the background noise are estimated so that the noise can be removed from the speech signal using filtering or subtraction techniques. A simple analog version of this approach is used in automatic low-frequency reduction circuits that were discussed earlier. In that case, the decision is made that sounds above the activation threshold are composed of primarily low-frequency energy. Thus, the high pass is filter-activated to remove this portion of the signal. A more sophisticated analog version of this technique was commercially available for several years in the late 1980s and was known as the ZETA Noise Blocker (Graupe, Grosspietsch, and Taylor, 1986). An assumption underlying the Zeta algorithm was that the spectrum of background noise tends to be more steady, whereas the spectrum of speech varies rapidly. This circuit design would monitor the stability of the input signal in several different frequency bands; any band with a spectrum determined to be "stable" was reduced in amplitude. This circuit, however, is no longer available in commercial hearing aids.

More sophisticated digital noise estimation techniques have been evaluated in the laboratory. One approach is to estimate the spectrum of the noise during nonspeech periods and then to subtract the assumed noise spectrum from that of the speech-plus-noise signal. The difficulty with this and all other noise estimation techniques is that many common "noise" situations consist of a background of other talkers so that the spectra of speech and noise are quite similar. It is extremely difficult to use filtering or subtraction techniques to separate one voice from another.

## Automatic Speaker Identification

The second promising area of development involves the use of automatic speaker identification. If an electronic device could identify and track the speech of one talker and separate it from the speech of other talkers in the same environment, then that particular voice could specifically be modified either through filtering or amplification (Summerfield and Stubbs, 1990). Unfortunately, widespread commercial application of such technology is not currently possible because an electronic device is not available that can accurately differentiate one voice from that of background talkers *in real time*. Attempts have been made, for example, to track the fundamental frequency of a particular talker and estimate the formant and harmonic structure in the higher frequencies based on the fundamental frequency. After this estimation has taken place, filtering or subtraction techniques are used to separate the intended speech target from the competing speech targets. Again, however, practical application of such an algorithm is likely years away.

## Multiple Microphone Arrays

The third major area of promise is the use of multiple microphone arrays. As discussed earlier, the normal binaural hearing system is dependent on the ability of the brain to compare the inputs from two different sides of the auditory periphery in an attempt to make use of slight spectral differences in the signals to extract the intended speech from the competition. Computer algorithms have been developed to replicate, in part, this comparison. However, such a system requires inputs from more than one microphone. Multiple microphones can essentially be set to focus on one particular point in space and cancel out sound arising from other places in the environment. Speech intelligibility improvements using such designs have been significant (Peterson, Durlach, Rabinowitz, and Zurek, 1987; Harris, Brey, Robinette, Chabries, Christiansen, and Jolley, 1988). The major disadvantage to widespread application of such a design is cosmetic concerns of wearers. The benefits of multiple microphone arrays increase as the physical distance between the multiple microphones are increased. Clearly, there are limitations to how much microphone separation can be obtained with hearing aids in a cosmetically acceptable manner.

## *Conclusion*

The audiologist fitting hearing aids is faced with the decision as to which hearing aid strategy should be used to address the concerns about poor performance of hearing aids in noise. It is clear from the literature that current technology cannot completely solve the difficulty that persons with sensorineural hearing loss have in noisy situations. However, recent advances in technology are promising, and it is generally well accepted that current hearing aids perform better in some difficult listening situations than hearing aids 5, 10, or 15 years ago. When attempting to make decisions about which circuitry or clinical strategies should be used to help minimize the effects of noise on understanding speech, the following considerations should be made by the audiologist.

First, many studies on the effectiveness of circuitry designed to improve speech understanding in noise have demonstrated wide intersubject variability. It has not been uncommon in studies for some subjects to show no difference between performance with one circuit or another. However, several individual subjects may demonstrate a clear preference and/or benefit for using one particular technology. Figure 8–24 represents the individual subject results from a study by Schum (1990). In that study, the investigator evaluated the effect on speech understanding in noise using an adaptive technique. Four noise reduction strategies [binaural hearing aids (H), directional microphones (D), ASP processing (A), and Zeta processing (Z)] were evaluated and compared to linear (L) amplification. In that study, there was a general effect for all four noise reduction strategies to improve understanding of speech in noise. Also, minimal differences were found between the group means for the four noise reduction strategies. However, as indicated by the data reproduced in Figure 8–24, some individual subjects showed clear benefit from one noise reduction strategy in comparison to the others. For example, subject 1 showed a clear benefit for the ASP technology,

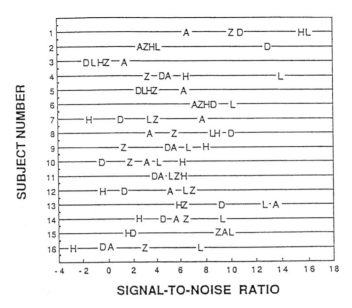

**Figure 8–24.**   Data from Schum (1990) indicating the individual results for a group of 16 hearing-impaired individuals using four different noise control strategies and also linear amplification (L = linear, H = high-pass, D = directional microphone, A = ASP or automatic low-frequency reduction, Z = Zeta noise reduction). (Figure used with permission.)

whereas subject 6 showed equal performance across all four noise reduction strategies (+7 to +10 dB). These findings are similar to the findings reported by Kuk, Tyler, and Mims (1990).

The implications of intersubject variability are that the clinician may need to find strategies to comparatively evaluate a variety of different noise strategies on any given patient. However, there are clear problems in achieving this goal, however. First, it has proven difficult to develop reliable and valid comparative hearing aid evaluation procedures that can be done in a clinical setting. Second, it may take a significant amount of time for benefit from a circuit to be revealed (e.g., Erdman and Sedge, 1981; Cox and Alexander, 1992; Gatehouse, 1992). Third, there are financial implications to performing a long comparative process of different circuits for a given patient. Very few audiology facilities can afford to support extended trials with several different hearing aid circuits on every patient. Finally, custom (in-the-ear, in-the-canal, and completely in-the-canal) hearing aid fittings are over 80% of the hearing aids fit. True comparative field trials of hearing aids, however, are typically done using behind-the-ear units. Many patients may not be interested in even a trial use of a behind-the-ear unit. Given these limitations, the audiologist may choose, instead, to use comparative trial periods only on a certain number of patients. Such patients may be, for example, those who have previously experienced significant difficulties in everyday environments using more traditional circuitry.

Conventional broadband hearing aids with low distortion that allows as much speech as possible to be audible have served the audiology community very well for many years. It has been difficult to experimentally prove the advantage for any number of nonlinear approaches in reducing the effect of noise (e.g., Bentler et al. 1993a, 1993b). Technical improvements are always being made to widen the bandwidth and decrease the distortion and internal noise of hearing aids. Thus, for many reasons, there is value in using linear amplification as a baseline fitting for patients who express a concern about understanding speech in noise. The use of more advanced circuitry in an attempt to specifically minimize the effects of noise may be reserved as a "back-up" when linear amplification does not appear to be successful.

As far as current nonlinear noise reduction strategies are concerned, the strongest evidence appears to support the use of multiple compression. Selectively processing input levels in different frequency regions appears to provide some benefit for certain listeners in some situations. However, the potentially modest improvements afforded by such technology need to be balanced against the potential dollar cost to the patient for the use of such technology. The most advanced programmable multiband hearing aids often cost two to three times the conventional amplification. Although it is difficult to balance financial versus performance concerns, especially when the specific effect of the technology is difficult to predict for any given patient, the audiologist does need to take the responsibility of describing the advantages and disadvantages, both performance and financial, to the user.

The jury is still out on high-frequency amplification, especially as implemented in automatic low-frequency reduction circuitry. Some results have been negative and others have been relatively positive. However, the most accurate finding is probably that there are true intersubject differences in subjective and objective benefits. The ability of this technology to provide benefits to a large number of patients still needs to be clearly demonstrated in the literature.

Finally, the audiologist should keep abreast of the technologies under development, some of which certainly hold promise for better performance for a larger number of patients. However, the practical uses of emerging technologies need to be clearly demonstrated using studies.

## References

Bacon SP, Viemeister NF. (1985). Temporal modulation transfer functions in normal-hearing and hearing-impaired listeners. *Audiology* 24:117–134.

Bentler RA, Niebuhr DP, Getta JP, Anderson CV. (1993a). Longitudinal study of hearing aid effectiveness. I: Objective measures. *Speech Hear Res* 36:808–819.

Bentler RA, Niebuhr DP, Getta JP, Anderson CV. (1993b). Longitudinal study of hearing aid effectiveness. II: Subjective measures. *Speech Hear Res* 36:820–831.

Bronkhorst AQ, Plomp R. (1990). A clinical test for the assessment of binaural speech perception in noise. *Audiology* 29:275–285.

Brooks DN, Bulmer D. (1981). Survey of binaural hearing aid users. *Ear Hear* 2:220–224.

Byrne D. (1980). Binaural hearing aid fitting: Research findings and clinical application. In: Libby ER, ed. *Binaural Hearing and Amplification.* Chicago: Benetron, Inc.

Byrne D, Dillon H. (1986). The National Acoustics Laboratories' (NAL) new procedure for selecting the gain and frequency response of a hearing aid. *Ear Hear* 1:257–265.

Carhart R. (1965). Monaural and binaural discrimination against competing sentences. *Int Audiol* 4(3):5–10.

Carhart R, Tillman TW. (1970). Interaction of competing speech signals with hearing losses. *Arch Otolaryngol (Stockh)* 91:273–279.

Carhart R, Tillman TW, Greetis ES. (1969). Perceptual masking in multiple sound backgrounds. *Acoust Soc Am* 45:694–703.

Cohen RL, Keith RW. (1976). Use of low-pass noise in word-recognition testing. *Speech Hear Res* 19:48–54.

Cooper JC, Cutts BP. (1971). Speech discrimination in noise. *Speech Hear Res* 14:332–337.

Cox RM, Alexander GC. (1992). Maturation of hearing aid benefit: Objective and subjective measurements. *Ear Hear* 13:131–141.

Cox RM, Alexander CC, Gilmore C. (1987). Development of the Connected Speech Test (CST). *Ear Hear* 8:119S–126S.

Crandell CC. (1993). Speech recognition in noise by children with minimal degrees of sensorineural hearing loss. *Ear Hear* 14:210–216.

Danaher EM, Pickett JM. (1975). Some masking effects produced by low-frequency vowel formants in persons with sensorineural hearing loss. *Speech Hear Res* 18:261–271.

Dempsey JJ. (1987). Effect of automatic signal-processing amplification on speech recognition in noise for persons with sensorineural hearing loss. *Ann Otol Rhinol Laryngol* 96:251–253.

Dirks DD, Bower DR. (1969). Masking effects of speech competing messages. *Speech Hear Res* 12:229–245.

Dirks DD, Morgan DE, Dubno JR. (1982). A procedure for quantifying the effects of noise on speech recognition. *Speech Hear Dis* 47:114–123.

Erdman SA, Sedge RK. (1981). Subjective comparisons of binaural versus monaural amplification. *Ear Hear* 2:225–229.

Fabry DA, Stupulkowski. (1992). *Evaluation of Hearing Aid Fitting Procedures for Multiple-Memory Programmable Hearing Aids.* Paper presented at the annual meeting of the American Academy of Audiology, Nashville, TN.

Fabry DA, Van Tasell DJ. (1990). Evaluation of an articulation-index based model for predicting the effects of adaptive frequency response hearing aids. *Speech Hear Res* 33:676–689.

Festen JM, Plomp R. (1986). Speech-reception threshold in noise with one and two hearing aids. *Acoust Soc Am* 79:465–471.

Fitzgibbons PJ, Wightman FL. (1982). Gap detection in normal and hearing-impaired listeners. *Acoust Soc Am* 72:761–765.

Fortune TW, Preves DA. (1992a). Hearing aid saturation and aided loudness discomfort. *Speech Hear Res* 35:175–185.

Fortune TW, Preves DA. (1992b). Hearing aid saturation, coherence, and aided loudness discomfort. *Am Acad Audiol* 3(2):81–93.

French-St. George M, Engebretson AM, O'Connell MP. (1992). Behavioral assessment of CID's benchtop (version 2) digital hearing aid: Noise reduction. *Am Acad Audiol* 3:132–141.

Gagné JP. (1988). Excess masking among listeners with a sensorineural hearing loss. *Acoust Soc Am* 83:2311–2321.

Gatehouse S. (1992). The time course and magnitude of perceptual acclimatization to frequency responses: Evidence from monaural fitting of hearing aids. *Acoust Soc Am* 92:1258–1268.

Gengel RW. (1971). Acceptable speech-to-noise ratios for aided speech discrimination by the hearing impaired. *Speech Hear Res* 11:219–222.

Gordon-Salant S. (1984). Effects of reducing low-frequency amplification on consonant perception in quiet and noise. *Speech Hear Res* 27:483–493.

Gordon-Salant S. (1987). Effects of acoustic modification on consonant recognition by elderly hearing-impaired subjects. *Acoust Soc Am* 81:1199–1202.

Gordon-Salant S, Sherlock LP. (1992). Performance with an adaptive frequency response hearing aid in a sample of elderly hearing-impaired listeners. *Ear Hear* 13:255–262.

Graupe D, Grosspietsch JK, Taylor R. (1986). A self adaptive noise filtering system. Part 1: Overview and description. *Hear Instrum* 37(9):29–34.

Groen JJ. (1969). Social hearing handicap; Its measurement by speech audiometry in noise. *Int Audiol* 8(1):182–183.

Hannley M, Dorman MR. (1983). Susceptibility to intraspeech spread of masking in listeners with sensorineural hearing loss. *Acoust Soc Am* 74:40–51.

Harris RW, Brey RH, Robinette MS, Chabries DM, Christiansen RW, Jolley RG. (1988). Use of adaptive digital signal processing to improve speech communication for normally hearing and hearing-impaired subjects. *Speech Hear Res* 31:265–271.

Hawkins DB, Yacullo, WS. (1984). Signal-to-noise ratio advantage of binaural hearing aids and directional microphones under different levels of reverberation. *Speech Hear Dis* 49:278–286.

Hogan C, Walton J, Frisina RD, Frisina DR, Bancroft, B. (1993). *Improvement in Speech Recognition in Noise Using a Novel, Adaptive ITE Hearing Aid Circuit.* Paper presented at the American Academy of Audiology Convention, Phoenix, AZ, April.

Horwitz AR, Turner CW, Fabry DA. (1991). Effects of different frequency response strategies upon recognition and preference of audible speech stimuli. *Speech Hear Res* 34:1185–1196.

Humes LE. (1982). Spectral and temporal resolution by the hearing impaired. In: Studebaker GA, Bess FH, eds. *The Vanderbilt Hearing-Aid Report, State of the Art Research Needs.* Upper Darby, PA: Monographs in Contemporary Audiology, pp. 16–31.

Humes LE. (1991). Understanding the speech-understanding problems of the hearing impaired. *Am Acad Audiol* 2:59–69.

Hygge S, Rünnberg J, Larsby B, Arlinger S. (1992). Normal-hearing and hearing-impaired subjects' ability to just follow conversation in competing speech, reversed speech, and noise backgrounds. *Speech Hear Res* 35:208–215.

Jerger JF, Speaks C, Trammell JL. (1968). A new approach to speech audiometry. *Speech Hear Dis* 33:318–328.

Jerger JF, Tillman TW, Peterson JL. (1960). Masking by octave bands on noise in normal and impaired ear. *Acoust Soc Am* 32:385–390.

Kalikow DN, Stevens KN, Elliott LL. (1977). Development of a test of speech intelligibility in noise using sentence materials with controlled word predictability. *Acoust Soc Am* 61:1337–1351.

Kamm C, Dirks D, Bell T. (1985). Speech recognition and the articulation index for normal and hearing-impaired listeners. *Acoust Soc Am* 27:281–288.

Kiessling J, Steffens T. (1991). Clinical evaluation of a programmable three-channel automatic gain control amplification system. *Audiology* 30:70–81.

Killon MC. (1985). The noise problem: There's hope. *Hear Instrum* 36(11):26–32.

Killon MC. (1993). The K-amp hearing aid: An attempt to present high fidelity for persons with impaired hearing. *Am Audiol* July:52–74.

Klein AJ, Mills JH, Adkins WY. (1990). Upward spread of masking, hearing loss, and speech recognition in young and elderly listeners. *Acoust Soc Am* 87:1266–1271.

Kuk FK. (1993). Clinical considerations in fitting a multimemory hearing aid. *Am Audiol* 2(3):23–27.

Kuk FK, Tyler RS, Mims L. (1990). Subjective ratings of noise-reduction hearing aids. *Scand Audiol* 19:237–244.

Lamb ST, Owens E, Schubert ED. (1983). The revised form of the hearing performance inventory. *Ear Hear* 4:152–157.

Larsby B, Arlinger S. (1994). Speech recognition and just-follow-up conversation tasks for normal-hearing and hearing-impaired listeners with different maskers. *Audiology* 33:165–176.

Lewis HD, Benignus VA, Muller KE, Malott, CM, Barton CN. (1988). Babble and random-noise masking of speech in high and low context cue conditions. *Speech Hear Res* 31:108–114.

Maré MJ, Dreschler WA, Verschuure H. (1992). The effects of input-output configuration in syllabic compression on speech perception. *Speech Hear Res* 35:675–685.

Martin ES, Pickett JM. (1970). Sensorineural hearing loss and upward spread of masking. *Speech Hear Res* 13:426–437.

Montgomery A, Edge R. (1988). Evaluation of two speech enhancement techniques to improve intelligibility for hearing-impaired adults. *Speech Hear Res* 31:386–393.

Moore BJ. (1987). Design and evaluation of a two-channel compression hearing aid. *Rehab Res Dev* 24:181–192.

Moore BJ, Johnson JS, Clark TM, Pluvinage V. (1992). Evaluation of a dual channel full dynamic range compression system for people with sensorineural hearing loss. *Ear Hear* 13:349–370.

Ono H, Kanzaki J, Mizoi K. (1983). Clinical results of hearing aid with noise-level-controlled selective amplification. *Audiology* 22:494–515.

Papso CF, Blood IM. (1989). Word recognition skills of children and adults in background noise. *Ear Hear* 10:235–236.

Pearsons KS, Bennett RL, Fidell S. (1977). *Speech Levels in Various Noise Environments.* Washington, DC: U.S. Environmental Protection Agency Contract No. 68 01-2466.

Peterson ME, Feeney MP, Yantis PA. (1990). The effect of automatic gain control in hearing-impaired listeners with different dynamic ranges. *Ear Hear* 11:185–194.

Peterson PM, Durlach NI, Rabinowitz WM, Zurek PM. (1987). Multimicrophone adaptive beamforming for interference reduction in hearing aids. *Rehab Res Dev* 24(4):103–110.

Plomp R. (1988). The negative effect of amplitude compression in multichannel hearing aids in the light of the modulation-transfer function. *Acoust Soc Am* 83:2322–2327.

Preves DA. (1992). The K-AMP circuit. *Am J Audiol* 1(2):15–16.

Punch JL, Beck LB. (1980). Low-frequency response of hearing aids and judgments of aided speech quality. *Speech Hear Res* 23:325–335.

Punch JL, Beck LB. (1986). Relative effects of low-frequency amplification on syllable recognition and speech quality. *Ear Hear* 7:57–62.

ReSound Corporation. (1993). *ReSound's Fitting Session Protocol and Fitting Guide.* Redwood City: ReSound.

Ricketts TA, Bentler RA. (1992). Comparison of two digitally programmable hearing aids. *Am Acad Audiol* 3:101–112.

Rittmanic PA. (1962). Pure-tone masking by narrow-noise bands in normal and impaired ears. *Aud Res* 2:287–304.

Scharf B, Florentine M. (1982). Psychoacoustics of elementary sounds. In: Studebaker GA, Bess FH. eds. *The Vanderbilt Hearing-Aid Report, State of the Art Research Needs*. Upper Darby, PA: Monographs in Contemporary Audiology, pp. 3–15.

Schum D. (1990). Noise reduction strategies for elderly, hearing-impaired listeners. *Am Acad Audiol* 1:31–36.

Schum D. (1994). *Older Adults' Expectations Concerning the Benefits of Hearing Aids*. Paper presented at the Audiologic Management of the Elderly workshop, Iowa City, IA, June.

Schum D, Matthews LJ, Lee F. (1991). Actual and predicted word-recognition performance of elderly hearing-impaired listeners. *Speech Hear Res* 34:636–641.

Sigelman J, Preves DA. (1987). Field trials of a new adaptive signal processor hearing aid circuit. *Hear J* 40(4):24–29.

Souza PE, Turner CW. (1994). Masking of speech in young and elderly listeners with hearing loss. *Speech Hear Res* 37:665–661.

Stach BA, Speerschneider JM, Jerger JF. (1987). Evaluating the efficacy of automatic signal processing hearing aids. *Hear J* 40(3):15–19.

Stelmachowicz PG, Lewis DE, Carney E. (1994). Preferred hearing-aid frequency responses in simulated listening environments. *Speech Hear Res* 37:712–719.

Stone MA, Moore BCJ. (1992). Spectral feature enhancement for people with sensorineural hearing impairment: Effects on speech intelligibility and quality. *Rehab Res Dev* 29(2):39–56.

Studebaker GA, Cox RM, Formby C. (1980). The effect of environment on the directional performance of head-worn hearing aids. In: Studebaker GA, Hochberg I, eds. *Acoustical Factors Affecting Hearing Aid Performance*. Baltimore: University Park Press.

Stypulkowski PH. (1993). Fitting strategies for multiple-memory programmable hearing instruments. *Am J Audiol* July:19–28.

Summerfield Q, Stubbs RJ. (1990). Strengths and weaknesses of procedures for separating simultaneous voices. *Acta Otolaryngol (Stockh)* 469S:91–100.

Suter, AH. (1985). Speech recognition in noise by individuals with mild hearing impairments. *Acoust Soc Am* 78(3):887–900.

Ter-Horst K, Byrne D, Noble W. (1993). Ability of hearing-impaired listeners to benefit from separation of speech and noise. *Aust Audiol* 15(2):71–84.

Trammell JL, Speaks C. (1970). On the distracting properties of competing speech. *Speech Hear Res* 13:438–448.

Tyler RS. (1986). Frequency resolution in hearing-impaired listeners. In: Moore B, ed. *Frequency Selectively in Hearing*. London: Academic Press Inc., pp. 309–371.

Tyler RS, Kuk FK. (1989). The effects of "noise suppression" hearing aids on consonant recognition in speech-babble and low-frequency noise. *Ear Hear* 10:243–249.

Tyler RS, Summerfield Q, Wood EJ, Fernandes MA. (1982). Psychoacoustic and phonetic temporal processing in normal and hearing-impaired listeners. *Acoust Soc Am* 72:740–752.

Van Dijkhuizen JN, Festen JM, Plomp R. (1991). The effect of frequency-selective attenuation on the speech-reception threshold of sentences in conditions of low-frequency noise. *Acoust Soc Am* 90:39–48.

Van Tasell DJ. (1980). Perception of second-formant transitions by hearing-impaired persons. *Ear Hear* 1:130–136.

Walden B, Demorest M., Hepler E. (1984). Self report approach to assessing benefit derived from amplification. *Speech Hear Res* 27:49–56.

Walker G, Byrne D, Dillon H. (1984). The effects of multichannel compression/expansion amplification on the intelligibility of nonsense syllables in noise. *Acoust Soc Am* 76:746–756.

*Webster's Ninth New Collegiate Dictionary*. (1990). Springfield, MA: Merriam-Webster, Inc.

Zurek PM, Delhorne LA. (1987). Consonant reception in noise by listeners with mild and moderate sensorineural hearing impairment. *Acoust Soc Am* 82:1548–1559.

# 9

# Amplification and the Central Auditory Nervous System

## Frank E. Musiek
## Jane A. Baran

## Introduction

A chapter on this topic in a book devoted to hearing aids is rare. The main reason a chapter on the central auditory nervous system (CANS) appears here is because of recent reports addressing the issue of how hearing aids may play a role in the maintenance of auditory function (Silman, Gelfand, and Silverman, 1984; Silverman and Emmer, 1993). Some reports have even shown that amplification may improve speech recognition scores over time (Gatehouse, 1992; Silverman and Emmer, 1993). Given our stage of knowledge, it is clear that the maintenance and/or improvement of auditory function must involve the CANS. Because of this, professionals who are involved with the selection and fitting of hearing aids are becoming increasingly interested in how the CANS and amplified sound interact. It now appears there may be an additional and important reason for people with hearing loss to wear hearing aids—to help preserve their hearing.

Considerable time, effort, and financial resources have been spent over the past several years on developing hearing aids with enhanced electroacoustic capabilities. At the same time there have been a number of recommendations for changes in protocols for the evaluation and fitting of hearing aids. However, there has been a paucity of information about how amplification may influence the function of the CANS. Also, from another perspective, it is important to know how the integrity of the CANS may affect the success of a given hearing aid fitting. Many times, an individual whose hearing aid is ineffective may have a disproportionate amount of CANS compromise. In most cases, CANS compromise is not entertained by the audiologist as a reason for the individual's poor response to amplification. It seems reasonable that a comprehensive hearing aid evaluation and fitting is one that attempts to account for central and peripheral deficits in hearing. This becomes most relevant in attempting to fit hearing aids to the elderly. It is well known that there are increasing numbers of elderly people and that many of these people have hearing losses and/or neurologic problems. Willott (1991), in a comprehensive review of a number of studies, reports that between 30 and 40% of individuals 61 to 70 years of age have audiometrically measured hearing losses. Nadeau (1989) reports that nearly 2% of the elderly suffer strokes. These reports indicate significant incidences of audiologic and neurological problems in the elderly.

It is known that aging can affect both the auditory periphery and the CANS (Schuknecht, 1964). Which of these two parts of the auditory system is more commonly affected in presbyacusis is currently a topic of much debate. However, it is safe to say that in some individuals the CANS is more involved than the periphery and, in others, just the reverse situation exists.

The audiologist who is aware of CANS compromise in a given client can make better judgments about amplification and management than the audiologist who is unaware of higher auditory processing deficits. Awareness of CANS function and dysfunction will become increasingly important to the professional committed to providing the best care to his or her hearing-impaired clientele.

A concept that should motivate aggressive efforts at fitting clients of all ages is that of brain plasticity. This concept will be discussed in greater detail later; however, its influence pervades this chapter and, thus, a brief definition is offered here. Brain plasticity in terms of the present discussion refers to the ability of the neural tissue in the CANS to reorganize and change function in response to auditory stimulation.

The concept of associating amplification with CANS integrity and plasticity is a valuable one, but the application of this concept is difficult. There is much we do not know about how the normal and abnormal CANS handles increases in the intensity of a stimulus. Moreover, our central auditory test procedures—especially those used with individuals with hearing loss—must be further developed and refined to minimize the confounding effects of peripheral hearing impairment. Finally, the concept of auditory plasticity is, unfortunately, foreign to many audiologists, yet the understanding of this concept is critical to the realization of long-term benefits for hearing aid users.

In this chapter, a brief overview of the anatomy of the CANS is provided. Attention is then directed toward defining the hearing aid candidate who has considerable CANS involvement. This will be accomplished in two ways: (1) by highlighting information that can be obtained though history taking, and (2) by demonstrating the use of assessment techniques to measure central auditory function in individuals with peripheral involvement. We also discuss the concepts of auditory deprivation, auditory stimulation, and brain plasticity as they pertain to the use of hearing aids. Finally, future directions in the area of amplification and their potential for interaction with the CANS are presented.

## Anatomy of the CANS

It is beyond the scope of this chapter to discuss the functional anatomy of the CANS in detail; however, a brief orientation is appropriate for those not familiar with this sensory system (Fig. 9–1). The CANS begins with the cochlear nucleus complex, which is located at the posterior and lateral aspect of the caudal pons. The cochlear nucleus receives direct input from the auditory nerve and is composed of several cell types that are capable of modifying the input from the auditory nerve. Information is conveyed from the cochlear nucleus to the superior olivary complex via the acoustic stria. The superior olivary complex is composed of several major groups of nuclei and is located deep in the caudal pons. The superior olivary complex receives both ipsilateral (weaker) and contralateral (stronger) inputs; hence, at this level of the CANS, representation from both ears is available. This provides the basis for localization and other differential time processing. Fibers leaving the superior olivary complex join a major ascending pathway in the brainstem known as the lateral lemniscus. The lateral lemniscus has nuclei of its own located at the rostral pons. The lateral lemniscus pathway inputs to the largest auditory nuclei in the brainstem, the inferior colliculus. The inferior colliculus is located in the midbrain and is responsible for much complex processing. This is also true for the medial geniculate body, which receives ipsilateral

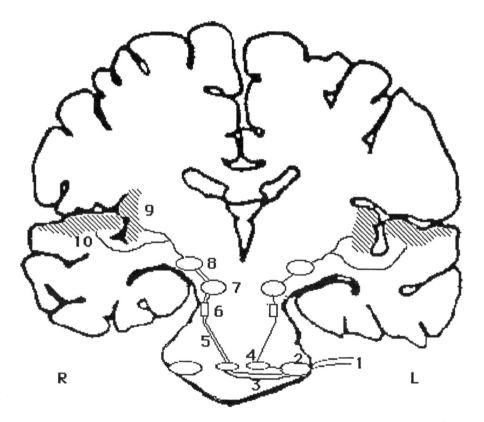

**Figure 9–1.** A drawing of a coronal section of the brain showing the auditory pathway. Key: 1 = auditory nerve, 2 = left cochlear nucleus, 3 = acoustic stria, 4 = left superior olivary complex, 5 = right lateral lemniscus tract, 6 = nuclei of the right lateral lemniscus, 7 = right inferior colliculus, 8 = right medial geniculate, 9 = right insula, 10 = right Heschl's gyrus.

input from the inferior colliculus via its brachium of the inferior colliculus. The medial geniculate body is located on the underside of the thalamus and sends fibers to the auditory cortex via a complex course. The auditory cortex and its association areas cover major portions of the cerebrum. Two of the more focal regions of auditory activity in the cortex include the insula, located medial to the mesial temporal lobe, and Heschl's gyrus, located on the superior temporal plane. The auditory areas in each hemisphere are connected by the corpus callosum to allow interhemispheric communication.

The CANS (both brainstem and cerebrum) is organized tonotopically to permit excellent frequency identification and discrimination. Generally, the brainstem fibers are capable of responding much more rapidly than cortical neurons, which may provide insight as to the nature of what these different areas do. There are far more fibers in the auditory cortex than in the brainstem and there is much intrahemispheric and interhemispheric communication involved in higher auditory processing. The large number of fibers and multiple connections provide the basis for a highly redundant system. Because of this redundancy, special test procedures are required to reveal deficits in the CANS.

## CANS Factors in the Client's History

Considerable information can be gleaned from a carefully obtained client history, and this information can implicate CANS involvement or the potential for CANS involvement. The information can be crucial to the successful fitting of hearing aids and/or some other type of assistive listening device to the individual with CANS involvement.

### Age of the Individual

Age is a factor that may work for or against a successful hearing aid fitting. Of particular interest to the present discussion is either end of the age spectrum. In the infant or young child, maturation of the central nervous system (CNS) is not complete and the effects of auditory deprivation may be of great consequence. This would be especially true for the young child who has been hearing impaired since birth. In this case, the auditory stimulation necessary for development of the CANS is compromised at best, and may be lacking completely, as in the case of profound hearing impairment. However, in spite of the potential deleterious effects of auditory deprivation, the young brain is "plastic" and can be changed with appropriate stimulation (Lenneberg, 1967). Obviously, the implication for fittings at this age is timely amplification so that one can capitalize on the brain's plasticity, which is known to lessen with advancing age.

On the other end of the spectrum is the elderly individual. As a person ages, senescent changes occur along the entire auditory pathway. Although changes in cochlear function are commonly recognized as one of the major physiological changes associated with aging, changes in the CANS also occur and are often overlooked by the audiologist working with the elderly client. Yet these changes are at least as important to the client's potential for successful use of amplification as are changes in cochlear function. Take, for example, the elderly client who perceives less benefit from amplification than does a younger client with comparable auditory thresholds. The loss of perceived benefits in the older client is likely caused by increases in the distortion of the signal associated with increased intensity. This inappropriate processing of intensity may be related to what is known as the "rollover" phenomenon, often noted in individuals with CANS involvement. At least one subgroup of the elderly with hearing losses have a disproportionate amount of central presbyacusis and, thus, may be expected to demonstrate "rollover." These individuals may hear poorly at higher intensities and, therefore, will perceive amplification as ineffective. It should be remembered, however, that the less-than-optimal handling of intensity could also be related to cochlear dysfunction (Henderson, Salvi, Boettcher, and Clock, 1994).

Finally, changes in the CANS may provide an explanation for the deterioration of aided performance over time in some previously successful hearing aid users. Most audiologists have encountered the successful hearing aid user who becomes more frustrated and has less success with amplification as the individual's age increases. In many of these people, routine pure-tone tests of peripheral auditory function reveal little, if any, change but word recognition scores, particularly if assessed under adverse listening conditions, suggest major deterioration in function. Moreover, central auditory tests reveal a significant reduction in CANS performance. Such CANS changes may signal the need to experiment with a hearing aid that is capable of complex signal processing, or to consider the use of an assistive listening device as an alternative to the traditional hearing aid fitting.

### Duration of Hearing Loss

The longer an individual has had a hearing loss, particularly if it is unaided, the poorer the prognosis for success. Ample evidence suggests that both morphological and physiological changes occur throughout the CANS as the result of a lack of auditory stimulation imposed by peripheral hearing loss (Morest, 1983). The nature and mechanisms underlying these changes are discussed in greater detail later in this chapter. Of importance to the present discussion is the recognition that such changes do occur, and that the longer the auditory deprivation exists, the greater the potential for significant changes in CANS function. On a more positive note, with the reintroduction of auditory stimulation some enhancement of CANS function may occur (Webster, 1988; Recanzone, Schreiner, and Merzenich, 1993). Therefore, timely selection and fitting of amplification is essential, as this will minimize deterioration of the central auditory structures in clients of all ages and will increase the potential for significant changes afforded by brain plasticity, particularly in the younger client.

### Severity of Hearing Problems

Obviously, the more severe the hearing loss, the greater the effects of auditory deprivation, because little or no stimulation of the CANS will occur. Although the negative effects of auditory deprivation are likely to be more significant the greater the loss, one must keep in mind the negative effects of even mild hearing loss on central auditory function (Webster and Webster, 1977; Gunnarson and Finitzo, 1991). This is particularly true in the young brain, where development of the CNS is dependent upon stimulation (Kalil, 1989). There may be a trade-off among several of the factors discussed thus far. For example, a mild hearing loss of short duration may be more devastating to the development of the CANS in a young child than a moderate hearing loss of longer duration to the maintenance of CANS function in a mature adult whose CANS has already matured.

A second consideration relating to severity of hearing problems is the situation where the client's hearing complaints appear to be disproportionate to his or her hearing loss. Many clients report that they seem to hear okay, but they have trouble following conversations. Such statements may herald central auditory system involvement. Here, again, identification of the CANS involvement is essential, because this may lead to different fitting strategies and to the ability to establish realistic expectations for aided improvement for the client.

### Neurological Involvement

One key aspect in the history of a child or adult who is a hearing aid candidate is the presence/absence of a history of neurological involvement. It is important to check for history of head trauma, mass or vascular lesions, CNS surgery, neural degenerative problems, drugs or medications that may have affected the CNS, and any indications of learning disabilities. If there is an indication that there is or has been neurological involvement, it would be valuable to determine if the CANS specifically has been involved. Sometimes this requires locating where the injury or disorder is localized in the brain. One may have to consult previous medical records to help determine if the auditory areas of the brain have been compromised. It is also worthwhile to ask the client if he or she noticed any change in auditory abilities because of the neurological condition.

If the client's history is positive for some type of neurological involvement, it may prove worthwhile to perform some central auditory tests. As will become apparent later in this chapter, the presence of a CANS disorder may have profound implications for the fitting of hearing aids. Useful tests are discussed in the next segment of this chapter, but it is important to note here that the interpretation of the central auditory test results may depend a great deal on the neurological history. For example, if a client had received a right temporal lobe injury, one might look for a left-ear deficit on various types of behavioral central tests.

### *CANS Assessment*

### Effects of Peripheral Hearing Loss

The evaluation of the central auditory system in the individual with peripheral hearing loss is problematic. It is well known that peripheral hearing loss often causes not only a loss of sensitivity, but also an increase in the distortion of a signal (see Chapters 7 and 8). Such distortion typically results in reduced speech recognition scores which, in turn, can affect central test performance. Because many of the available central auditory tests use speech materials as test stimuli, these tests must be used with caution. Although the presence of a peripheral hearing loss may appear to be an insurmountable hurdle, careful selection and interpretation of test results can help avoid these pitfalls and lead to appropriate diagnosis.

## Central Tests Resistant to Cochlear Effects

A number of tests have been shown to be relatively resistant to the effects of cochlear distortion. These include the temporal ordering tasks, selected dichotic speech tests, and some of the electrophysiological procedures. The following provides a brief overview of some of the tests shown to be resistant to the effects of peripheral hearing impairment. For more information regarding test administration and scoring for the tests reviewed, see Musiek, Baran, and Pinheiro (1994). This reference also provides information on central auditory tests not reviewed in this chapter.

TEMPORAL PATTERNING TASKS

Two tests in this category that have been used clinically include the Auditory Duration Patterns Test and the Frequency Pattern Sequences Test. In each of these tests, sequences consisting of three tones are presented to the individual who is asked to describe the sequences heard using the words *high* and *low* in the case of the Frequency Pattern Sequences Test, and *long* and *short* in the case of the Auditory Duration Patterns Test. In the Frequency Pattern Sequences Test 2 different tones are presented in a series of three, where one tone is always different from the remaining two tones. On one commonly used version of the test, the low tone is 880 Hz (L) and the high tone is 1122 Hz (H). The protocol permits the generation of six sequences: HHL, HLL, HLH, LLH, LHH, and LHL. The test sequences are typically presented monaurally to each ear at 50 dB re: SRT and the client is asked to describe the sequences heard using the words *high* and *low*. A percentage correct identification score is derived for each and compared to norms. Musiek and Pinheiro (1987) reported that the test was highly sensitive to cerebral compromise and that the false-positive rate was relatively low. Clinical experience with the test suggests that it can be used with individuals with mild to moderate conductive, mixed, or sensorineural hearing losses and that it is less likely to be adversely affected by flat as opposed to sloping sensorineural hearing losses. Although only one version of this test is currently available, advances in computer technology make it relatively easy for audiologists to generate their own test stimuli, which would permit the generation of sequences using other test frequencies. When assessing an individual who has a significant hearing loss at either of the standard test frequencies, it may be prudent to use sequences employing test frequencies for which the individual's hearing is normal or near normal.

The Auditory Duration Patterns Test is similar to the Frequency Pattern Sequences Test, except that in this test the tones within the sequences are of different duration. There is a long (L) tone (500 millisecond) and a short (S) tone (250 millisecond). Similar to the frequency pattern sequences, the test sequences are constructed so that two of the tones are identical while the third tone differs within the temporal or duration domain. Here again, six different sequences are permissible: LLS, LSS, LSL, SSL, SLL, and SLS. The client simply describes the sequences using the words *short* and *long*. The test has been highly sensitive to cerebral abnormalities while being largely unaffected by hearing losses through the moderately severe hearing loss range (Musiek et al., 1990). The attractive feature of this test is that only one frequency is used; in the currently available test the frequency is 1000 Hz. Because frequency does not change, the detrimental effects of frequency distortion are minimized. The only requirement would be that the hearing threshold at 1000 Hz be sufficiently low so that the test stimulus could be presented at a suprathreshold level. Commonly 50 dB re: SRT is used; however, if recruitment is a problem, the most comfortable loudness level can be used. Also, test stimuli using other test frequencies can be generated easily with readily available computer technology so that, if an individual's hearing loss is sufficiently severe at 1000 Hz to prohibit assessment with the current test, an alternate form can be used.

DICHOTIC SPEECH TESTS

Although speech tests are more likely to be prone to the effects of cochlear distortion, at least two of the tests in this category have been shown to be relatively resistant to these effects. The two tests that fall into this category include the Dichotic Digits Test and the Dichotic Sentence Identification Test. In one commonly used version of the Dichotic Digits Test (Musiek, 1983) the numbers from one to 10, excluding seven, are presented dichotically, with two digits presented to each ear (i.e., 4 digits per test items). The test stimuli are presented at 50 dB re: SRT to the respective ears and the client is asked to repeat all numbers heard. Percentage correct identification scores are derived for each ear and compared to normative data. Musiek and several investigators report that this version of the digits test is highly sensitive to compromise of auditory portions of the cerebral cortex and the interhemispheric fibers, and that is also has good specificity for individuals with mild to moderate sensory (i.e., cochlear) hearing losses (Speaks, Niccum, and Van Tassel, 1985; Musiek, Gollegly, Kibbe, and Verkest-Lenz, 1991).

Likewise, the Dichotic Sentence Identification Test (Fifer, Jerger, Berlin, Tobey, and Campbell, 1983), a modification of the Synthetic Sentence Identification Test (Jerger and Jerger, 1974), has been shown to be quite sensitive to compromise of the auditory portions of the cortex, while being largely unaffected by mild to moderate cochlear hearing losses. In the original test, 10 third-order approximations to English sentences were used as test stimuli while a competing message was presented to the contralateral ear for dichotic testing. In the modification of the test, six of the original 10 synthetic sentences were used as stimuli but, in this test, the sentences were combined in pairs and presented dichotically (one to each ear). Typically, the client is asked to indicate the sentences presented by picking the numbers of the sentences heard from a printed form containing six numbered sentences. For the Dichotic Sentence Identification Test, the test stimuli are presented at equal sensation levels (e.g., 50 dB re: SRT) to the two ears. With the Synthetic Sentence Identification Test, the message-to-competition ratio is often varied (Jerger and Jerger, 1974) and the client is provided a list of 10 numbered sentences from which to indicate a response.

ELECTROPHYSIOLOGICAL TESTS

The middle latency response and the late auditory-evoked responses can be affected by significant peripheral hearing loss; however, in individuals with mild to moderate hearing losses, these potentials may be evident in spite of the peripheral involvement (Hall, 1992). It is safe to assume that if the auditory brainstem response is present and normal, abnormalities in the later potentials are more likely to be related to central auditory system compromise as opposed to peripheral involvement. For more information on electrophysiological test procedures see Hall (1992).

The preceding discussion highlights some of the tests shown to be somewhat resistant to the effects of cochlear hearing loss. The discussion of these tests to the exclusion of other central tests should not be taken as an indication that other tests cannot be used with clients with peripheral hearing losses. Many of these central tests can provide valuable information if interpretation of the test results is performed cautiously. To demonstrate the utility of the central auditory assessment we highlight below three cases evaluated in our clinic. For a comprehensive review of all the central tests used, see Musiek, Baran, and Pinheiro (1994).

### Interpretation of Test Results

Although peripheral hearing loss can affect test performance and interpretation, there are a number of unique patterns that, if present, are a potential indication of CANS compromise or pathology.

*If the hearing loss is symmetrical and the performance of one ear is markedly poorer than that of the other ear on central auditory tests, CANS is indicated.* This case is one of a 71-year-old man who had sustained a right-sided cerebrovascular accident a number of years earlier. Hearing loss was found to be symmetrical, as were speech recognition scores (Fig. 9–2). However, asymmetrical findings were evident on a number of the central auditory tests administered (Fig. 9–3). Bilateral, but clearly asymmetrical deficits were noted on both monaural low redundancy tests (Compressed Speech and Low Pass Filtered Speech), with left-ear scores significantly more depressed than right-ear scores. On two dichotic speech tests (Dichotic Rhymes and Dichotic Digits), severe left-ear deficits were evident with normal right-ear scores, and on two temporal patterning tasks (Frequency Pattern Sequences and Auditory Duration Patterns), bilateral deficits were noted.

As mentioned earlier, extreme caution must be used when interpreting central test data in cases with peripheral hearing loss. However, the pattern of results in this case points clearly to central and peripheral involvement. A significant hearing loss is clearly present in both ears, but the loss is bilaterally symmetrical and word recognition scores are equivalent. Given these findings, the asymmetrical results noted on the dichotic and monaural speech tests cannot be explained solely on the basis of a peripheral hearing loss. The peripheral involvement may be the basis for some of the deficits noted on the monaural speech tests, as both ears are depressed to some extent; however, in spite of the bilaterally depressed scores on these tests there is evidence of a "contralateral ear effect," because the left-ear scores are noticeably lower than the right-ear scores on both tests. A similar ear difference is obvious on the dichotic speech tests where right-ear performance was normal and significant left-ear deficits were noted. Finally, the observation of bilaterally depressed scores (such scores are expected with unilateral CANS involvement) on both patterning tests is significant, especially in light of evidence

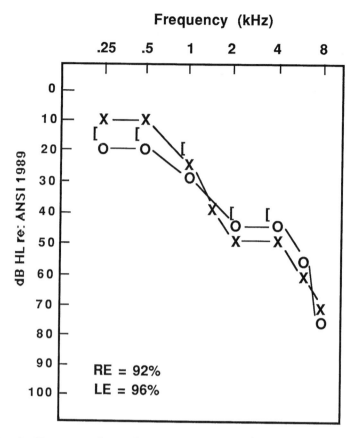

**Figure 9–2.**  Audiogram and speech recognition scores for a 71-year-old man with a right-sided cerebrovascular accident. (From Baran J, Musiek F, 1995. Reprinted with permission.)

demonstrating that at least one of these tests, the Auditory Duration Patterns Test, is largely unaffected by mild to moderate hearing losses (Musiek et al., 1990). On these patterning tests one cannot completely rule out some contribution of peripheral compromise; however, the extent of the deficits appears to be inconsistent with the degree of hearing loss and, therefore, CANS compromise must be questioned. The pattern of test results in this case appears to suggest both peripheral auditory compromise and right auditory hemisphere involvement. This CANS compromise is not unlikely, given the client's history of a right-sided cerebrovascular accident.

   The identification of these deficits has several implications for the management of this client. If the client is to be fit with amplification, the central effects must be considered. One must question whether binaural amplification will help, given the test findings. Monaural amplification may be preferable, as there is the potential for binaural interference in this individual. If the client is to be fit monaurally (which often occurs for financial reasons if not for audiological considerations), then selection of the optimal fitting would point to a right-ear fitting in this case.

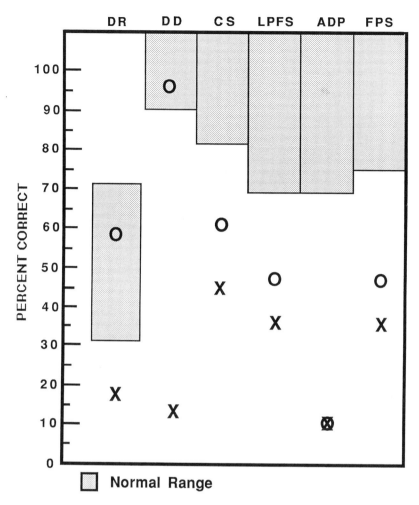

**Figure 9–3.** Central test data for the case presented in Figure 9–2. Test results are presented for the right (O) and left (X) ears on the following behavioral tests: DR = Dichotic Rhymes, DD = Dichotic Digits, CS = Compressed Speech, LPFS = Low-Pass Filtered Speech, ADP = Auditory Duration Patterns, and FPS = Frequency Pattern Sequences. (From Baran J, Musiek F, 1995. Reprinted with permission.)

However, without the results of the CANS assessment, the advantage of a right-ear fitting would not be obvious.

*If the hearing loss is asymmetrical and the performance of the better ear is significantly poorer than that of the poorer ear, CANS involvement should be suspected.* This case is one of a 62-year-old man who presented with significant auditory complaints. Specifically, he complained of significant hearing difficulties, particularly when listening in noise. He also had a history of a fronto-parietal tumor, which was surgically removed. The audiogram (Fig. 9–4) revealed an asymmetrical hearing loss with essentially normal hearing sensitivity in the low to midfrequencies in the left ear, and a mild to moderate high-frequency sensorineural hearing loss in

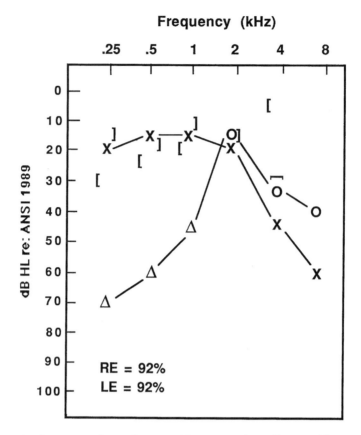

**Figure 9–4.** Audiogram and speech recognition scores for a 62-year-old man with a history of surgical removal of a meningioma of the right hemisphere.

that same ear. In the right ear, a moderately severe mixed hearing loss was noted in the low frequencies, which rose to within normal limits at 2000 Hz and then dropped to a mild high-frequency hearing loss. Central auditory test findings for this case are depicted in Figure 9–5.

Of interest here are the normal test findings for the poorer ear (i.e., right ear) on all three dichotic speech tests (Dichotic Digits, Competing Sentences, and Staggered Spondaic Words) and on the monaural low redundancy speech test (Low Pass Filtered Speech). The performance of the left ear on all these tests was depressed significantly, as were the scores for both ears on the Frequency Pattern Sequences Test. The significantly depressed scores noted for the left ear were disproportionate to the hearing loss in this ear, and as such argued for CANS compromise. As mentioned, this client had undergone surgical removal of a tumor (meningioma) located in the fronto-parietal region of the right hemisphere. The low-frequency hearing loss was primarily conductive in nature and was not surgically or medically correctable. Given the peripheral test results in this case, many audiologists might consider fitting the left ear, pending medical clearance, or possibly a binaural fitting. Here, again, the advisability of both fittings must

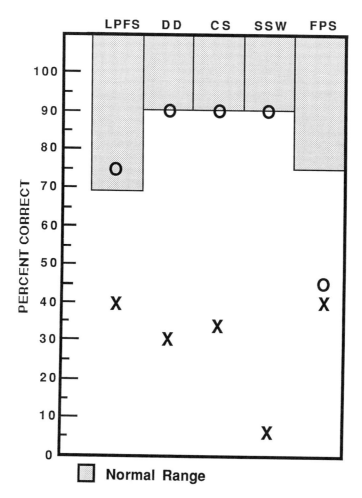

**Figure 9–5.** Central test data for the case presented in Figure 9–4. Test results are presented for the right (O) and left (X) ears on the following behavioral tests: LPFS = Low-Pass Filtered Speech, DD = Dichotic Digits, CS = Competing Sentences, SSW = Staggered Spondaic Words, and FPS = Frequency Pattern Sequences.

be questioned, given the central auditory results. In the case of a monaural fitting, the more advantageous fitting would appear to be a right-ear fitting, as long as there are no medical contraindications, because the scores for the central auditory tests were noticeably superior to those of the left ear. With a binaural fitting one must, again, question the possibility of binaural interference, which would need to be explored.

*If abnormal middle and/or late potentials are noted from electrodes over one hemisphere versus the other (i.e., a significant electrode effect), CANS involvement should be suspected.* This patient in this case is a 57-year-old man with a history of a left caudate stroke. Pure-tone threshold testing revealed a somewhat asymmetrical high-frequency hearing loss with bilaterally poor speech recognition scores (Fig. 9–6).

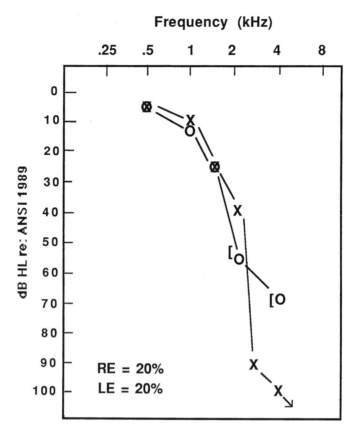

**Figure 9–6.** Audiogram and speech recognition scores for a 57-year-old man with an infarct of the left caudate. (From Musiek et al., 1994. Reprinted with permission.)

Late auditory evoked potentials and P300s were derived for both right-ear (Fig. 9–7) and left-ear (Fig. 9–8) stimulation with electrodes positioned at C3, C4, and both earlobes. For both right-ear and left-ear presentations, the amplitudes of the N1 and P2 responses (see frequent tracings) are substantially reduced in size for the electrode recordings over the lesioned side of the brain (C3-left side), as compared to the corresponding responses from the C4 electrode. Moreover, significant differences in the P300 responses are noted when the C3 and C4 recordings are compared. These results are consistent with the client's history of CANS compromise. In individuals such as this patient, the finding of significant CANS compromise may signal the need to consider a monaural (i.e., ipsilateral ear) fitting or an additional assessment prior to finalizing a binaural fitting. The discussion on binaural interference following the case presentations may provide a rationale for the need to pursue further testing in some of these clients.

*If significant ear effects are noted on electrophysiological testing in the presence of symmetrical hearing loss, the possibility of CANS involvement should be entertained.* This final case is a 69-year-old woman with auditory complaints and possible multiple sclerosis, which was suspected but not confirmed. The audiogram

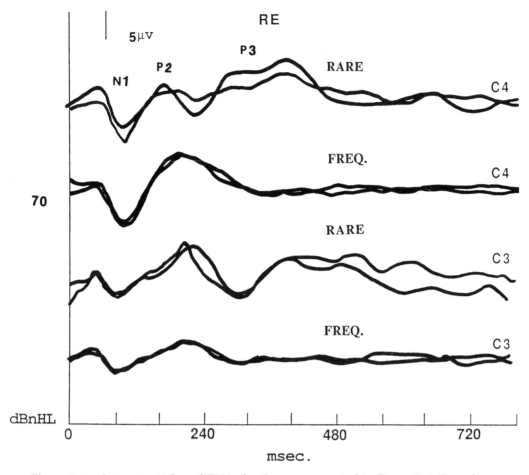

**Figure 9–7.**  Late potentials and P300s for the case presented in Figure 9–6. Recordings were derived from the right ear at two electrode sites (C3 and C4). (From Musiek et al., 1994. Reprinted with permission.)

revealed a bilaterally symmetrical high-frequency sensorineural hearing loss with excellent speech recognition scores for both ears (Fig. 9–9). Auditory brainstem responses (ABR) were derived for both ears, with results showing a normal response for the right ear, a normal Wave I for the left ear, a delayed Wave III, and an absent IV/V complex (Fig. 9–10). Although not shown, behavioral central tests were also administered, and significant left-ear deficits were evident on two dichotic speech tests (Dichotic Digits and Competing Sentences) and one monaural low redundancy speech test (Compressed Speech). This case provides an excellent example of the importance of careful case history taking and the need for CANS assessment. Given the peripheral test results, there was no clear indication of any potential central effects. However, the suspicion of multiple sclerosis prompted further assessment, which lead to the identification of the CANS involvement. A computed tomography scan revealed a tumor in the hypothalamus and thalamus that extended toward the brainstem. The abnormal ABR findings for the left side

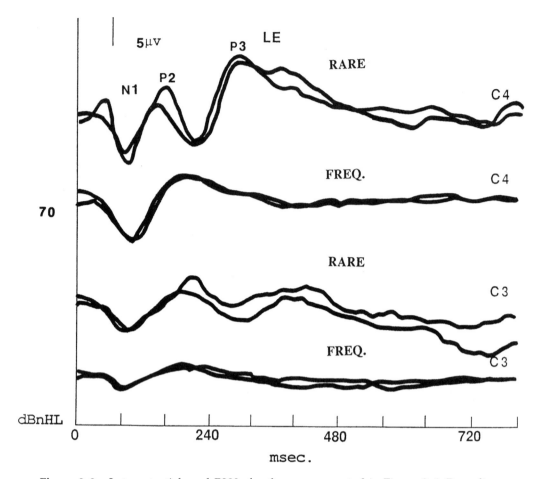

**Figure 9–8.** Late potentials and P300s for the case presented in Figure 9–6. Recordings were derived from the left ear at two electrode sites (C3 and C4). (From Musiek et al., 1994. Reprinted with permission.)

suggested compromise of the upper pons area, which was likely due to the effects of indirect pressure to the pons or possibly demyelination related to multiple sclerosis. The left-ear deficits may have been secondary to the ABR results or may have been a manifestation of compromise introduced by the tumor itself. Regardless of the cause, significant central and peripheral involvement is present in this case and, as in previous cases, should be considered when decisions regarding fittings are made for this individual.

### Binaural Interference

It is now commonly accepted that binaural fittings are preferable to monaural fittings. An extensive body of research has documented binaural advantages for a number of objective and subjective test measures (Bryne, 1980; Hawkins, 1986; Mueller and Hawkins, 1990). Clearly, binaural advantages are evident for sound

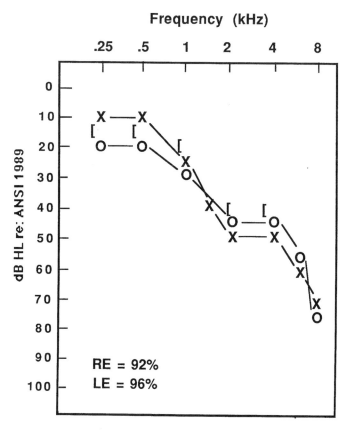

**Figure 9–9.**   Audiogram and speech recognition scores for a 69-year-old woman with a tumor of the thalamus and hypothalamus which extended into the brainstem. (From Musiek et al., 1994. Reprinted with permission.)

localization, ease of listening, perception of "balanced hearing," hearing in noise, and hearing at increased distances. The evidence of such auditory benefits has prompted the fitting of binaural hearing aids, even in individuals with asymmetrical hearing loss who would have previously had a monaural fitting. This supports the idea that "two ears are better than one" and, all things being equal, this statement is true; however, a growing body of evidence suggests that binaural fittings may not always be preferable to monaural fittings, even though binaural summation and other desirable features are presumed to exist. Specifically, one needs to consider the possible detrimental effects of binaural interference, i.e., a condition where binaural performance is actually poorer than monaural performance of the "better" ear.

Recently, Jerger and his colleagues reviewed four cases where evidence of binaural interference was provided (Jerger, Silman, Lew, and Chmiel, 1993). The binaural interference phenomenom was demonstrated in terms of speech recognition performance and/or electrophysiological measures. In three of the four cases speech recognition scores were presented. In each case, the word recognition scores of the two ears were largely discrepant, despite the fact that the hearing

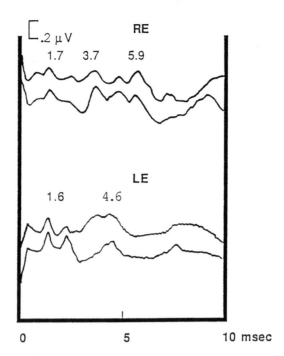

**Figure 9–10.**    ABR for the case presented in Figure 9–9. The latencies for waves I, III, and V for the right ear and waves I and III for the left ear are indicated on the tracings. (From Musiek et al., 1994. Reprinted with permission.)

loss in each case was essentially symmetrical. Word recognition performance was measured under three conditions: monaural right ear aided, monaural left ear aided, and binaurally aided. In all three cases the performance of the better ear was substantially superior to the performance of the poorer ear but, interestingly, the binaural performance was poorer than the performance of the better ear (Fig. 9–11). Typically, the expectation would be either an enhancement of the binaural score over the monaural score or a binaural score that at least equals the better monaural score. The fact that the binaural score in each of these cases was considerably lower than the better score suggests that the poorer ear interfered in some manner with the processing of the information presented to the better ear. Although the mechanisms underlying this type of binaural interference are not known, it does appear that some type of competition is introduced by distortion arising at either the peripheral or central system. Jerger, Silman, Lew, and Chmiel (1993) suggest that the poorer ear may inhibit or suppress the performance of the better ear. Although there is no evidence to contradict this hypothesis, an alternative explanation would be that some type of compromise of the auditory pathways comprises the CANS and, when stimulation arises from both ears, there is a competition for healthy neural tissue as the CANS attempts to process auditory information arriving from two ears. A similar compromise for healthy tissue in a client with CANS involvement has been suggested previously by Musiek, Reeves, and Baran (1985).

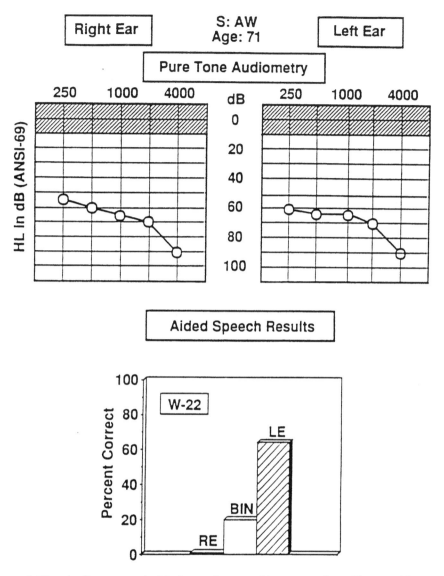

**Figure 9–11.** Audiogram and aided speech recognition scores for a 71-year-old woman showing poorer speech recognition ability for a binaurally aided test condition than for the better ear monaurally aided test condition. (From Jerger et al., 1993. Reprinted with permission.)

Jerger, Silman, Lew, and Chmiel (1993) also provide electrophysiological evidence of the binaural interference phenomena. Topographic maps and/or traditional middle latency response (MLR) recordings were derived for three of their four subjects. In all three cases, MLRs were derived monaurally for both the right and left ears and then binaurally. In each of the three cases the amplitude of the NaPa wave complex from one of the ears (better ear) was noticeably larger and/or more normally distributed over the scalp than was the response derived from the second ear (poorer ear). Of interest was not so much the difference of the response between the two ears, but the fact that with binaural stimulation the response was again found to be "poorer" than the response of the better ear, suggesting some type of binaural interference. A representative case is presented in Figure 9–12. It appears that the presence of the electrophysiological input from the poorer (left) ear interfered with the input from the better (right) ear in such a way that the binaural response was negatively affected. The presence of such binaural interference effects are likely to have profound implications for the successful fitting of at least some potential hearing aid clients. It may be that two ears are not better than one. Additional testing may, therefore, be indicated, particularly if a binaural fitting appears to provide less benefit than expected.

An issue that may be related to binaural interference, yet may exist on its own, is that of less-than-optimal binaural processing. To take advantage of binaural amplification, binaural processes in the auditory system must work appropriately. The brainstem and the cortex are involved in binaural processing, and it may be reasonable to attempt to screen for some of these binaural processes, especially in people who do not do as well as expected with binaural amplification. Tests are

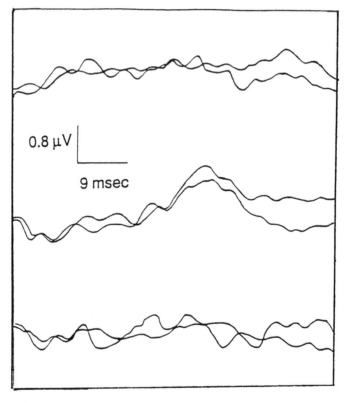

**Figure 9–12.** Middle latency responses (MLRs) for right ear stimulation, left ear stimulation, and binaural stimulation for an 81-year-old man. Amplitude of the response is less in the binaural condition than in the right ear condition. (From Jerger et al., 1993. Reprinted with permission.)

available that can provide, at least on a theoretical basis, insight to binaural integrity of the brainstem and/or cortex. Two brainstem tests that require little time to administer include the Binaural Masking Level Difference and Binaural Fusion (Wilson, Zizz, and Sperry, 1994; Wilson, 1994). These tests provide information on how well the brainstem (although not exclusively) can use phase differences to help hear in noise (Binaural Masking Level Difference) and to integrate and combine acoustic inputs from each ear (Binaural Fusion). Binaural interaction measures with the ABR may also provide valuable information, but they may take too long to administer and may be too expensive to use as a routine screening procedure.

Binaural integrity is more difficult to document at the cortical level. This is because most tests used for assessment at this level are influenced by the brainstem; hence, it is difficult to interpret a deficit as having a brainstem or cortical basis. However, if "brainstem tests" are normal, it may be reasonable to administer some dichotic listening tasks, such as those suggested above, to assess neural integrity and binaural integration of information at the cortical level.

### Additional Comments

As mentioned, any history of neurological insult or compromise should be given serious consideration when considering a hearing aid fitting. Such a history can provide both insight on the need for further testing and an explanation for many of the results noted above. For example, consider the second case presented. The history of surgical removal of a meningioma should herald the possibility of a central auditory processing deficit. Documenting the central deficit in this case should lead to a better fitting rationale. The significant left-ear deficits, despite the fact that this ear had the better peripheral hearing status, might implicate the "poorer" right ear as the ear to be fitted in this case. Although some audiologists might be inclined to recommend against a hearing aid fitting in this case, the central data may argue in favor of a fitting. Given the facts in this case—the hearing in the left ear is normal through 2000 Hz, the gentleman is retired, and he has good word recognition ability at levels approximating normal conversational levels—many audiologists may decide against amplification in this case; however, his central test data clearly indicate the potential benefits of amplification. Although speech recognition ability is good under quiet conditions, under conditions of competition performance in the "better" left ear is actually poor. Though we did not test specifically for performance in noise, the evidence seems to suggest that similar problems would also be evident in these conditions. Thus, the central data in this case may indicate the potential benefits of amplification in an individual who may not otherwise be considered a good candidate for amplification.

### *Amplification: Links to Neuroauditory Function and Brain Plasticity*

As mentioned, one of the main reasons the CANS is discussed within the framework of this book devoted to hearing aids is that there appears to be a positive influence of amplification on measures of speech recognition. More specifically, it has been reported that people who have hearing loss can maintain or improve their speech recognition scores with the use of amplification. Conversely, if amplification is needed but not used, speech recognition scores tend to become gradually worse over time (Silman et al, 1984). Stubblefield and Nye (1989) showed decrements over several years in the speech recognition scores of unaided ears in individuals with hearing loss, while ears that were aided did not show these decrements in performance. Other studies have shown that in individuals with symmetrical hearing loss when one ear was aided and the other not, poorer speech recognition scores were found in the unaided ears (Fig. 9–13) (Gelfand and Ross, 1987; Gatehouse, 1992; Hurley, 1993). Moreover, research findings illustrate that the decrements in speech recognition scores evolving over several years have been reversed by applying amplification (Fig. 9–14) (Boothroyd, 1993; Silverman and Emmer, 1993).

Hattori (1993) used a dichotic listening task (nonsense syllables) to assess the long-term effects of monaural and binaural amplification on children. This study used two groups of children—one with monaural hearing aids, the other with binaural or alternating amplification (a time period with amplification to one ear and then the other ear). In the group with monaural amplification, scores improved approximately 20% for the aided ear, but there was no significant change in the unaided ear. An Interaural Difference Score (IDS) was also measured for the two groups of subjects. This index was computed by comparing the scores obtained from each of the ears from the two groups. The monaural group showed a significant change in the IDS upon retest, but the binaurally aided group did not. In the monaural group, the aided ear increased in performance but the unaided ear did not; hence, a large IDS. The binaurally aided group

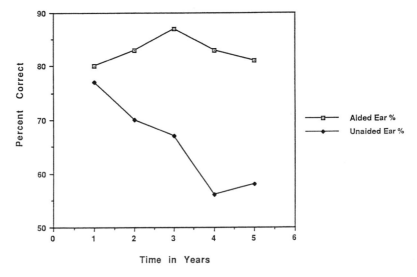

**Figure 9–13.** Speech recognition scores recorded over 5 years from an individual who had a bilateral symmetrical hearing loss and similar speech recognition scores in both ears prior to being fitted monaurally. (Adapted from Hurley, 1993; with permission from the publisher.)

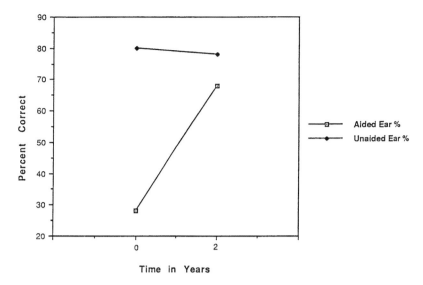

**Figure 9–14.**   Speech recognition scores for an individual with a unilateral hearing loss, which was stable over time. Marked improvement in speech recognition performance was noted when the ear with the hearing loss was aided. (Figure constructed from the data of Silverman and Emmer, 1993.)

improved in both ears over time. Thus, there was little difference between ears in regard to performance on the dichotic task. This study provides some important insights. The study tested a population of children, and the results are critical for comparison to adults. Also, the use of a dichotic speech paradigm has been aligned with central auditory function.

Most studies on the effects of amplification on speech recognition scores have been retrospective in nature and, therefore, it is difficult to know the length of time required before positive changes are noted. Gatehouse and Killion (1993) report that the brain may take six weeks or more to make use of new acoustic information supplied by a hearing aid. This is often approximately the length of time necessary for people to "get used to" a new hearing aid.

Many of the above studies show a decrement in speech recognition over time in ears with hearing loss that have not received amplification. This type of change has been viewed as a type of auditory deprivation (Silman et al., 1984). Auditory deprivation is not a new term, as scientists have studied deprivation effects in sensory systems for many years. Most deprivation studies take one of two approaches. One approach is to alter the environment, such as by placing an animal in a sound-treated chamber for a period of time. The other approach is to alter the sensory apparatus so a stimulus cannot reach the CNS, or if it does reach the CNS, the sound level is much reduced. This usually means ablating the cochlea, cutting the auditory nerve or impairing middle-ear function.

Studies have shown a reduced neural density of central (brainstem) auditory neurons after long-term sound isolation (Webster and Webster, 1977; Webster, 1983). Experimentally inducing conductive hearing losses has also resulted in a decrease in neural density and cell size of brainstem auditory structures (Webster, 1983). Damage to the cochlea by ablation, noise, and ototoxicity has resulted in transsynaptic degeneration of the auditory brainstem nuclei (Morest, 1983; Tucci, Born, and Rubel, 1987). Transsynaptic degeneration related to damaging the periphery on one side generally results in most effects noted at the ipsilateral cochlear nucleus, the contralateral superior olive, and the contralateral inferior colliculus (Morest, 1983). These morphological changes due to lack of stimulation seem to have a greater effect if they occur at "critical periods" of development. However, the effects have also been noted in "adult" animals.

Some recent physiological findings pertaining to the inferior colliculus are interesting and rather curious. Henderson, Salvi, Boettcher, and Clock (1994) reported that after intense noise exposure experimental animals lost hearing sensitivity. Input-output functions of the amplitude of evoked potentials showed decreased maximum amplitude at the auditory nerve and cochlear nucleus. However, recordings from the inferior colliculus showed a larger evoked response than preexposure recordings (Fig. 9–15). This finding indicates an enhancement of the evoked potential. This enhancement takes place within 24 hours after exposure and seems to actually become greater when measured at 30 days. Recent communication with Dr. Salvi indicates this evoked potential enhancement at the inferior colliculus has remained for several months.

The effects of acoustic deprivation on the auditory cortex appear to be different from those of the low brainstem. Schwaber, Garraghty, and Kaas (1993) demonstrated that the tonotopic maps of the auditory cortex changed at the frequencies where cochlear damage occurred. That is, the cortical representation of the damaged region (high frequency) of the cochlea shifted to adjacent lower frequencies, but still remained viable (Fig. 9–16). This means there was a larger anatomical region of the cortex responding to the lower frequency region adjacent to the

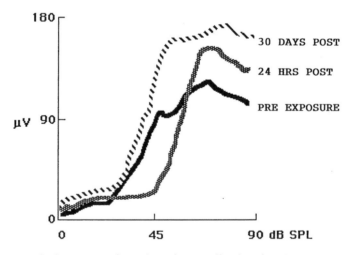

**Figure 9–15.** Evoked responses from the inferior colliculus showing greater amplitude at higher intensities of stimulation for postnoise exposure conditions. (Adapted from Henderson et al., 1994.)

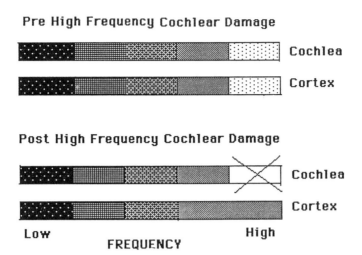

**Figure 9–16.** The corresponding frequency maps of the cochlea and primary auditory cortex. The portion of the drawing showing the high-frequency cochlear damage shows how the cortical region, which previously responded to high frequencies, has shifted to a lower frequency to match the segment of the cochlea that has not been damaged.

high-frequency area that represented the cochlea. There is a possibility, unlike in the brainstem, that the cortical tissue remains intact and does not degenerate. These changes in frequency maps of the auditory cortex manifest in the hemisphere contralateral to the lesioned cochlea. It also appears that this cortical tissue that has assumed different tonotopicity has neurons with characteristic frequency thresholds similar to those of normal regions (Rajan, Irvine, Wise, and Heil, 1993). This remapping may be what happens at the inferior colliculus. Another theory is that perhaps the neurons needed to switch frequency are already present but are not expressed until certain neural tissue is damaged.

In addition to the anatomical changes just mentioned, there are physiological effects of auditory deprivation. For example, Clopton and Silverman (1978) reported delayed latencies of responses from the inferior colliculus in animals auditorily deprived by induced conductive losses. The long-term effects of otitis media on children have been reflected in delayed latencies of the later ABR wave components, which is consistent with brainstem dysfunction (Gunnarson and Finitzo, 1991).

A number of important factors are related by the aforementioned studies on the anatomical and physiological effects of auditory deprivation. First, it is important to consider that auditory deprivation can take many forms ranging from environmental alterations to various degrees of hearing loss. Regardless of the form of acoustic deprivation, the auditory system does undergo changes, and these changes result in the system functioning less than optimally. Clearly the concept of "use it or lose it" is relevant to the auditory system. In most cases of hearing loss, however, the CANS, or at least some portions of the CANS, are not used because peripheral hearing loss prevents the appropriate stimulation of groups of neurons. This may make a difference in regard to how the neurons function as well as to their functional interactions with other neurons. These interactions, or lack of interactions, may be the basis for the subtle auditory malfunctions that manifest themselves in difficult listening situations.

If acoustic deprivation results in changes in the functional morphology of the CANS, what would be the effect of increased acoustic stimulation? This question is important to the field of hearing aids because amplification can be looked at as a way of providing increased stimulation to the auditory system. This is especially true for the individual who for some time has had significant hearing loss but has not pursued amplification. As mentioned early in this section, amplification has been shown to improve speech recognition scores in people with sensorineural hearing loss who have worn a hearing aid for a period of time. Another view of this kind of effect is reported by Hall, Grose, and Pillsbury (1990). These investigators measured masking level differences (MLDs) in adults with otosclerosis before surgery, 1 month after surgery, and 1 year after surgery. Masking level differences improved over each of the sequential tests to near normal levels for the majority of subjects. A control group of normal-hearing individuals showed no change in their MLDs over the same time period. One could view the Hall, Grose, and Pillsbury (1990) study as showing the effect of increased acoustic stimulation on the auditory system. Because these studies are on human subjects, certain questions cannot be answered in terms of underlying anatomic and physiological mechanisms. However, there are animal studies that seem to corroborate the kinds of findings noted in people who use hearing aids. Some of the animal studies also show a rather dramatic effect of acoustic stimulation on the auditory system similar to the findings of Hall, Grose, and Pillsbury (1990).

A relevant study on deprivation/stimulation of the auditory system is one by Webster (1988). As mentioned earlier, Webster demonstrated in mice that conductive hearing loss early in life results in reduced auditory nuclei volume in the brainstem. This neural reduction can be offset by piping amplified sounds into the immediate environment of mice with conductive hearing losses. Another important study was done with newborn rats (Hassmannova, Myslivecek, and Novokova, 1981). One group of rats were subjected daily to systematic presentations of various sounds, while the other group of rats were raised in a normal environment. After several weeks, near field cortical evoked potentials were obtained from the control and experimental groups. The experimental group showed significantly shorter latency of auditory evoked potentials when compared to the control group. A more recent study on primates also demonstrated a positive effect of acoustic stimulation on the auditory cortex (Recanzone et al., 1993). These animals were trained with frequency discrimination tasks within a restricted frequency range. The animals improved their frequency discrimination (most notably within the first 10 days of training), and the cortical area representing the frequency range under training reorganized to provide a larger tissue base. In other words, the frequency map of a selected frequency became larger with training on a discrimination task. This study represents a situation in which the behavioral improvement on an auditory behavioral task had an anatomical correlate.

The aforementioned studies are examples of brain plasticity. When word recognition scores improve from using amplification, we believe this also is a form of plasticity. Gatehouse (1992), however, uses the term *acclimatization* for hearing improvement secondary to wearing amplification. A definition of plasticity is, indeed, difficult. Based in part on a definition by Lund (1978) and on our own embellishment of this definition, the following is offered: "Neural form and connections take on a predictable pattern, probably genetically determined, which is termed neural specificity." Exceptions to this predictable neural pattern in certain circumstances, such as accommodation to environmental influences, is neural plasticity. Gatehouse's (1992) linking of acclimatization to higher intensity presentation of acoustic signals via amplification is not inconsistent with our view of plasticity. Plasticity can have as its basis many neural functions, including morphological, physiological, and biochemical activities. We submit that when a person "adjusts" to a hearing aid so that he or she perceives benefit, part of the process of the "adjustment" is related to the process of neural plasticity. The neural plasticity may involve the auditory system as well as other systems that may interact with the auditory system. We would expect that cognitive and emotional aspects (in addition to auditory) of behavioral change may come into play when an individual "adjusts" to a hearing aid. However, when hearing improves, there are probably changes in the auditory system consistent with this change. In the future it will be important that changes in hearing related to neural plasticity be documented carefully by both electrophysiological and psychophysical measures.

## Future Directions

The future directions in the area of the effects of amplification on central auditory function could take many courses. One direction is to develop a better understanding of deprivation effects on the auditory system. Some of the key questions might include the following: how much hearing is required for deprivation effects to be evident, or at least measurable? (Some studies mentioned earlier indicate that conductive losses of a mild degree can have effects.) Do deprivation effects increase with the magnitude and duration of the hearing loss? What about congenitally deaf children? Do these children have compromised or underdeveloped auditory systems related to a lack of stimulation? If the CANS is not fully developed in a child with a profound congenital hearing loss, does it have to undergo extensive reorganization before sound can be properly used by the brain? Some animal research shows that there may be critical time periods for maximum deprivation effects to be realized (Webster, 1988; Knudsen, 1988). What are these critical time periods and can amplification prevent and/or reverse these negative effects?

If we need to learn more about acoustic deprivation effects on the CANS, we also need more knowledge on the effects of acoustic stimulation. Is late onset acoustic deprivation different than early onset deprivation? To what degree can stimulation offset early and late onset acoustic deprivation? At which times in life is the brain most plastic? What kinds of plastic changes are made by the neurons when they are stimulated over long periods of time? What are the effects of binaural versus monaural amplification on CANS anatomy and physiology? What kinds of acoustic signals can provide the best overall stimulation effects? What factors play a role in individual differences in regard to improved hearing from stimulation? Is the acoustic stimulation provided by hearing aids optimal for improving hearing or should other types of amplification be considered?

Another major direction regarding hearing aids and the CANS is the development and use of central auditory tests. Clearly, both electrophysiological and behavioral approaches will have to be used and integrated. By combining evoked potentials and behavioral tests insights into functional relationships can be gained that can be useful in both the diagnosis and management of candidates for hearing aids. Both evoked potential and behavioral central tests will need improvement for use with clients for whom hearing aids will be prescribed. Tests with good reliability and validity, and which do not require extensive time to administer, will be in demand. Tests that provide insight on the relative involvement of the central versus peripheral systems will help the audiologist better evaluate and counsel the client in need of a hearing aid. Test strategies for the use of screening procedures for denoting significant CANS involvement may be necessary. There are several scenarios for including a screening central test for the evaluation of hearing aid candidates (Fig. 9–17). One approach would be to

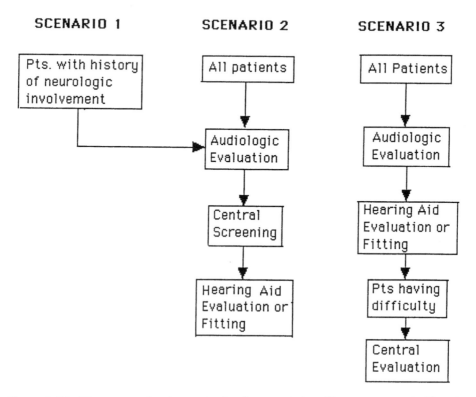

**Figure 9–17.**   Three scenarios demonstrating how central auditory assessment of hearing aid candidates could be included in the overall evaluation of these clients.

include a central screening test for all hearing aid candidates. Another would be to include a central test for only those that have a positive history of neurological involvement. A retrospective approach would be to use central tests on those people whose hearing aids are ineffective or who prefer a monaural over a binaural fitting.

Because there has been little research on testing hearing aid candidates with central auditory tests, it is difficult to recommend which tests should be used for this purpose. As mentioned earlier, there are a few tests currently available that are easy and quick to administer and that are relatively resistant to mild or moderate degrees of peripheral hearing loss. The Dichotic Sentence Identification Test (Fifer et al., 1983), the Dichotic Digits Test (Speaks et al., 1985; Musiek et al., 1991), the Frequency Pattern Sequences Test, and the Auditory Duration Patterns Test (Musiek, 1994) have all been shown to have good sensitivity and specificity in differentiating cochlear from central involvement. However, future clinical research is necessary to demonstrate the value of these tests in predicting proportions of central versus peripheral involvement in hearing aid candidates.

The pediatric population is another area of future research regarding the CANS, hearing loss, and amplification. Children who are candidates for amplification present several interesting factors in terms of their CANS. It is known that the CANS does not reach maturation until adolescence (Musiek, Verkest, and Gollegly, 1988). We also know that the younger the brain, the more plastic it is. Young brains can recover from insults that older brains cannot (Lenneberg, 1967). Given this information, investigations on the pediatric population could center around comparisons to adults in terms of increments in central function secondary to applied amplification for peripheral hearing loss. Do children with peripheral loss, even though they are aided, develop central deficits? If so, are the deficits related to the degree of hearing loss, the age of the child, or the adequacy of the type of amplification? Can amplification used on an intermittent basis offset the auditory effects of early otitis media reported by Gunnarson and Finitzo (1991) and others?

The recent and future research into amplification and the CANS highlights some important concepts in hearing. Foremost is the concept that the peripheral and central auditory systems work together and are interdependent. The two systems have differing capabilities but, for these capabilities to be fully expressed, both systems must function optimally. Another concept is that amplification may have an additional role in regard to hearing. One obvious goal of amplification is to improve communication skills, but the maintenance or improvement of auditory function is now a possibility. Another worthwhile concept is that amplification affects both the peripheral and central auditory systems and both systems must appreciated in the evaluation process.

## References

Boothroyd A. (1993). Recovery of speech reception performance after prolonged auditory deprivation: Case study. *J Am Acad Audiol* 4:331–336.

Bryne D. (1980). Binaural hearing aid fitting: Research findings and clinical application. In: Libby E, ed. *Binaural Hearing Aid Amplification*. vol. 1. Chicago: Zenetron, pp. 23–74.

Clopton B, Silverman N. (1978). Changes in latency and duration of a neural responses following developmental auditory deprivation. *Exp Brain Res* 32:39–47.

Fifer R, Jerger J, Berlin C, Tobey E, Campbell J. (1983). Development of a dichotic sentence identification test for hearing impaired adults. *Ear Hear* 4:300–305.

Gatehouse S. (1992). The time course and magnitude of perceptual acclimatization to frequency response: Evidence for monaural fitting of hearing aids. *J Acoust Soc Am* 92:1258–1268.

Gatehouse S, Killion M. (1993). HABRAT: Hearing aid brain rewiring accommodation time. *Hear Instrum* 44(10):29–32.

Gelfand S, Ross L. (1987). Long-term effects of monaural, binaural, and no amplification in subjects with bilateral hearing loss. *Scand Audiol* 16:201–207.

Gunnarson A, Finitzo T. (1991). Conductive hearing loss during infancy: Effects on later auditory brainstem electrophysiology. *J Speech Hear Res* 34:1207–1215.

Hall J. (1992). *Handbook of Auditory Evoked Responses*. Boston: Allyn and Bacon.

Hall J, Grose J, Pillsbury H. (1990). Predicting binaural hearing after stapedectomy from pre-surgery results. *Arch Otolaryngol Head Neck Surg* 116:946–950.

Hassmannova J, Myslivecek J, Novokova B. (1981). Effects of early auditory stimulation on cortical centers. In: Syka J, Aitkin L, eds. *Neuronal Mechanisms of Hearing*. New York: Plenum Press, pp. 355–359.

Hattori H. (1993). Ear dominance for nonsense syllable recognition ability in sensorineural hearing impaired children: Monaural versus binaural amplification. *J Am Acad Audiol* 4:319–330.

Hawkins D. (1986). Selection of hearing aid characteristics. In: Hodgson W, ed. *Hearing Aid Assessment and Use in Audiologic Habilitation*. 3rd ed. Baltimore: Williams and Wilkins, pp. 128–151.

Henderson D, Salvi R, Boettcher F, Clock A. (1994). Neurophysiologic correlates of sensorineural hearing loss. In: Katz J, ed. *Handbook of Clinical Audiology*. Baltimore: Williams and Wilkins, pp. 37–55.

Hurley R. (1993). Monaural hearing aid effect: Case presentations. *J Am Acad Audiol* 4:285–295.

Jerger J, Jerger S. (1974). Auditory findings in brainstem disorders. *Arch Otolaryngol* 99:342–350.

Jerger J, Silman S, Lew H, Chmiel R. (1993). Case studies in binaural interference: Converging evidence from behavioral and electrophysiologic measures. *J Am Acad Audiol* 4: 122–131.

Kalil R. (1989). Synapse formation in the developing brain. *Sci Am* Dec.:76–85.

Knudsen E. (1988). Experience shapes sound localization in auditory unit properties during development in the barn owl. In: Edelman G, Gall W, Cowan W, eds. *Auditory Function: Neurobiological Basis of Hearing*. New York: John Wiley & Sons, pp. 137–152.

Lenneberg E. (1967). *Biological Foundations of a Language*. New York: John Wiley & Sons.

Lund R. (1978). *Development in Plasticity of the Brain*. New York: Oxford University Press, pp. 5–6.

Morest K. (1983). Degeneration of the brain following exposure to noise. In: Hamernik R, Henderson D, Salvi R, eds. *New Perspectives on Noise Induced Hearing Loss*. New York: Raven Press, pp. 87–94.

Mueller H, Hawkins D. (1990). Three important considerations in hearing aid selection. In: Sandlin R, ed. *Handbook of Hearing Aid Amplification*. Vol. II. Boston: College-Hill Press, pp. 31–60.

Musiek F. (1983). Assessment of central auditory dysfunction: The dichotic digit test revisited. *Ear Hear* 4:79–83.

Musiek F. (1994). Frequency (pitch) duration pattern tests. *J Am Acad Audiol* 5:265–268.

Musiek F, Baran J, Pinheiro M. (1990). Duration pattern recognition in normal subjects and subjects with cerebral and cochlear lesions. *Audiology* 29:304–313.

Musiek F, Baran J, Pinheiro M. (1994). *Neuroaudiology: Case Studies*. San Diego: Singular Publishing Group, Inc.

Musiek F, Gollegly K, Kibbe K, Verkest-Lenz S. (1991). Proposed screening test for central auditory disorders: Follow-up on the dichotic digits test. *Am J Otolaryngol* 12:109–113.

Musiek F, Pinheiro M. (1987). Frequency patterns in cochlear, brainstem, and cerebral lesions. *Audiology* 26:79–88.

Musiek F, Reeves A, Baran J. (1985). Release from central auditory competition in the split-brain patient. *Neurology* 35:983–987.

Musiek F, Verkest S, Gollegly K. (1988). Effects of neuromaturation on auditory evoked potentials. *Semin Hear* 9:1-13.

Nadeau S. (1989). Stroke. *Med Clin North Am* 73:1351–1369.

Rajan R, Irvine D, Wise L, Heil P. (1993). Effect of unilateral partial cochlear lesions in adult cats on the representation of lesioned and unlesioned cochleas in primary auditory cortex. *J Comp Neurol* 338:17–49.

Recanzone G, Schreiner C, Merzenich M. (1993). Plasticity in the frequency representation of primary auditory cortex following discrimination training in adult owl monkeys. *J Neurosci* 13:87–103.

Schuknecht H. (1964). Further observations and a pathology of presbycusis. *Arch Otolaryngol* 80:369–382.

Schwaber M, Garraghty P, Kaas J.(1993). Neuroplasticity of the adult primate auditory cortex following cochlear hearing loss. *Am J Otolaryngol* 14:252–258.

Silman S, Gelfand S, Silverman C. (1984). Late onset auditory deprivation: Effects of monaural versus binaural hearing aids. *J Acoust Soc Am* 76:1357–1362.

Silverman C, Emmer M. (1993). Auditory deprivation in recovering adults with asymmetric sensorineural hearing impairment. *J Am Acad Audiol* 4:338–346.

Speaks C, Niccum N, Van Tassel D. (1985). Effects of stimulus materials on the dichotic listening performance of patients with sensorineural hearing loss. *J Speech Hear Res* 28:16–25.

Stubblefield J, Nye C. (1989). Aided and unaided time related differences in word discrimination. *Hear Instrum* 40(9):38–43.

Tucci D, Born D, Rubel H. (1987). Changes in spontaneous activity in CNS morphology associated with conductive and sensorineural hearing loss in chickens. *Ann Otol Rhinol Laryngol* 96:343–350.

Webster D. (1983). A critical period during postnatal auditory development in mice. *Int J Pediatr Otorhinolaryngol* 6:107–118.

Webster D. (1988). Sound amplification negates central effects of neonatal conductive hearing loss. *Hear Res* 32:192–195.

Webster D, Webster M. (1977). Neonatal sound depravation affects brainstem auditory nuclei. *Arch Otolaryngol* 103:392–396.

Willott J. (1991). *Aging and the Auditory System.* San Diego: Singular Press, pp. 1–8.

Wilson R. (1994). Word recognition with segmented-alternated CVC words: Compact disc trials. *J Am Acad Audiol* 5:255–258.

Wilson R, Zizz C, Sperry J. (1994). Masking level difference for spondaic words in 2000-msec bursts of broadband noise. *J Am Acad Audiol* 5:236–242.

# *Index*